D0806017

INFANTS, TODDLERS, AND FAMILIES IN POVERTY

INFANTS, TODDLERS, AND FAMILIES IN POVERTY

Research Implications for Early Child Care

Edited by
Samuel L. Odom
Elizabeth P. Pungello
Nicole Gardner-Neblett

THE GUILFORD PRESS
New York   London

3/27/13
Lan
$ 60 -

© 2012 The Guilford Press
A Division of Guilford Publications, Inc.
72 Spring Street, New York, NY 10012
www.guilford.com

All rights reserved

No part of this book may be reproduced, translated, stored in a retrieval
system, or transmitted, in any form or by any means, electronic, mechanical,
photocopying, microfilming, recording, or otherwise, without written permission
from the publisher.

Printed in the United States of America

This book is printed on acid-free paper.

Last digit is print number: 9   8   7   6   5   4   3   2   1

Library of Congress Cataloging-in-Publication Data

Infants, toddlers, and families in poverty : research implications for early child
care / edited by Samuel L. Odom, Elizabeth P. Pungello, Nicole Gardner-Neblett.
    p. cm.
  Includes bibliographical references and index.
  ISBN 978-1-4625-0495-4 (hardcover : alk. paper)
  1. Poor families—United States. 2. Infants—Services for—United
States. 3. Toddlers—Services for—United States. 4. Child welfare—United
States. 5. Early childhood education—United States. I. Odom, Samuel
L. II. Pungello, Elizabeth Puhn. III. Gardner-Neblett, Nicole.
  HV699.I48 2012
  362.77′690973—dc23
                                                            2012019369

About the Editors

Samuel L. Odom, PhD, is Director of the Frank Porter Graham Child Development Institute (FPG) and Professor in the School of Education at the University of North Carolina at Chapel Hill. He is the author or coauthor of over 100 refereed journal articles and editor or coeditor of seven books on early childhood intervention and developmental disabilities. Dr. Odom's research interests include preschool prevention and school readiness, effectiveness of programs for children and youth with autism spectrum disorders, and early intervention for infants and toddlers with or at risk for disability. He has served on many national advisory committees related to early education, including the National Academy of Sciences Committee on Educational Interventions for Children with Autism. In 2007, Dr. Odom received the Special Education Research Award from the Council for Exceptional Children. Currently, he and a team from FPG edit the *Society for Research in Child Development Social Policy Report*.

Elizabeth P. Pungello, PhD, is a Scientist at FPG, a Research Associate Professor in the Developmental Psychology Program at the University of North Carolina at Chapel Hill, and a Mentor Faculty member at the Center for Developmental Science. Her research focuses on closing the achievement gap between at-risk and other children. More specifically, her current work includes the investigation of the long-term outcomes of the Abecedarian Project (an early educational intervention for children at high risk for poor cognitive and academic outcomes); the exploration of the associations among race, income, parenting, child care quality, and language development and school readiness; and the examination of factors that influence why and how parents search for and select child care. In addition, she is helping lead the FPG Infant/Toddler Child Care Initiative in the development and evaluation of a model of high-quality center care for infants and toddlers raised in poverty.

Nicole Gardner-Neblett, PhD, is an Investigator at FPG at the University of North Carolina at Chapel Hill. Her main focus is the FPG Infant/Toddler Child Care Initiative, where she works to design and implement a model for infant/toddler care to promote the early learning, development, and health of children living in poverty. Her principal research interests are the effects of parenting practices and the classroom context on children's language and literacy development.

Contributors

Lawrence Aber, PhD, is Distinguished Professor of Applied Psychology and Public Policy at New York University and board chair of its Institute of Human Development and Social Change. An internationally recognized expert in child development and social policy, he is Chair of the Board of Directors of the Children's Institute, University of Cape Town, South Africa, and of the Forum for Youth Investment in Washington, DC. Dr. Aber's basic research examines the influence of poverty and violence, at the family and community levels, on the social, emotional, behavioral, cognitive, and academic development of children and youth.

Kathleen Baggett, PhD, is Associate Research Professor at Juniper Gardens Children's Project at the University of Kansas. Her research interests are social–emotional health promotion and child maltreatment prevention for young children, especially those with or at risk for disabilities. One focus of her research is the translatability of evidence-based interventions for web-based delivery to improve home visitor implementation fidelity and reach of interventions aimed at improving parent–child interaction and preventing child maltreatment. Another focus is adapting effective web-based parent–caregiver interventions for authentic delivery in child care centers via teacher professional development programs aimed at promoting infant social–emotional development for typically developing children as well as those with and at risk for disabilities.

John E. Bates, PhD, is Professor in the Department of Psychological and Brain Sciences at Indiana University, Bloomington. His primary research interests concern developmental origins of behavior problems and social competencies in children, adolescents, and adults. He is especially interested in longitudinal research that considers factors such as temperament, specific genes, sleep patterns, family environment, and their interactions.

Patricia J. Bauer, PhD, is Senior Associate Dean for Research and the Asa Griggs Candler Professor of Psychology at Emory University. Her research focuses on the development of memory from infancy through childhood, with special emphasis on the determinants of remembering and forgetting; and links between social, cognitive, and neural developments and age-related changes in autobiographical or personal memory.

Lisa J. Berlin, PhD, is Associate Professor at the University of Maryland School of Social Work. Her research integrates developmental psychology, social work, and public health. She is especially interested in integrating attachment theory, research, and intervention with public health initiatives for infants and young children, such as Early Head Start, and home visiting services to prevent early abuse and neglect. In several ongoing projects she is examining the effects of intensive home visiting on infant–mother attachment; the extent to which mothers' own attachment security can moderate the effectiveness of home visiting and Early Head Start services; and the efficacy of an attachment-based intervention for new mothers with substance use disorders. Dr. Berlin also directs Project M.O.M., a prospective, longitudinal study of the associations between mothers' prenatal psychosocial risks and assets and their later parenting.

Daniel Berry, EdD, is Postdoctoral Research Associate in the Neuroscience and Education Lab in the Department of Applied Psychology at New York University. His research interests are in normative and individual differences in children's self-regulation development.

Clancy Blair, PhD, is Professor in the Department of Applied Psychology at New York University. Dr. Blair is known for his research on school readiness and self-regulation. His research focuses primarily on executive functions in early childhood and the ways in which stress in children's lives can promote or impede the development of executive functions. He is currently conducting longitudinal studies designed to identify early influences on self-regulation and to determine the effect of innovative preschool curricula on self-regulation development and early academic achievement.

Caitlin C. Brez, PhD, is Research Associate and Postdoctoral Trainee at the Schiefelbusch Institute for Life Span Studies at the University of Kansas. Her research interests focus on the development of quantitative abilities in infants and young children and the translation of this research to other disciplines, such as science, technology, engineering, and mathematics (STEM) education.

Jeanne Brooks-Gunn, PhD, is the Virginia and Leonard Marx Professor of Child Development at Teachers College and the College of Physicians and Surgeons at Columbia University and Co-Director of the National Center for Children and Families at Columbia. A developmental psychologist, she focuses on charting the trajectories of children from birth through early adulthood, with a special interest in low-income and low-education families. She designs and tests prevention programs for children and adolescents. Dr. Brooks-Gunn is a member of the Institute of Medicine, National Academies, and the National Institute of Education.

Jay Buzhardt, PhD, is Associate Research Professor at Juniper Gardens Children's Project at the University of Kansas. His interests focus on investigating factors that impact the implementation and effectiveness of technology-based intervention, assessment, and training. He has directed and co-directed several federally funded research projects from the National Institutes of Health, the Institute of

Education Sciences, the Office of Special Education Programs, the National Institute on Disability and Rehabilitation Research, and local foundations. Examples of Dr. Buzhardt's work include the development and experimental evaluation of web-based progress monitoring and decision-making tools for early childhood service providers, the OASIS distance training program to teach applied behavior analysis to parents of young children with autism, a web-based foster parent training program, and technology-enhanced inservice professional development and coaching for K–8 teachers.

Natasha J. Cabrera, PhD, is Associate Professor of Human Development at the University of Maryland. Dr. Cabrera arrived at the University of Maryland with several years of experience as an Expert in Child Development with the Demographic and Behavioral Sciences Branch of the National Institute of Child Health and Human Development. Her current research topics include the role of father involvement with children; theoretical frameworks related to father involvement; children's developmental trajectories in low-income and minority families; ethnic and cultural differences in fathering and mothering; the role of mother–father relationship quality in father involvement and children's outcomes; and the mechanisms that link early experience to children's later development. She has published in peer-reviewed journals on policy, methodology, theory, and the implications of father involvement on child development.

Judith J. Carta, PhD, is Director of Early Childhood Research at the Juniper Gardens Children's Project, Senior Scientist in the Schiefelbusch Institute for Life Span Studies, and Professor of Special Education at the University of Kansas. She is Principal Investigator or Co-Principal Investigator on several research projects funded by the Institute of Education Sciences (IES), the National Institute of Child Health and Human Development, and the Centers for Disease Control and Prevention, and is the Co-Director of the IES-funded Center for Response to Intervention in Early Childhood. Her research career has focused on finding evidence-based approaches to support the growth and development of young children growing up in poverty. Specific research areas have included developing intervention strategies for promoting children's language, literacy, and social–emotional outcomes; validating parenting interventions focused on vulnerable populations; and developing tools for monitoring progress of young children.

Rachel Chazan-Cohen, PhD, is Associate Professor of Applied Developmental Psychology at George Mason University. Previously, she was the Coordinator of Infant and Toddler Research in the Office of Planning Research and Evaluation in the Administration for Children and Families, U.S. Department of Health and Human Services, where she was involved in the evaluation of the federal Early Head Start program. Dr. Chazan-Cohen is particularly interested in the biological, relational, and environmental factors influencing the development of at-risk children, and, most especially, in the creation, evaluation, and refinement of intervention programs for families with infants and toddlers.

John Colombo, PhD, is Professor of Psychology and Director of the Schiefelbusch Institute for Life Span Studies at the University of Kansas. His interests are in early cognitive development, with a special focus on the development of attention in infancy and early childhood. Dr. Colombo has conducted research on the basic biobehavioral aspects of attention, the long-term consequences of early attention for later cognition, the use of attentional and autonomic functions for early identification of intellectual and developmental disabilities, and the effects of various interventions on early cognitive and language outcomes. He serves on several editorial boards and is an Associate Editor for *Child Development*.

Allison H. Friedman, EdM, is a doctoral student in applied psychology at New York University.

Nicole Gardner-Neblett, PhD (*see* "About the Editors").

Roberta Michnick Golinkoff, PhD, holds the H. Rodney Sharp Chair in the School of Education at the University of Delaware, with joint appointments in the Department of Psychology and the Department of Linguistics and Cognitive Science. An Associate Editor of *Child Development*, she is also Co-Director (with Kathy Hirsh-Pasek) of the Center for Re-imagining Children's Learning and Education (CiRCLE) at Temple University and one of the co-founders of the Ultimate Block Party, designed to share the science of learning with parents, practitioners, and educators. Her research focuses on how children learn language, preschool education and the value of play, and children's knowledge of geometric forms. The recipient of a John Simon Guggenheim Fellowship and a James McKeen Cattell Sabbatical Award, Dr. Golinkoff is also a spokesperson for research in developmental science and is frequently featured in print and electronic media.

Rachel A. Gooze, MPH, is a PhD student in public health at Temple University. Her research interests are at the intersection of developmental psychology, public health, and early childhood education. She is particularly interested in how young children's health and well-being are influenced by their socioemotional development and their relationships with adults such as parents and teachers. In the years following her undergraduate education, Ms. Gooze worked as a research assistant to a developmental psychologist at the University of New Hampshire and with a team of health psychologists and pediatricians at Trousseau Children's Hospital in Paris, France. She came to Temple University in 2007 and completed a master's degree in public health while working with Dr. Robert Whitaker on obesity prevention issues in early childhood, with a focus on Head Start families and staff.

Charles Greenwood, PhD, is Director of the Juniper Gardens Children's Project and Professor of Applied Behavioral Science at the University of Kansas. He is the author of over 100 scholarly articles and books related to education and special education. Dr. Greenwood is nationally known for his expertise in developing and evaluating innovative instructional intervention procedures for use in schools, especially urban PreK–12 classrooms. In 2009 he received the Irvin Youngberg Research Achievement Award in the Applied Sciences from the University of Kansas.

Kathy Hirsh-Pasek, PhD, is the Stanley and Debra Lefkowitz Professor in the Department of Psychology at Temple University, where she serves as Director of the Infant Language Laboratory and Co-Director (with Roberta Michnick Golinkoff) of the Center for Re-imagining Children's Learning and Education (CiRCLE). Her research in the areas of early language development, literacy, and infant cognition has been funded by the National Science Foundation, the National Institute of Child Health and Human Development, and the Department of Education, resulting in 11 books and over 100 publications. She is a recipient of the American Psychological Association's Bronfenbrenner Award for lifetime contribution to the science of developmental psychology in the service of science and society and its Award for Distinguished Service to Psychological Science.

Erika Hoff, PhD, is Professor of Psychology at Florida Atlantic University. She studies early monolingual and bilingual development and its relations to properties of children's language exposure. She is the author of *Language Development*, coeditor of the *Blackwell Handbook of Language Development* and *Childhood Bilingualism: Research on Infancy through School Age*, and editor of *Research Methods in Child Language*.

Brenda Jones Harden, PhD, is Associate Professor in the Early Childhood Education Program of the Department of Human Development at the University of Maryland, College Park. Her work has spanned the early childhood policy, practice, and research arenas, and has focused on the developmental and mental health needs of young children at environmental risk, with a specific emphasis on preventing maladaptive outcomes in these populations through early childhood intervention programs. Dr. Jones Harden is the author of numerous empirical articles and chapters on young children at environmental risk and early intervention programs, and the author or coauthor of several books on child welfare.

Kathleen N. Kannass, PhD, is Associate Professor of Psychology at Loyola University of Chicago. Her expertise is in cognitive development in infancy and early childhood, and her primary research interests lie in the development of attention and distractibility in infancy, toddlerhood, and the preschool years. She is also part of interdisciplinary research teams that use our basic understanding of attention to address applied issues such as how nutrition affects cognitive development.

Ellen Eliason Kisker, PhD, is President and Managing Partner of Twin Peaks Partners, LLC (TPP). She has extensive experience conducting policy and evaluation research on early childhood care and education programs, as well as other types of education and welfare programs. Dr. Kisker has led several large randomized controlled trials, and, more recently, she has provided leadership in reviewing the literature on the effects of early childhood education programs and in providing technical assistance to other researchers conducting randomized controlled trials. She co-directed the Early Head Start Research and Evaluation Project.

John M. Love, PhD, provides independent consulting in early care and education research and policy for Mathematica Policy Research, Los Angeles County's First 5 LA program, Arizona's First Things First program, and others. He has been involved in teaching, research, and evaluation studies of programs for children from birth to age 5 and their families since the mid-1960s as a principal investigator for multiple Head Start national evaluations, the Bill and Melinda Gates Foundation's Early Learning Initiative in Washington state, and a multisite experimental study of preschool curricula for the U.S. Department of Education. Dr. Love serves on the Research Advisory Committee for Oregon's Healthy Start America Program, the U.S. Department of Health and Human Services' Advisory Committee on Head Start Research and Evaluation, and the Board of Directors of Zero to Three.

Colleen Monahan, BA, is a doctoral student in the Human Development Program at the University of Maryland, College Park. Her research interests center on the impact of environmental risk factors on young children's developmental trajectories. Ms. Monahan has worked as a research assistant in the psychophysiology lab at the University at Buffalo, examining the brain functioning of individuals with substance use disorders using electroencephalogram/event-related potential technology.

Samuel L. Odom, PhD (*see* "About the Editors").

Silvia Place, MA, is a PhD candidate in the Department of Psychology at Florida Atlantic University. Her research interests include the influence of the sociolinguistic environment on bilingual language acquisition.

Elizabeth P. Pungello, PhD (*see* "About the Editors").

Helen Raikes, PhD, is Professor in the Department of Child, Youth and Family Studies at the University of Nebraska–Lincoln. Her research has focused on infants, toddlers, and preschool-age children at greatest risk; early language and social–emotional development; and parenting, with an emphasis on understanding influences on the developmental trajectories of vulnerable children that are amenable to intervention. Another strand of research focuses on state and federal programs and policies that affect young children's developmental outcomes. She was a Society for Research in Child Development Social Policy Fellow at the Administration for Children, Youth, and Families when the Early Head Start Research and Evaluation Study began.

Cheri A. Vogel, PhD, is a senior researcher with more than 10 years of experience conducting evaluations of early childhood education programs and developing and adapting infant/toddler measures for use in large-scale research projects. She currently directs the Early Head Start Family and Child Experiences Survey (Baby FACES). Baby FACES, a 6-year longitudinal cohort study of a nationally representative sample of 89 programs and two cohorts of children, is examining the experiences of low-income families and children, and measuring child outcomes, service receipt, quality, and program implementation. Dr. Vogel also has interests in home visitation programs and is currently involved in a national cross-site evaluation of home visiting programs to prevent child maltreatment.

Dale Walker, PhD, is Associate Research Professor at Juniper Gardens Children's Project at the University of Kansas. Her research addresses early childhood communication and language intervention, professional development, and intervention implementation, as well as assessment practices for infants and toddlers at risk and with special needs. She directs and co-directs research projects related to early communication intervention, progress monitoring, and accountability. Dr. Walker serves on the editorial boards of the *Journal of Early Intervention*, *Early Childhood Research Quarterly*, *Topics in Early Childhood Special Education*, and *Young Exceptional Children*.

Robert C. Whitaker, MD, MPH, is Professor of Public Health and Pediatrics at Temple University. His research interests are in the childhood antecedents of adult chronic disease. He has conducted much of his research on childhood obesity, including studies on the epidemiology of childhood obesity, parent–child feeding interaction, and obesity prevention strategies in low-income preschool children. His work has also focused on the determinants of social and emotional well-being in children. Dr. Whitaker served on the Institute of Medicine's Committee on the Prevention of Obesity in Children and Youth and on its Committee on Obesity Prevention Policies for Young Children. Prior to joining Temple University, he was a Senior Fellow at Mathematica Policy Research and a Senior Visiting Research Scholar at the Center for Health and Wellbeing at Princeton University.

Meryl Yoches, BA, is a doctoral student in Human Development, with a specialization in Developmental Science and a concentration in Early Childhood, at the University of Maryland, College Park. Her research interests include the intersection of child development and public policy, specifically child care and preschool programs for low-income families.

Barry S. Zuckerman, MD, is the Joel and Barbara Alpert Professor of Pediatrics and Public Health at Boston University School of Medicine/Boston Medical Center. He is also co-founder of Reach Out and Read (ROR), a national childhood literacy program; founder of the Medical–Legal Partnership for Children (MLPC); and developer of the Healthy Steps Program for Young Children. Dr. Zuckerman has authored more than 200 scientific publications emphasizing the impact of biological and social factors on children's health and development and is an editor of four books. He was a member of the National Commission on Children and the Carnegie Commission on Young Children and consults nationally and internationally. Among his awards are the C. Anderson Aldrich Award from the American Academy of Pediatrics, the Robert F. Kennedy Embracing the Legacy Award for MLPC, and the Confucius Award for ROR.

Preface

More than 40 years ago, pioneering efforts to address the developmental disparity of infants and toddlers living in poverty resulted in early childhood intervention programs such as the Abecedarian Project and the Perry Preschool Project. Findings from these early experiments demonstrate the positive outcomes of early educational programs, which can extend well into adulthood. In the decades following these pioneering programs, research on children's health and development has expanded. A great deal has been learned about children's brain development, the early developmental underpinnings of language acquisition, cognitive development, social competence, the linguistic and cultural contexts of development, and early childhood intervention. To summarize this wealth of literature and distill implications for infant/toddler care, in May 2010 we convened a 3-day working meeting at the Frank Porter Graham Child Development Institute (FPG) in Chapel Hill, North Carolina, involving leading researchers in developmental science, health, and early child care and education. These individuals summarized the most current developmental, health, and education science in their areas and offered implications for a program for infants/toddlers and their families living in poverty. For each paper, experts on the paper's topic area provided commentary, which was followed by discussion among the small group of participants. It was a heady event! Presenters agreed to summarize their presentations in papers, which then became the chapters of this book.

The book opens with an introduction to the scope of the problem of poverty. Next, the material presented during the FPG working conference is organized into six main sections. The first four cover current understanding of the basic science within four areas of development: cognition (with the main focus on attention and memory development in early childhood), language development (covering both general language acquisition and dual language learning), social–emotional development (considering the constructs of self-regulation, temperament, and attachment and early relationships), and health/physical development (reviewing important issues within nutrition and physical activity as well as general physical health). The next two sections are more applied in nature, with one focused on families (considering important issues surrounding cultural diversity as well as poverty) and another reporting recent findings concerning infant/toddler care and education (presenting findings from Early Head Start studies and other interventions addressing individual differences). The chapter authors all presented and/or served as discussants at the FPG working conference, each providing a definition of the topic area, a summary of the most relevant scientific findings from that area, and the implications of these scientific findings for designing and delivering effective infant/toddler interventions and care for children and families living in poverty. The concluding chapter draws together these implications to describe possible new models of early care and education.

We hope that our readers—be they researchers, practitioners, academics, other professionals, or students seeking to promote the early development of children and families facing economic adversity—will find the content to be "cutting-edge" science and a useful resource. In addition, we intend for the book to be provocative, stimulating further discussion and thought about how to provide the optimal early care and educational environments for young children.

This book would not have been possible without the assistance of many people. We were very fortunate to have the renowned experts who presented at the conference contribute the chapters that make up the bulk of the book. In addition, the advisory committee for the FPG Infant/Toddler Child Care Initiative—Peg Burchinal, Frances Campbell, Kathleen Gallagher, Iheoma Iruka, Kirsten Kainz, Jonathan Kotch, and Steve Reznick—helped plan the conference and select the speakers. Sarah Henderson and Marie Huff assisted with the organization. Other discussants were Vonnie McLoyd, Peter Ornstein, Linda Watson, Dina Castro, Martha Cox, Dianne Ward, Olson Huff, Cristina Gillanders, Peg Burchinal, Donna Bryant, and Lawrence Aber. Last, we are very grateful for a planning grant from the Office of the Vice Chancellor for Research at the University of North Carolina at Chapel Hill, which supported the conference and the beginning activities of this initiative.

Contents

INTRODUCTION

CHAPTER 1

Poor and Low-Income Families, Infant/Toddler Development, and the Prospects for Change

Back to the Future

Lawrence Aber

There are more than 12 million children under the age of 3 who live in the United States. Shockingly, 24% of these infants and toddlers live in "poor" families (with incomes below the federal poverty line, which was $22,050 for a family of four in 2010). Another 22% live in "low-income" families (with incomes between 100% and 200% of the federal poverty line). Consumer expenditure research by the Economic Policy Institute (EPI) clearly indicates that a family income of at least 200% of the poverty line (about $44,000/year on average for a family of four) is necessary to meet a family's basic needs (for food, shelter, clothing, essential services, and other necessities) (Allegretto, 2005). That means that 46% of America's youngest children—5.9 million infants and toddlers—live in families with incomes that are insufficient to ensure their health and development.

This book is about these infants and toddlers from poor and low-income families. Specifically, this book will describe recent advances in the developmental and health sciences on the first 3 years of life and the implications of these advances for the care and education of poor and low-income infants and toddlers. One goal of the book is to generate new, creative ideas about how to harness those advances in the service of designing and creating better care for poor and low-income infants and toddlers. The goal for this introductory chapter is to provide a context for the rest of the book. First, I describe how the conditions under which young children grow up in the United States vary greatly by critical factors like family income, race, and residence. Second, I summarize some of what we know about how low family income and related conditions affect young children's health and development. In keeping with the holistic view of the child in context that this book embodies, I use examples from health and physical development (obesity), cognitive–intellectual development (language delay), and social–emotional development (insecure attachment). Each of these features is negatively influenced by poverty and forecasts future life chances. They are among the many candidates for critical factors that may mediate the influence of poverty during early childhood on later life chances; and so, they are also among the potential targets of change through improved infant and toddler care, education, and development. Third, I locate the recent work on infant and toddler care in the decades-long efforts to use science to enhance early development of poor young children. Fourth and finally, I highlight a few key policy challenges that our field must face in any efforts to use science to improve infant and toddler care.

The Demographic Context: What Is Early Childhood Poverty in 21st-Century America? And Who Are America's Youngest Poor?

Of course, poverty and near poverty can be defined in many ways. Depending on the definition, our understanding of its root causes, its impacts on development, and preferred program and policy interventions to tackle poverty will vary as well (Aber, Jones, & Raver, 2007). The U.S. government's official definition is considered an "absolute" measure of poverty because it is measured against an absolute (but very outdated) standard of the costs of meeting a family's basic material needs. European governments, in contrast, use a "relative" measure of poverty, namely, how far a family's income is from the national median for families. Families with incomes less than 0.5 or 0.6 of national median family income are considered poor. "Subjective" poverty, a third definition of poverty, takes family perceptions and local economic conditions into effect because it is based on adults' answers to the question, "How much income does it take for a family of four to just barely get by in your community?" Finally, as noted earlier, a fourth definition of poverty is income that is too low to meet a family's basic needs without relying on external, government, or charitable support (EPI's "family self-sufficiency" standard). Today, the family self-sufficiency standard is approximately twice the poverty line. The relative and subjective poverty lines fall in between the official U.S. poverty line and the family self-sufficiency standard. So the figures I noted at the start of the chapter, 24% of poor infants and toddlers and another 22% of low-income infants and toddlers combine to offer an upper bound of 46% of America's youngest children as the foci of this book. Said another way, nearly half of America's infants and toddlers start life in or near poverty, in families facing the daily stress that their income is inadequate to meet their basic needs. This means that early childhood poverty is *not* a small problem but a massive one, deserving of our society's most creative thinking, urgent calls to action, and collective problem solving.

Who are "America's Youngest Poor" (National Center for Children in Poverty, 1996)? As is well known, poverty is not distributed evenly across peoples or places (Chau, Thampi, & Wright, 2010). In the United States, the poverty rate (less than 100% of the poverty line) is 15% among white infants and toddlers and 42% and 34% among black and Hispanic infants and toddlers, respectively. The poverty plus low-income rates (from 0 to 200% of the poverty line) are 32%, 68%, and 64% for white, black, and Hispanic young children. Similarly, rates of poor and low-income young children are higher for children of parents who are younger, less educated, and under- or unemployed. Poverty rates vary greatly by states: five states experience poverty rates above 25% (Arkansas, the District of Columbia, Kentucky, Mississippi, and New Mexico), and 13 states have infant and toddler poverty rates under 15%. In short, young children's poverty status is strongly associated with their parents' situation (race/ethnicity, education, and employment) and also with their family's place of residence. This variation of poor and low family incomes is a deep and enduring reality and one which a re-visioning of infant and toddler care for the poor must confront in all its complexities.

Infant and toddler poverty is not only a problem for just some races and places in the United States. Even among the young children of white parents, educated parents, and working parents, and even in our best states, child poverty in the United States is very high by international comparative standards (UNICEF, 2000). Indeed, among 22 "rich nations" studied by UNICEF, the U.S. rate is second highest. Only five other countries have child poverty rates above 15%. Sixteen of the 22 countries have child poverty rates for their entire country that are better than the poverty rate the United States has for its white children or in its best states.

Clearly, child poverty "U.S. style" has some unique causes and dynamics that account for the United States being an outlier. Cross-national studies rule out the normal, pat answers as to why America is an outlier. Careful research has demonstrated that our exceptionally high child poverty rates are *not* due primarily to differences with other countries in the racial/ethnic composition of young families, nor to young parents' education and employment levels, nor to our relatively high rates of single-parent families (Garfinkel, Rainwater, & Smeeding, 2006). Rather, the biggest reason for our high poverty rates is the nature of our public policies in support of low-income families with children. Our "tax and transfer" system is much less effective in reducing child poverty than are the tax and transfer systems of other rich nations (UNICEF, 2000; Garfinkel et al., 2006).

Finally, of particular relevance to this volume is the question of how family income is associated with the types and qualities of nonparental care that young children receive. The data to address this issue for infants and toddlers are a bit dated; but the general findings are likely to still hold true (Kreader, Ferguson, & Lawrence, 2005). Among children born in 2001, those from poor families were less likely to be in nonparental care arrangements by age 2 than those in higher-income families (43% vs. 52%; Cappizano & Adams, 2003). Even among the under-3-year-olds with employed mothers, those from low-income families were less likely to be in a regular nonparental care arrangement than those from higher-income families (62% vs. 68%). Finally, among those infants and toddlers in nonparental care, the type of care varied by family income. Infants and toddlers from low-income families were more likely to be in relative care (32% vs. 26%) and less likely to be in center-based care (16% vs. 21%) and family child care (11% vs. 15%). Because quality center-based and family child care have consistently been associated with developmental advantages for low-income infants and toddlers (Shonkoff & Phillips, 2000; Love et al., 2003), these figures on different child care experiences by family income tell a sobering story of inequality in care and education opportunities well before children reach the schoolhouse door.

The Developmental Implications:
How Do Poor and Low Family Incomes (and Related Risk Factors) Affect Young Children's Health and Development?

How exactly do poor and low family incomes set off a chain of processes that lead to less optimal outcomes across the full spectrum of developmental domains? Serious scholarship on this issue is nearly a half-century old, and several colleagues and I have summarized that history elsewhere (Aber et al., 2007). The take-home message of this history is that as both theory and research methods have advanced over the decades, we are more and more clear about these chains of processes. Recent work emphasizes different pathways by which different features of poverty (and its many cofactors) impact childhood health and development. One pathway, from low family income to low parental investments of time and money into their children's development, appears to be especially influential on children's cognitive, language, and academic development. Another pathway runs from material hardship (a correlate of but not identical to income poverty) through family stress to harsh and unresponsive parenting and appears especially influential on children's social–emotional learning and development (Gershoff, Aber, Raver, & Lennon, 2007; Yeung, Linver, & Brooks-Gunn, 2002). A third perspective has also been very important in advancing knowledge about how poverty and other risk factors impact child development. Often referred to as "risk and resilience" theory, it emphasizes how the cumulative effects of multiple risks (including poverty) are more important than any single risk in affecting outcomes (see the groundbreaking work of Sameroff [Sameroff, Seifer, Barocas, Zax, & Greenspan, 1987], Garmezy [Garmezy & Rutter, 1983] and Rutter [1987]). More recently, there is mounting evidence that certain children in some contexts are relatively resilient in the face of risk, adversity, and threat. Masten and Powell (2003), Cicchetti and Blender (2006), and others have emphasized how resilience processes at multiple levels of the human ecology (from the genetic and biological through the individual to the familial and broader ecological levels) help explain the enormous heterogeneity in children's responses to risks like poverty and many other adverse experiences that are highly correlated with or potentiated by poverty.

These three models—the family investment model (informed by Gary Becker's [1976] economic theory of the family), the family stress model (informed by Rand Conger's family stress theory [Conger & Conger, 2008; Conger, Rueter, & Conger, 2000]), and the risk and resilience model (informed by the theories of developmental psychopathology of Garmezy & Rutter [1983], Rutter [1987], Masten & Powell [2003], and Cicchetti & Blender [2006]) help organize much of what we've learned to date about poverty, and poverty cofactors, and their impact on child development, including early child development.

To illustrate, I briefly draw on several chapters in this volume to describe in more detail current thinking about how family poverty is associated with impairments in infant and toddler health and development, and by what processes poverty influences these early childhood outcomes.

Social–Emotional Development: Security of Attachment

Attachment theory and research is over half a century old (Bowlby, 1969, 1973, 1980; Ainsworth, 1973) and has spawned an extremely rich set of empirical findings (Thompson, 2008). Security of attachment refers to the young child's ability to use the parent/caregiver to gain protection and comfort in times of danger and distress and his or her use of the attachment figure as a secure base to confidently explore and learn from his or her environment. Security of attachment in early childhood has been shown to forecast a wide range of social and emotional competencies through adolescence (Allen & Land, 1999; Allen, McElhaney, Kuperminc, & Jodi, 2004). Berlin (Chapter 8, this volume) describes how family poverty and low socioeconomic status (SES) are associated with more insecure infant and toddler attachments, both to parents and to nonparental caregivers. Further, she points out that the main predictor of secure attachments, parent and caregiver sensitivity and responsivity to the young child, is less predictive of security among poor dyads than nonpoor dyads. She reasons that this may be due to the infant and/or toddler (and his or her caregivers) being overwhelmed by other cofactors of poverty. Finally and hopefully, Berlin cites evidence from an emerging set of intervention studies that demonstrate that both parent and caregiver responsiveness *and* child security attachment are malleable, a point to which I return below.

Cognitive–Intellectual Development: Early Language Development

The first 3 years of life are a critical period in the emergence of language and cognition. Infants and toddlers grow rapidly in features of linguistic and communicative competence like phonemic awareness, vocabulary, and grammar (among other features of early language development), each of which have been shown to predict school readiness and later school achievement. Hirsh-Pasek and Golinkoff (Chapter 4, this volume) describe the dramatically different language environments of poor and nonpoor infants and toddlers, the significant delays in early language and cognitive development associated with poverty and impoverished early language environment, and the processes that help explain SES differences in very early language learning. As with Berlin (Chapter 8, this volume), Hirsh-Pasek and Golinkoff also argue strenuously that children's early trajectories of language and cognitive development are malleable. They articulate a set of six evidence-based principles as guides to direct how to intervene to ensure positive language trajectories for *all* young children. And like Berlin, they leave us with a road map for practitioners who work with young children and their families.

Given the large portion of Hispanic children living in poverty cited earlier in the chapter, Hoff and Place (Chapter 5, this volume) address the critical issue of bilingual language learning. Learning two languages at the same time affects the rate at which each language is acquired. Thus, infants and toddlers of language-minority parents need extra language support. Hoff and Place discuss several implications for the work of caregivers (e.g., the value of one-on-one conversations). The chapters by Colombo, Kannass, Walker, and Brez (Chapter 2, this volume) and Bauer (Chapter 3, this volume) describe important work on other key aspects of early cognitive development. Colombo et al. discuss the development of attention— a system that research shows is very important for learning and school readiness and appears to be influenced by the context of poverty. Bauer presents work on early memory development that is also critical for learning. Both Colombo et al. and Bauer describe research that has clear implications for how to promote both cognitive development in young children and the kinds of activities that should be done to promote these cognitive capabilities.

Physical Health and Development: Obesity

Obesity is the most common health consequence of poor nutrition among poor children in the United States (Karp, Cheng, & Meyers, 2005). Obesity, an excess of body fat that is associated with physical and psychological morbidity, is defined by the Centers for Disease Control and Prevention (CDC) as at or above the 95% of body mass index (BMI) by earlier historical standards for age and gender. Obesity is not formally diagnosable until age 24 months, but by that age, 10.4% of toddlers in the United States currently meet this (historically defined) standard (Ogden, Carroll, Curtin, Lamb, & Flegal, 2010).

Building on these concepts and definitions, Whitaker and Gooze (Chapter 9, this volume) note the co-occurrence of poverty, food insecurity, and obesity in early childhood and later life. Food insecurity is defined as "limited or uncertain availability of nutritionally adequate and safe foods, or limited or uncertain ability to acquire food in socially acceptable ways" (Bickel, Nord, Price, Hamilton, & Cook, 2000, p. 6). Directly relevant to this volume, in 2009, 46% of U.S. households with incomes below 130% of the federal poverty line *and* with young children (less than 5 years of age) were food insecure (Nord, Coleman-Jensen, Andrews, & Carlson, 2010). Again, Whitaker and Gooze reason that food insecurity is a likely mediator linking poverty and obesity, and that risk for obesity in early childhood is malleable because many of the determinants of obesity, like food insecurity, are malleable.

In short, the chapters of this volume summarize the state of the art in developmental and health science in our understanding of how poverty is associated with nonoptimal social–emotional (e.g., insecurity of attachment), cognitive–intellectual (e.g., language, attention, memory), and physical health (e.g., obesity) development and what is known about which processes mediate the influence of poverty on early childhood developmental outcomes and how malleable these processes and outcomes are. Each chapter makes singular contributions to our understanding in specific and important domains. And yet, the field cannot rest there. If we are to draw upon the best science to improve the care and education of poor and low-income infants and toddlers, we must begin to pull the literature and research on the complex domain-specific processes and outcomes into a more coherent picture of how the whole child in context, as a developing system, works. Fortunately, significant progress on these cross-domain syntheses of processes and outcomes is also being made. The Blair chapter (Chapter 6, this volume) is very interesting in that it crosses the social–emotional, cognitive, and physical domains with the focus on self-regulation. He describes how the stress of poverty seems to "get under the skin" by how it affects the stress response system that consequently influences self-regulation and in turn later executive function skills. This mechanism for how poverty affects development also helps to explain why kids raised in poverty seem to be differentially affected by high-quality early learning environments (i.e., why they effect kids in poverty more). The domain-specific work in this volume needs to be further integrated into work on influences of poverty across domains of development. By way of illustration, I refer to recent work by Martha Zaslow and colleagues (2009) that pull several of these strands together.

Using data from the Early Childhood Longitudinal Study–Birth Cohort (ECLS-B), Zaslow and colleagues (2009) have modeled the relationship among poverty, poverty cofactors and food insecurity (at 9 months of age in a young child's life), parent functioning and parenting (also at 9 months), and a set of early childhood outcomes (at 24 months). Figure 1.1 is my summary of their results from several independent analyses (Zaslow et al., 2009; Bronte-Tinkew, Zaslow, Capps, Horowitz, & McNamara, 2007). What Figure 1.1 illustrates are plausible (but not proven) pathways from poverty (not shown) through food insecurity (at 9 months) to cognitive–language, social–emotional, and physical health outcomes (at 24 months). The key point I wish to make is that food insecurity and nonpositive parenting are common pathways to three sets of nonoptimal early childhood developmental outcomes: low mental proficiency, insecure attachment (Zaslow et al., 2009) and obesity (Bronte-Tinkew et al., 2007).

Finally, it must be emphasized that there are a very broad range of other factors besides food insecurity that are correlated with poverty, are relatively common among infants and toddlers in the United States, and

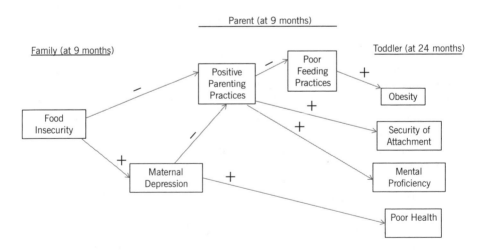

FIGURE 1.1. Plausible pathways from food insecurity to early childhood developmental outcomes. Based on Zaslow et al. (2009) and Bronte-Tinkew, Zaslow, Capps, Horowitz, and McNamara (2007).

are known to negatively influence early childhood development. These include exposure to child maltreatment (7.5% of infants and toddlers) and to parental substance abuse (9.8% of infants and toddlers) to name but two. As the work on cumulative risk and resilience clearly indicates, it is the accumulation of multiple risks associated with poverty that has the most powerful effect on early development and brain function and structure, mediated most likely by truly toxic levels of stress experienced by infants and toddlers and their caretakers (Shonkoff, Boyce, & McEwen, 2009).

This variation in levels of risk raises the issue of the great heterogeneity among the poor and how to tailor prevention and care strategies to address this heterogeneity. (See Cabrera [Chapter 11, this volume] and Jones Harden, Monahan, and Yoches [Chapter 12, this volume] for descriptions of the unique dynamics and needs of infants and toddlers in Hispanic families and in the highest-risk families; see also Carta, Greenwood, Baggett, Buzhardt, and Walker [Chapter 14, this volume] and Love et al. [Chapter 13, this volume] for important discussions of the value of and challenges to effectively tailoring prevention and care strategies to individuals and subgroups.)

In order to reach the goal of this book—to harness advances like those presented in the service of designing and creating better care for poor and low-income infants and toddlers—we must keep our scientific and programmatic eyes on the prize: that the young child in context is a developing system of multiple and interacting developing systems (physical, cognitive, social–emotional); that family poverty creates perturbations in each of these systems *and* their interactions; and that they do so through complex, precisely ordered sequences of processes in specific contexts and in real time. That means we must strive to understand these processes in contexts as well as we possibly can in order to create the most effective ways of changing these processes and contexts to put poor and low-income infants and toddlers on the best possible early life trajectory.

Using Developmental and Health Science to Improve the Life Trajectories of Infants and Toddlers in Poverty: Some Historical Context

The second decade of the 21st century is not the first time the United States has pursued this path to reform. At several earlier points in our history, we've endeavored to draw on the best of developmental and health science to inform program and policy design and evaluation for poor and low-income infants and toddlers. The first generation of work was led by initiatives like the Abecedarian Project (Campbell, Ramey, Pungello, Sparling, & Miller-Johnson, 2002) and the Infant Health and Development Project (McCormack et al., 2006). These efforts were designed to be implemented by well-trained and supervised service providers, and they assumed access to considerable financial resources to support the services model. Rigorous

randomized control trial (RCT) studies were mounted to test their efficacy under near-optimal conditions. They had largely positive short-term
effects, many of which were sustained or transferred to new domains of
functioning over time. We learned from this first generation of "existence
proofs" that we could create intensive (and thus expensive) interventions
with large effect sizes on key features of infant and toddler development.
But, needless to say, this first generation did not prove that we could obtain
this level of change with "regular" programs, delivered under more normal
conditions (and perhaps reliant on few financial resources).

Thus emerged a second generation of initiatives targeted on poor and
low-income infants and toddlers and their families. Again informed by the
best available developmental and health sciences, they varied broadly in
focus, design, auspice, cost, and impact. Each was rigorously evaluated via
RCTs. The Comprehensive Child Development Program (CCDP), an initiative targeted at multiple risk factors, had virtually no impact on early
childhood development (St. Pierre, Layzer, Goodson, & Bernstein, 1999).
The Early Head Start (EHS) initiative, targeted on a broadly defined range
of low-income youngsters and families and at the critical spheres of child
and parent development, but also at staff and community development, had
important impacts on children and parents by ages 3 and 5 but which largely
faded out by fifth grade (Love et al., Chapter 13, this volume). Finally, the
Nurse Home Visiting Program model, targeted to first-time parents at high
risk for the worst outcomes, appears to have reduced incidents of child
maltreatment and serious accidents and injuries (among young children)
and improved the economic status of their parents (Olds, 2006). From this
second generation of initiatives, we learned that we could undertake efforts
on a larger scale and could get positive results if we targeted key outcomes
with efficacious practices. But the outcomes were more modest and quite
variable, and the program models are too expensive to easily scale, at least
under the current political and economic conditions of the nation.

A third generation of initiatives has begun to emerge over the last
decade. Unlike the programs described above, they were not designed to be
intensive, costly, and sufficient in and of themselves. Rather, they are relatively brief (10 to 20 sessions over the course of infancy and toddlerhood),
low-cost interventions that nonetheless aspired to have the same or larger
impact on cognitive and/or social–emotional development as the earlier
initiatives. Examples of these initiatives include the Videotape Interaction
Project, an intervention delivered via primary pediatric care practices and
designed to enhance language development and reduce problem behaviors
among poor infants and toddlers (Mendelsohn et al., 2007); and the Family Check-Up, an intervention for poor toddlers at high risk for externalizing behavior problems that has been delivered via food supplementation
(e.g., Women, Infant and Children [WIC]) programs and can be adapted
to be delivered via primary care practices as well (Dishion et al., 2008).
Other promising early interventions designed to be relatively brief and

low in cost but equally high or higher in impact include Dozier's (Dozier, Lindhiem, & Ackerman, 2005; Dozier et al., 2009) attachment theory-based intervention (Attachment and Biobehavioral Catch-Up [ABC]) and Landry's parent-responsiveness intervention (Play and Learning Strategies [PALS]; Landry, Smith, & Swank, 2006; Landry, Smith, Swank, & Guttentag, 2008).

As the contents of this volume document, the early childhood field is now preparing to embark on a new generation of work that strives to use the best possible developmental and health science to improve the care and education of poor and low-income infants and toddlers. As the brief history of such efforts sketched above suggests, we have learned a lot about what works and what doesn't from both basic science and from science-informed rigorous program and policy evaluation. But as a nation, we are still light-years away from the goal of providing quality infant and toddler care and education to all youngsters regardless of family income. There are numerous challenges that face the early childhood field (in particular) and the nation (as a whole) if we are ever to reach our goal. In the last section of this introductory chapter, I focus on three policy challenges that seem to me to be the most important to address.

Key Policy Challenges

Like many in my field (and like most if not all of the contributors to this volume), I deeply believe that the science of early development can be used to improve practice and policy. But I also believe that we already know more scientifically than we've been able to use pragmatically. Why? Of course, there are many reasons. But the biggest and most determinative reasons, in my view, are an interrelated set of policy challenges.

Institutional/Organization Challenges

Perhaps the most concrete challenge facing the early childhood field is that there is no truly universal public platform on which to advance efforts to improve early learning and development for infants and toddlers in the United States. By right, all children in the United States are entitled to a free and equal education. Historically, that has been interpreted as K–12 education. Consequently, there is an overwhelming reliance on families not to only provide but "fund" children's care and education in the first 3 to 4 years of life. The only "near-universal" system of care and services for infants and toddlers in the United States is the health care system. It is funded by a combination of private and public insurance.

If science is to be used to improve the care and education of poor and low-income infants and toddlers, the nation must finally develop and maintain a universal platform for early learning and development beyond the family. Such a universal platform could be a truly national system for nonparental care like those in operation in many other economically advanced nations, for example, the crèche system in France (Kamerman, 2000). Indeed, such a universal system was envisioned 40 years ago by many of the nation's leading child care advocates when then-Senator Walter Mondale introduced the "Comprehensive Child Development Bill of 1972." Congress passed the bill in 1971. But President Nixon vetoed it in 1972, calling it a "communal approach to child-rearing" that had "family-weakening implications." If the bill had become law, it would have begun to fund a national child care system designed explicitly to make it easier for mothers to work and care for their children. But if the United States is still not ready for a truly universal voluntary system of nonparental care for infants and toddlers, perhaps the only other "near-universal" system, the health care system, could be used to more effectively advance infant and toddler development.

Funding/Equity Challenges

I believe that the nation is well beyond Nixon's concerns that a universal early care and education system is a danger to the American family. But even if the nation agrees that such a system would be valuable, perhaps especially for our poorest young children, the question of funding continues to present a major challenge. There are numerous ways to meet such a challenge, but first it is necessary to decide what the goal should be. As a place to start, I've proposed the goal of achieving "developmental equity" in public funding of early care and education (Aber, 2007). Currently, the United States spends between $9,000 and $15,000/year in per pupil expenditures on K–12 education (depending on the states and local districts). In New York City, it is estimated that the public sector invests no more than $4,000/year in children before they reach kindergarten. I propose that the United States put itself on a course of closing this developmental equity gap by investing approximately the same amount in public funds per infant and toddler per year in his or her care and education. Options to invest range from supply-side investments in quality center-based and family child care to demand-side strategies like vouchers for use in quality programs *or* a dramatic expansion of the Child Tax Credit. The key point is that it is irrational to make such a small public investment in the first 3 years of life when the quality of care and education is inadequate and the potential returns on investment are at their highest (Heckman, 2006).

Political/Fiscal Challenges

Now in 2012, several years after the "Great Recession" hit the United States (and much of the globe), when the U.S. economy is still stuck in a bad place and there is a bipartisan call to cut government spending in order to cut deficits, it is a tough time to call for a universal system of early care and education and funding of the first 3 years that is comparable to funding during the K–12 years. But as Ajay Chaudry and I argue in a recent paper, it is also a critically important time to do so as well (Aber & Chaudry, 2010). It is beyond the scope of this chapter to go into detail, but suffice it to say that our current plans about how to deal with the recession can and must be reconciled with our long-term goals for the future. For nearly 50 years, the United States has endeavored to use science to improve early development. For nearly 40 years, we have known that nothing less than a comprehensive child development plan was necessary to do so. For the last 30 years, we have made important progress in working out how the science of early child development could improve practice and policy, but we have not worked out clear and viable answers to the three big policy challenges necessary to create change at population level: a universal platform, sufficient and equitable public funding, and the political will to make progress even in the face of severe fiscal constraints. This book offers insight and optimism on the science and practice fronts. But the future outlook on the policy and political fronts are dangerously unclear.

REFERENCES

Aber, J. L. (2007, December). Changing the climate on early childhood [special report]. *The American Prospect,* pp. A4–A6.

Aber, J. L., & Chaudry, A. (2010). *Low-income children, their families and the great recession: What next in policy?* Urban Institute. Retrieved from *www. urban.org/publications/412069.html.*

Aber, J. L., Jones, S. M., & Raver, C. C. (2007). Poverty and child development: New perspectives on a defining issue. In J. L. Aber, S. J. Bishop-Josef, S. M. Jones, K. T. McLearn, & D. A. Phillips (Eds.), *Child development and social policy: Knowledge for action* (pp. 149–166). Washington, DC: American Psychological Association Press.

Ainsworth, M. D. S. (1973). The development of infant–mother attachment. In B. Caldwell & H. Ricciuti (Eds.), *Review of child development research* (Vol. 3, pp. 1–94). Chicago: University of Chicago Press.

Allegretto, S. (2005, August 30). *Basic family budgets: Working families' incomes often fail to meet living expenses around the U.S.* (Briefing paper). Washington, DC: Economic Policy Institute.

Allen, J. P., & Land, D. (1999). Attachment in adolescence. In J. Cassidy & P. R. Shaver (Eds.), *Handbook of attachment: Theory, research, and clinical applications* (pp. 319–335). New York: Guilford Press.

Allen, J. P., McElhaney, K. B., Kuperminc, G. P., & Jodi, K. M. (2004). Stability and change in attachment security across adolescence. *Child Development,* 75(6), 1792–1805.

Becker, G. S. (1976). *The economic approach to human behavior.* Chicago: University of Chicago Press.

Bickel, G., Nord, M., Price, C., Hamilton, W., & Cook, J. (2000). *Guide to measuring household food security, revised 2000.* Retrieved July 11, 2011, from *www.fns.usda.gov/fsec/FILES/FSGuide.pdf.*

Bowlby, J. (1969). *Attachment and loss. Vol. 1. Attachment.* New York: Basic Books.

Bowlby, J. (1973). *Attachment and loss. Vol. 2. Separation: Anxiety and anger.* New York: Basic Books.

Bowlby, J. (1980). *Attachment and loss. Vol. 3. Loss: Sadness and depression.* New York: Basic Books.

Bronte-Tinkew, J., Zaslow, M., Capps, R., Horowitz, A., & McNamara M. (2007). Food insecurity works through depression, parenting, and infant feeding to influence overweight and health in toddlers. *Journal of Nutrition, 137*(9), 2160–2165.

Campbell, A. C., Ramey, C. T., Pungello, E., Sparling, J., & Miller-Johnson, S. (2002). Early childhood education: Young adult outcomes from the Abecedarian project. *Applied Developmental Science, 6*(1), 42–57.

Capizzano, J., & Adams, G. (2003). *Snapshots of American families: Children in low-income families are less likely to be in center-based child care* (Report No. 16). Washington, DC: Urban Institute.

Chau, M., Thampi, K., & Wright, V. R. (2010). *Basic facts about low-income children, 2009: Children under age 3.* New York: National Center for Children in Poverty, Columbia University, Mailman School of Public Health.

Cicchetti, D., & Blender, J. A. (2006). A multiple-levels-of-analysis perspective on resilience: Implications for the developing brain neural plasticity, and preventive interventions. *Annals of New York Academy of Sciences, 1094,* 248–258.

Conger, K. J., Rueter, M. A., & Conger, R. D. (2000). The role of economic pressure in the lives of parents and their adolescents: The family stress model. In L. J. Crockett & R. J. Silbereisen (Eds.), *Negotiating adolescence in times of social change* (pp. 201–233). Cambridge: Cambridge University Press.

Conger, R. D., & Conger, K. J. (2008). Understanding the processes through which economic hardship influences families and children. In D. R. Crane & T. B. Heaton (Eds.), *Handbook of families and poverty* (pp. 64–81). Thousand Oaks, CA: Sage.

Dishion, T. J., Shaw, D. S., Connell, A., Gardner, F., Weaver, C., & Wilson, M. (2008). The family check-up with high-risk indigent families: Outcomes of positive parenting and problem behavior from ages 2 through 4. *Child Development, 79*(5), 1395–1414.

Dozier M., Lindhiem, O., & Ackerman, J. P. (2005). Attachment and biobehavioral catch-up. In L. J. Berlin, Y. Ziv, L. Amaya-Jackson, & M. T. Greenberg (Eds.), *Enhancing early attachments: Theory, research, intervention and policy* (pp. 178–194). New York: Guilford Press.

Dozier, M., Lindhiem, O., Lewis, E., Bick, J., Bernard, K., & Peloso, E. (2009). Effects of a foster parent training program on young children's attachment behaviors: Preliminary evidence from a randomized clinical trial. *Child and Adolescent Social Work Journal, 26*(4), 321–332.

Garfinkel, I., Rainwater, L., & Smeeding, T. M. (2006). A reexamination of welfare state and inequality in rich nations: How in-kind transfers and indirect taxes change the story. *Journal of Policy Analysis and Management, 25*(4), 855–919.

Garmezy, N., & Rutter, M. (1983). *Stress, coping and development in children.* New York: McGraw-Hill.

Gershoff, E. T., Aber, J. L., Raver, C. C., & Lennon, M. C. (2007). Income is not enough: Incorporating material hardship into models of income associations with parenting and child development. *Child Development, 78*(1), 70–95.

Heckman, J. J. (2006). Skill formation and the economics of investing in disadvantaged children. *Science, 312*(5782), 1900–1902.

Kamerman, S. B. (2000). Early childhood education and care: An overview of developments in OECD countries. *International Journal of Educational Research, 33*(1), 7–29.

Karp, R. J., Cheng, C., & Meyers, A. F. (2005). The appearance of discretionary income: Influence on the prevalence of under- and over-nutrition. *International Journal for Equity in Health, 4*(10), 1–7.

Kreader, J. L., Ferguson, D., & Lawrence, S. (2005). *Infant and toddler child care arrangement.* Child Care and Early Education Research Connections No. 1, New York: Columbia University National Center for Children in Poverty.

Landry, S., Smith, K. E., & Swank, P. R. (2006). Responsive parenting: Establishing early foundations for social, communication, and independent problem-solving skills. *Developmental Psychology, 42*(4), 627–642.

Landry, S., Smith, K. E., Swank, P. R., & Guttentag, C. (2008). A responsive parenting intervention: The optimal timing across early childhood for impacting maternal behaviors and child outcomes. *Developmental Psychology, 44,* 1335–1353.

Love, J. M., Harrison, L., Sagi-Schwartz, A., van Ijzendoorn, M. H., Ross, C., Ungerer, J. A., et al. (2003). Child care quality matters: How conclusions may vary with context. *Child Development, 74,* 1021–1033.

Masten, A. S., & Powell, J. L. (2003). A resilience framework of research, policy, and practice. In S. S. Luthar (Ed.), *Resilience and vulnerability: Adaptation in the context of child adversities* (pp. 1–25). New York: Cambridge University Press.

McCormick, M. C., Brooks-Gunn, J., Buka, S. L., Goldman, J., Yu, J., Salganik, M., et al. (2006). Early intervention in low birth weight premature infants: Results at 28 years of age for the Infant Health and Development Program. *Pediatrics, 117*(3), 771–780.

Mendelsohn, A. L., Valdez, P. T., Flynn, V., Foley, G. M., Berkule, S. B., Tomopoulos, S., et al. (2007). Use of videotaped interactions during pediatric well-child care: Impact at 33 months on parenting and on child development. *Journal of Developmental and Behavioral Pediatrics, 28,* 206–212.

National Center for Children in Poverty. (1996). *One in four: America's youngest poor.* New York: Columbia University National Center for Children in Poverty.

Nord, M., Coleman-Jensen, A., Andrews, M., & Carlson, S. (2010). *Household food security in the United States, 2009,* ERR-108, U.S. Department of Agriculture, Economic Research Service. Available at *www.ers.usda.gov/Publications/ERR108/ERR108.pdf.*

Ogden, C. L., Carroll, M. D., Curtin, L. R., Lamb, M. M., & Flegal, K. M. (2010). Prevalence of high body mass index in U.S. children and adolescents, 2007–2008. *Journal of the American Medical Association, 303*(3), 242–249.

Olds, D. L. (2006). The nurse-family partnership: An evidence-based preventive intervention. *Infant Mental Health Journal, 27*(1), 5–25.

Rutter, M. (1987). Psychosocial resilience and protective mechanisms. *American Journal of Orthopsychiatry, 57*(3), 316–331.

Sameroff, A. J., Seifer, A., Barocas, R., Zax, M., & Greenspan, S. (1987). Intelligence quotient scores of 4-year-old children: Social–environmental risk factors. *Pediatrics, 79*(3), 343–350.

Shonkoff, J. P., Boyce, W. T., & McEwen, B. S. (2009). Neuroscience, molecular biology, and the childhood roots of health disparities building a new framework for health promotion and disease prevention. *Journal of the American Medical Association, 301*(21), 2252–2259.

Shonkoff, J., & Phillips, D. (2000). *From neurons to neighborhoods: The science of early child development.* Washington, DC: National Academy of Sciences Press.

St. Pierre, R. G., Layzer, J. I., Goodson, B. D., & Bernstein, L. S. (1999). The effectiveness of comprehensive case management interventions: Evidence from the National Evaluation of the Comprehensive Child Development Program. *American Journal of Evaluation, 20*(1), 15–34.

Thompson, R. A. (2008). Early attachment and later development: Familiar questions, new answers. In J. Cassidy & P. R. Shaver (Eds.), *Handbook of attachment: Theory, research and clinical applications* (2nd ed., pp. 348–365). New York: Guilford Press.

UNICEF. (2000). *A league table of child poverty in rich nations.* Innocenti Report Card, No.1. Florence, Italy: Innocenti Research Centre.

Yeung, J., Linver, M., & Brooks-Gunn, J. (2002). How money matters for young children's development: Parental investment and family processes. *Child Development, 73*, 1861–1879.

Zaslow, M., Bronte-Tinkew, J., Capps, R., Horowitz, A., Moore, K. A., & Weinstein, D. (2009). Food security during infancy: Implications for attachment and mental proficiency in toddlerhood. *Maternal and Child Health Journal, 13*(1), 66–80.

PART I

COGNITIVE DEVELOPMENT

CHAPTER 2

The Development of Attention in Infancy and Early Childhood

Implications for Early Childhood and Early Intervention

John Colombo, Kathleen N. Kannass, Dale Walker, and Caitlin C. Brez

Attention is a central concept in psychology and a major area of study for human cognition and cognitive development. As an applied concept (Parasuraman & Wilson, 2008), the phenomenon of attention has been useful in improving practices in human–computer interaction (Lee & Seong, 2009), transportation (Shinar, 2008), and medicine (Sutton et al., 2010).

The impact of the concept of attention in the realm of education, however, has been relatively constrained. Recently, attention has gained some purchase in the area of early psychoeducational assessment (Greenwood, Walker, Hornbeck, Hebbeler, & Spiker, 2007). Measures of attention have begun to be considered in predictive models of educational attainment (Auerbach et al., 2005; Hart et al., 2004; Ohgi, Takahashi, Nugent, Arisawa, & Akiyama, 2003) and in parent–child interactions during early childhood (Hart et al., 2004; Ohgi, Akiyama, & Fukuda, 2005). Within the literature in early childhood education (ECE) and early childhood intervention (ECI), the concept of attention has attracted consideration with respect to disorders such as attention-deficit disorder (ADD) and autism. In addition, the concept of joint attention, which refers to concurrent or shared attention during play, reading, or social interaction, has been a focus of work within the promotion of communicative and language development and intervention in typically developing children (Carpenter, Nagell, & Tomasello, 1998; Hockenberger, Goldstein, & Haas, 1999; Morales et al., 2000; Richman & Colombo, 2007) and children with intellectual and developmental disabilities (Brady & Warren, 2003; Kaiser & Trent, 2007; McBride & Peterson, 1997; Stone, Coonrod, & Ousley, 2000; Toth, Munson, Meltzoff, & Dawson, 2006; Yoder & Warren, 2001a, 2001b). However, relative to the ubiquity and centrality of the concept within the fields of developmental and cognitive science, the extant literature on the neurodevelopment and nature of attention has had relatively constrained impact on either procedures or policy in ECE and ECI (Rieger et al., 2004).

There may be several reasons for this, not the least of which may be confusion in professional and academic circles about what attention actually is, and what it does. Another reason may be that the existing academic research on attention has not been particularly amenable to translation to more applied settings. This unfortunate state of affairs, common to many concepts in cognitive science, is one that this volume hopes to address.

Our purpose here is to clarify attention, as a construct, and its function in the cognitive system. We also present current scientific information about the nature of attention in infancy and early childhood and translate the implications of that knowledge for the areas of ECE and ECI.

Attention and Its Functions

The Varieties of Attention

Most modern scholars reference William James (1890) for the first systematic definition of attention:

> Everyone knows what attention is. It is the taking possession by the mind of one out of what seem several simultaneously possible objects or trains of thought. Focalization, concentration, of consciousness is of its essence. It implies withdrawal from some things in order to deal effectively with others, and is a condition that has a real opposite in the confused, dazed, scatterbrained state which in French is called *distraction* and in German *Zerstreutheit*. (pp. 403–404)

Prescient passages like this make one wonder about the nature of modern progress in the behavioral sciences. Over a century ago, James (1890) correctly identified attention as a *condition* or a *state,* and articulated the critical implication that attention involves processes in which the organism *focuses* or *concentrates* (i.e., selects) certain objects or events in the environment for special emphasis or processing. Furthermore, in *Principles,* James made reference to the existence of several types, or "varieties" of attention. Indeed, in the years since James's definition, many phenomena have been identified as attention in the literature on human cognition.

We have previously described (Colombo, 2001a, 2002) four broad categories of phenomena that have been classified as attention. Again, it is worth noting that the common thread that links them all is *selection of stimuli from the environment*:

- *The attentional state.* This is a state of receptivity or readiness for stimulation, often linked to alertness or arousal. These processes are thought to be mediated by ascending brain stem systems that are identified with specific neurotransmitters (Aston-Jones, 2005; Aston-Jones, Chen, Zhu, & Oshinsky, 2001; Aston-Jones & Cohen, 2005; Everitt & Robbins, 1997; Robbins et al., 1998).
- *Visual–spatial ("visuospatial") orienting.* This involves the simple detection of stimuli or events in space and the direction of sensory receptors to that locus (Posner & Petersen, 1990).
- *Object perception.* These are processes through which the content of stimuli or events detected after spatial orienting are processed and organized (Desimone & Duncan, 1995; Posner & Driver, 1992).
- *Voluntary/endogenous attention.* These are processes through which the other three forms are controlled in a top-down fashion (Posner & Dehaene, 1994; Pribram & McGuinness, 1975).

The nature of the science of object perception is more relevant to basic visual processing, and its path to contributing to the realm of education is unclear, and so we do not include it in this discussion. However, we believe the other three (the attentional state, visual–spatial orienting, and voluntary/endogenous attention) are especially relevant to considerations for ECE and ECI. In the following sections, we briefly review the literatures on the nature of these three varieties of attention, and what is known about them in infancy and early childhood. We also attempt to articulate the implications that we believe this research holds for applications and practice in ECE and ECI.

The Attentional State

As noted above, the attentional state is likely mediated by brain stem systems that modulate higher-order structures in the brain through specific neurotransmitters (Robbins & Everitt, 1995). These brain stem systems, however, also mediate other vital physiological and autonomic functions, such as the function and responsiveness of cardiac, pupillary, and respiratory systems, and the modulation of sleep–wake cycles and states. It is for this reason that attention has so often been linked with the concept of arousal (Pribram & McGuinness, 1975; Yerkes & Dodson, 1908), that sleep has so often been observed to be integrally linked with cognitive function (Dujardin, Guerrien, & Leconte, 1990; Hobson & Pace-Schott, 2002; Paller & Voss, 2004) and why autonomic indicators are excellent convergent measures of attention (Colombo, Richman, Shaddy, Greenhoot, & Maikranz, 2001; Richards & Cameron, 1989).

During the attentional state, properties of the attended-to stimulus or event are enhanced or amplified (Blaser, Sperling, & Lu, 1999; Yeshurun & Carrasco, 1998), and such enhancement is detectable in central nervous system (CNS) neurons involved in processing the stimulus or event (Treue, 2001). Such enhancement may be due to the reduction or dampening of other neural activity in the CNS (Dosher & Lu, 2000; Lu & Dosher, 1998). In addition to this enhancement, it is becoming increasingly clear that the attentional state is associated with increases in coordinated neural activity (Mishra, Fellous, & Sejnowski, 2006; Niebur, 2002; Niebur, Hsiao, & Johnson, 2002; Roy, Steinmetz, Hsiao, Johnson, & Niebur, 2007; Steinmetz et al., 2000; Ward, Doesburg, Kitajo, MacLean, & Roggeveen, 2006) that is the putative fundamental neural basis for many forms of associative learning (Eckhorn et al., 2004; Grossberg & Versace, 2008; Sanes, 2003; Usher & Donnelly, 1998; Virsu, Oksanen-Hennah, Vedenpaa, Jaatinen, & Lahti-Nuuttila, 2008).

To summarize, then, this form of attention is a neurally based organismic state that raises the probability of learning. The widely known phenomenon of joint attention (Carpenter et al., 1998) may be thought of as the simultaneous attainment of the attentional state by both child and caregiver such that social, symbolic, and communicative events taking place within the context of this state are more likely to be retained by the child.

The Attentional State in Infancy

For many years, attention was studied in infants through behavioral measures such as looking; more recently, measures of looking have been augmented with psychophysiological indices such as heart rate and respiration (Richards, 1985a, 1985b). The use of heart rate allows one to parse looking into various phases of attention, as infants' heart rate typically slows, or *decelerates*. Many studies indicate that the infant is engaged in meaningful cognitive activity during the decelerative period of the look, which has been called *sustained attention* (see Figure 2.1). It is generally presumed that this reflects the attainment of the attentional state (Graham & Clifton, 1966).

We included these measures of attention in a longitudinal study of visual attention and its consequences for preschool language and cognitive outcomes (Colombo, Shaddy, Richman, Maikranz, & Blaga, 2004). The results have been explicated in detail elsewhere (Blaga et al., 2009; Colombo & Mitchell, 2009; Colombo, Shaddy, Blaga, Anderson, & Kannass, 2009; Colombo, Shaddy, Blaga, Anderson, Kannass, et al., 2009; Colombo et al., 2010), and so we describe them only briefly here.

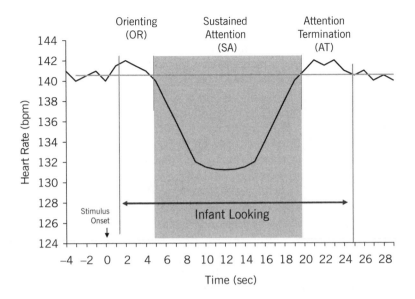

FIGURE 2.1. Heart-rate-defined phases of attention. From Colombo (2002, adapted from Richards and Casey, 1992). Copyright 2002 by Sage Publications. Reprinted by permission.

A sample of over 200 infants was recruited and tested monthly on a visual habituation protocol, which is a fairly simple perceptual learning task. Prior work had shown that duration of looking measured during habituation was modestly predictive of childhood intellectual outcomes; shorter looking is taken to reflect more rapid stimulus processing. However, looking variables have a complex developmental course across infancy; we reasoned that a careful measurement of the developmental course might yield more robust levels of prediction. As noted above, heart rate was also measured.

Results from this study suggested that the relationship between attention and later outcomes was complex, with best outcomes predicted for infants who showed steep declines in look duration over the course of the first 9 months, but who also maintained high and consistent levels of sustained attention. Infants with both of these characteristics scored more optimally on standardized tests of language and intellectual status up to 4 years of age (Colombo, Shaddy, Blaga, Anderson, Kannass, & Richman, 2009; Colombo, Shaddy, et al., 2004). Thus, better outcomes were observed for infants who consistently showed engagement in the attentional state, coupled with developmental improvements in speed of processing across the first year.

Implications for ECE and ECI

If the attainment and maintenance of the attentional state is related to optimal outcomes, it seems reasonable that we should seek manipulations or interventions that elicit it.

Using Stimulus Properties to Elicit and Hold Attention

There is considerable evidence to suggest that, during early infancy (e.g., from birth to 4 months of age), infants' attention can be captured and held by powerful visual properties such as high-contrast and moderately fine-grained patterns (Banks & Ginsburg, 1985; Gayl, Roberts, & Werner, 1983) and motion (Dannemiller, 1998; Hollich & Prince, 2009). These properties have already been used in the construction of commercially available toys and objects (e.g., mobiles) for use in infants' immediate environments, but such accessories for eliciting attention may be less frequently seen in low-socioeconomic status or higher-risk environments (Bradley et al., 1989), where there may be constrained resources.

In the arena of audition, the ability of infant-directed speech (Cooper, Abraham, Berman, & Staska, 1997; Fernald, 1985; Fernald & Kuhl, 1987) to capture and hold infant attention is well known. Along with its exaggerated pitch and slowed rate, "motherese" is often accompanied by exaggerated gestures (Iverson, Capirci, Longobardi, & Caselli, 1999) that likely contribute to its ability to elicit attention. Once again, this strategy for early stimulation in eliciting an attentional state is quite common among caregivers in low-risk environments, but research has shown that the use of infant-directed speech is not universal, and is in fact noticeably absent or tempered in stressed or depressed caregivers (Bettes, 1988; Murray, Kempton, Woolgar, & Hooper, 1993).

Contingency and Attention

Another property of experience that deserves consideration in eliciting the attentional state in young infants is contingency (Watson, 1966, 2001), where the infant's action is correlated with a subsequent consequence, for example, where pressing a button or activating a lever might produce a temporally contiguous visual or auditory event. Our own experience in using multimodal procedures with infants through the first year (Colombo & Bundy, 1981, 1983) suggests that contingency per se is a powerful means for eliciting attention. For example, when operant testing situations are arranged so that the infant can activate an auditory stimulus by looking at a stimulus or location (Coldren & Colombo, 1994; Colombo, Mitchell,

Coldren, & Atwater, 1990), infants remain attentive, engaged, and active far longer than one would expect based on the apparent reinforcement value of the auditory or visual stimuli per se. In social situations, contingency would translate to the concept of caregiver responsiveness, but given young infants' surprisingly acute sensitivity to timing (Colombo & Richman, 2002), the contiguity of consequences needs to be much quicker for younger infants. Toys and games that provide contingent consequences are also likely to be effective.

Synchrony and Attention

The last property that has been shown to elicit attention in a number of studies with young nonhumans (Best, Kemps, & Bryan, 2005) and humans (Black et al., 2004), and to improve performance on cognitive tasks (Flom & Bahrick, 2010) is the degree of redundancy across modalities or across stimulus properties (i.e., stimulus synchrony). Examples of this would be the temporal correspondence of speech sounds with lip or mouth movements that would be experienced with a talking caregiver, or the correlation between sounds and the visual image of a mallet hitting a drum or xylophone. As noted previously, synchronous neural activity is one of the by-products of the attentional state; some research suggests that the attentional state may itself be exogenously elicited by multimodal synchrony and produce long-term improvements in learning (Virsu et al., 2008).

Visual–Spatial Orienting

Visual–spatial orienting is a second type of attention that is pertinent to our discussion here. This type of attention is specific to vision, although it is suspected that there is a similar system for orienting to sound. Research on this phenomenon has largely converged on attributing the functions of this system to a pathway involving the visual cortex, superior colliculus, and the parietal cortex. This system, called the posterior attention system (Posner & Petersen, 1990), or the dorsal stream (Creem & Proffitt, 2001), is generally thought to detect the presence of a visual stimulus in a location, move (*shift*) the eyes to that location, and engage attention at that locus (Colombo, 1995). This system is also thought to control a separate function involved in disengaging attention from the stimulus; consistent with this notion is the fact that bilateral damage to the parietal lobes produces a condition called Balint's syndrome (Wojciulik & Kanwisher, 1998) that is characterized by extreme difficulty in disengaging attention away from one stimulus or location.

Measuring Visual–Spatial Orienting in Infancy

Measuring this system in preverbal infants is actually easier than one might expect, given that infants' attention is naturally drawn to the sudden appearance of stimuli in the visual field (Richards, 1997). The gap-overlap technique (Blaga & Colombo, 2006; Frick, Colombo, & Saxon, 1999) takes advantage of this tendency by first drawing the infant's fixation to the center of a visual display with a stimulus located at midline, and then presenting a visual stimulus in a location that is either in the infant's right or left peripheral visual field. This location must be far enough off the central stimulus to necessitate an eye movement on the part of the infant, yet within the limits of the infant's peripheral vision. The dependent measure is the infant's ocular reaction time, or *ocular latency,* to move toward the peripheral stimulus. One can manipulate whether the central stimulus remains when the peripheral stimulus appears (here, the central stimulus "overlaps" in time with the peripheral stimulus), or whether the central stimulus is withdrawn for some brief interval before the peripheral stimulus appears (hence, there is a brief time "gap" where no stimulus is present).

The logic of the procedure holds that when there is a "gap" between stimuli, the infant does not need to disengage from the central stimulus in order to make the response to the peripheral stimulus. However, when the peripheral and central stimuli overlap in time, the infant must first disengage attention before making an eye movement to the right or left. If the logic is correct, then ocular latencies should be longer in the overlap condition than in the gap condition, since the extra cognitive process of disengagement must be executed. Indeed, this result is uniformly reported in the literature.

Also commonly reported, however, is that younger infants—that is, infants younger than 6 months of age—are typically less able to disengage attention than older infants (see Figure 2.2). In addition, for infants at 3 and 4 months, ocular reaction time in the overlap condition is correlated with their length of looking to faces (Frick et al., 1999) and to geometric stimuli (Blaga & Colombo, 2006). This means that part of the prolonged patterns of looking seen in younger infants to visual stimuli (Colombo & Mitchell, 1990; Colombo, Mitchell, & Horowitz, 1988) is attributable to difficulties in disengagement and, by logical extension, to immaturity of the dorsal pathway or posterior attention system (Colombo, 1995, 2004).

Implications for ECE and ECI

The fact that young infants have difficulty in disengaging attention from objects or events has some interesting implications for applied practices in ECE and ECI. A common strategy advocated in some early childhood materials and curricula (e.g., prelinguistic milieu teaching) is to be sensitive

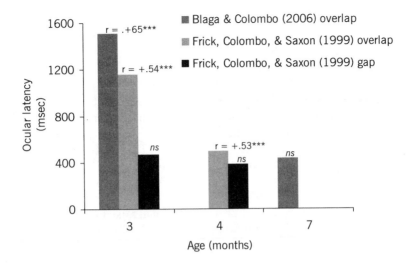

FIGURE 2.2. Ocular latencies across the first year, redrawn from two different studies conducted in our laboratory. Values listed at the top of the bars reflect the correlations between ocular latency and the length of infant looking in laboratory situations.

to the child's cues in terms of initiating social or stimulative interaction, and to "follow the child's lead" (Kaiser & Trent, 2007) based on cues that reflect where the child's attention may be directed. While it is certainly valid advice to be sensitive to such cues, the fact that young infants have difficulty disengaging attention from objects and stimuli suggests that caregivers may need to be more active in structuring and guiding infants' attention for the first 6–7 months. That is, the developmental data suggest that "follow your infant's lead" is perfectly appropriate for older infants, but younger infants may actually be attentionally "stuck on" or "captured by" a visual stimulus or event, in which case following the infant's "lead" may be less adaptive. Caregivers may instead be taught or advised to be sensitive to such circumstances with young infants, and to intervene by introducing new materials or initiating a social bid, rather than wait for a cue from the infant to do so. Indeed, research suggests that infants' attention is malleable in this way; when the looking of infants who had demonstrated longer processing was experimentally "shifted" across the stimulus, they performed as well as infants who had demonstrated faster processing (Jankowski, Rose, & Feldman, 2001).

Indeed, evidence suggests that caregivers are already sensitive to this point to some degree. Data from our own laboratory (Saxon, Colombo, Robinson, & Frick, 2000; Saxon, Frick, & Colombo, 1997) suggest that caregivers are often more directive and active with young infants than with older infants, and naturally make the transition from being more active in driving interactions earlier in infancy.

One final issue worthy of note is that measures of visual–spatial development, and measures of disengagement in particular, show great promise as a marker for autism and pervasive developmental disorders (Ciesielski & Harris, 1997; Elsabbagh et al., 2009; Fletcher-Watson, Leekam, Turner, & Moxon, 2006; Hughes & Russell, 1993; Ibanez, Messinger, Newell, Lambert, & Sheskin, 2008; Kawakubo et al., 2007; Landry & Bryson, 2004; van der Geest, Kemner, Camfferman, Verbaten, & van Engeland, 2001; Wainwright & Brown, 1996), as children with autism tend to show aberrant disengagement and shifting. Given that visual–spatial orienting is a nonverbal task, there is significant potential for its use in early identification for such disorders during infancy and early childhood.

Voluntary/Endogenous Attention

To this point, we have described forms of attention that are largely driven by factors external (*exogenous*) to the infant. We discussed how the infant's attentional state might be manipulated, and how the infant's sensory receptors are drawn to events and objects in visual space. However, as the infant progresses into the second half of the first postnatal year, some qualitative changes are typically observed that suggest that attention may be deployed or allocated as a function of factors internal (*endogenous*) to the infant.

One of the best examples of this comes from a simple but very compelling study of the ways in which infants attend to, and are distracted from, objects with which they are engaged (Oakes, Kannass, & Shaddy, 2002). In free-play situations, infants investigated both familiar toys (which had been shown to them prior to having access to them in the experimental session) and novel toys (which had not been seen previously). While infants were examining the toys, a television was activated and played a brief visual–auditory clip. In the first study, infants were tested longitudinally at 6.5 and 9 months of age, while in the second, infants were tested at either 6.5 or 10 months. In both experiments, older infants (9- to 10-month-olds) took longer to turn to the distractor when they were examining novel toys than when they were examining familiar toys. This is exactly what one might expect from a more mature subject: If one is more deeply engaged (as one might expect with a new object or event), one would be slower to be distracted from it. However, in both studies, younger infants (6 to 6.5 months) were just as distractible with a novel toy as they were with a familiar toy. This suggests that younger infants' attention is relatively more vulnerable to distraction.

What is especially interesting about this study is that the only thing that varied in terms of the toys being examined was whether or not infants had seen them before. As such, the study demonstrates that the attention of infants at 9–10 months of age can be held in check as a function of an internal (endogenous) cognitive process: memory. However, the attention of infants at 6 or 6.5 months of age did not show evidence of being controlled endogenously. It is almost as if, at the younger ages, attention and memory are disconnected, and that these functions become integrated a few months later on.

Indeed, we have elsewhere (Colombo & Cheatham, 2006) proposed that the emergence of what might be called "voluntary" or "executive" attention occurs as a result of the maturation of neural pathways that connect various cognitive processes with attentional functions. We have also proposed that the emergence of this endogenous form of attention represents the first step in the development of executive function. This notion also forms the basis for a substantial literature on executive function in human adults (Engle, 2002; Kane & Engle, 2002, 2003; Kane, Poole, Tuholski, & Engle, 2006).

This qualitative shift in the factors that control attention after 6 months of age is reflected in several other measures of cognition that are observable during infancy (Colombo, Shaddy, Blaga, Anderson, Kannass, et al., 2009). Look duration, which in early infancy is thought to reflect a combination of infants' processing speed (Colombo et al., 1988, 2001) and the facility of attentional disengagement (Blaga & Colombo, 2006; Frick et al., 1999), declines from 2 months to about 6 or 7 months of age (Colombo & Mitchell, 1990). However, after 6 months, the developmental function for looking time flattens out, and in some samples, actually *increases* with age (Colombo, 2002; Lansink & Richards, 1997; Saxon et al., 1997). This pattern of results (see Figure 2.3) suggests that either (1) infants are becoming worse at processing speed or disengagement with age, or (more likely) (2) the measure must be affected by some other cognitive processes. In terms of relations to later cognitive outcomes, measures of infants' processing speed during the first year show a negative relation to later cognitive functioning, such that shorter looking predicts more advanced cognitive functioning (Bornstein & Sigman, 1986; Colombo, 1993; Colombo, Shaddy, et al., 2004; Rose & Feldman, 1997), whereas measures of attention and persistence in the second year and beyond show a positive relation to later cognitive functioning; here, longer looking predicts more advanced cognitive functioning (Kannass & Oakes, 2008; Kopp & Vaughn, 1982; Ruff & Lawson, 1990; Sigman, Cohen, Beckwith, & Topinka, 1987).

A similar pattern is seen for ocular latencies (Colombo & Cheatham, 2006). Infants become progressively faster at ocular latencies with age until about 6 months; this is interpreted as an indication that they are increasingly

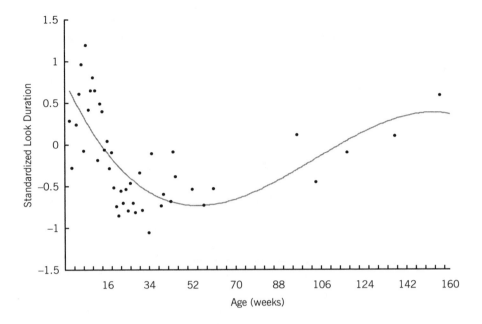

FIGURE 2.3. Developmental course of look duration, modeled from a meta-analysis of 53 studies. From Colombo and Cheatham (2006). Copyright 2006 by Elsevier. Reprinted by permission.

facile with both engagement and disengagement. However, after 6 months, there appears to be an increase in these latencies (see Figure 2.4). Once again, either infants are becoming less skilled, or something else (i.e., attention is being voluntarily held in the interest of taking in more information, or perhaps more complex information) is influencing the decision to make eye movements.

In each of the previous examples, we propose that the infant's determination to move attention from one stimulus to another is held in check by some other, centrally mediated process; that is, the decision to shift attention becomes predominantly endogenous.

The Consequences of Integrated Cognitive Processes

As cognitive components become integrated with one another in later infancy, a number of higher-order abilities become possible in early childhood (Banich, 2009; Fuster, 2002). The first and most simple of these is goal-directed behavior (Lippert, Logothetis, & Kayser, 2007; Willatts, 1999), where the infant can allocate attention and responses as a function of

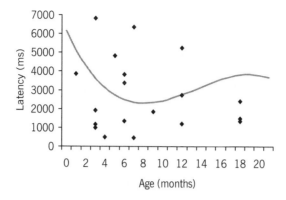

FIGURE 2.4. Ocular latency data across the first year, modeled from eight independent studies. From Colombo and Cheatham (2006). Copyright 2006 by Elsevier. Reprinted by permission.

some concrete object in working memory. Rule-based learning is also possible, as attention can be directed as a function of some abstraction, which can be accessed during responding (Coldren & Colombo, 2009; Vertes, 2004). As memory becomes more facile or flexible, the more adaptive the deployment of attention can become, thus leading to the active switching of responses when the application of rules for behavior is dynamic (Paller & Voss, 2004; Vertes, 2004); when switching is appropriate and repetition of prior responses is avoided, this is sometimes characterized as inhibition (Carlson, Moses, & Claxton, 2004; Durston et al., 2002), although one might wonder whether the additional construct of inhibition is necessary, separate from the failure of applying the appropriate rule. Finally, integrated cognitive components can result in strategic behavior or planning (Bishop, Aamodt-Leeper, Creswell, McGurk, & Skuse, 2001). One other phenomenon that might be attributable to the integration of cognitive processes is the development of interactive knowledge networks, where there are broader connections between acquired facts and concepts. Perhaps one example of this is in the area of categorization. Infants can be shown to categorize or generalize stimuli very early in the first year (Oakes & Madole, 2000), but there is little evidence that the perceptual categories acquired during this time are integrated or connected with any other information or behavioral responses that the infant exhibits. Knowledge gained from categorization that occurs later in the second year, however, readily spreads across concepts (e.g., form and function) and is connected to a number of other cognitive processes, especially word learning (Booth & Waxman, 2002, 2008; Waxman & Booth, 2003). We take this as at least preliminary evidence that, after the integration of these cognitive processes, acquired information readily enters interconnected networks. Interestingly, direct measures of brain coherence or coordination improve later in the first year and are related to performance on the types of tasks described here (Bell & Wolfe, 2007; Mundy, Fox, & Card, 2003), which lend further support to this contention.

Implications for ECE and ECI

The predominance of more endogenously driven attentional functions and behaviors in the second year bolsters the rationale for the long-advised strategy of having caregivers follow their infants' cues for initiating bids during social interactions. Coupled with suggestions derived from the data on visual–spatial orienting, caregivers would need to be advised of the shift from a more directive strategy for interaction during early infancy to the less directive strategy that should be adopted when endogenous attention emerges. Some data taken during the transition period suggest that caregivers are to some extent sensitive to the changes that signal this shift. For example, there is evidence that parents change their interactive styles as infants get older (Saxon et al., 2000), and that within ages, they adjust their interactive styles to the attentional skills of their infants (Saxon et al., 1997). Indeed, if the shift from "directing" to "being directed" that coincides with the emergence of endogenous attention does not happen, long-term outcomes appear to be at risk (Saxon et al., 2000), although it is not at all clear whether this is unilaterally due to caregivers' choice of action, or to their reaction to some aberrant aspect of their infants' attention. We have elsewhere (Colombo & Saxon, 2002) argued that child cognitive and language outcomes may be best under situations where infants' attentional profiles and caregivers' interactional styles are well matched or functionally complementary. This is similar to recommendations that encourage caregivers to communicate or interact with their child at the child's level, as in responsive interaction strategies. This lends support for why those strategies may work and supports use of those strategies. For example, outcomes for infants with more active or rapid processing capacities might be optimized with caregivers who are themselves active and willing to move quickly during interactions; outcomes for infants who are less active or slower to process might be better with parents whose personal styles are compatible with more slowly paced interactions.

The emergence of higher-order abilities during the second year suggest the importance of caregiver strategies that use attention to impact language, social skills, and other abilities (Buzhardt et al., 2010; Luze et al., 2001; Thompson & Trevathan, 2008), and the choice of activities that are commensurate with the level of those abilities and their integrative nature.

Summary and Additional Implications

In this chapter, we have provided an overview of how the construct and phenomenon of attention is relevant to considerations of ECE and ECI. In all of its forms, attention facilitates learning. Through the attentional state, it does so by preparing the CNS to receive input, emphasizing specific stimuli or environmental events, and promoting coordinated neural processes that likely underlie the formation of connections among neurons. Through visual–spatial orienting, attention facilitates learning by mediating overt (shifting) and covert (engagement and disengagement) motor actions that underlie the selection of stimuli or events for processing emphasis. Finally, in its endogenous form, attention is linked to other cognitive components (most notably memory), which forms the fundamental basis for the emergence of processes that will guide higher-order cognitive functions such as goal-directed behavior, rule following, strategies, inhibition, and planning.

Using Attention in ECE and ECI Domains

Along with the use of attention concepts in caregivers' crafting dimensions of the environment in early childhood, as described above, it should be noted for the consideration of ECE and ECI interests that various forms of attention (both behavioral and psychophysiological) are predictive of later outcome (Colombo, 1993; Colombo, Shaddy, Blaga, Anderson, & Kannass, 2009; Colombo, Shaddy, Blaga, Anderson, Kannass, et al., 2009; Colombo, Shaddy, et al., 2004). To summarize this literature, infants who show evidence of rapid/efficient processing and who show strong levels of sustained attention across the first year have higher IQs and more advanced vocabulary at preschool ages. There are two critical implications of this that follow.

Attention as an Indicator of the Effect of Early Interventions

Attention measures may provide a means for evaluating the effects of early childhood interventions in studies that do not extend into the preschool or school-age years. Therefore, in studies of parent training, infant stimulation, or other interventions, researchers in EI might be well advised to consider using assessments that tap into the domain of attention. Measures for infancy and toddlerhood are readily available; indeed, this strategy has been exploited quite widely in the field of nutrition, where such measures have been utilized in longitudinal designs (Colombo, 2001b) and have been found to document the effects of beneficial nutritional supplementation (Colombo et al., 2008; Colombo, Kannass, et al., 2004; Gustafson,

Colombo, & Carlson, 2008; Kannass, Colombo, & Carlson, 2009). In addition, more standardized and validated measures of attention in older children have been recently developed and disseminated (Rueda et al., 2004; Rueda, Posner, & Rothbart, 2005) for use in longitudinal designs, facilitating the inclusion of such measures as outcomes in studies of early intervention.

Attention as a Marker for Developmental Disabilities

Extant data suggest that measures of attention will also be sensitive to developmental disabilities. In keeping with a history of the use of attentional measures in the study of autism (Ming, Julu, Brimacombe, Connor, & Daniels, 2005; Schoen, Miller, Brett-Green, & Hepburn, 2008; Toichi & Kamio, 2003; Wainwright-Sharp & Bryson, 1993), recent work in our laboratory shows that autonomic measures related to the attentional state discriminate the presence of autism spectrum disorders in toddlers and preschoolers (Anderson & Colombo, 2009; Anderson, Colombo, & Shaddy, 2006), and we are currently investigating the validity of using these measures at earlier ages and in concert with other diagnostic criteria. It is likely that other disorders may be accessed through early assessment in this domain as well; a logical and obvious choice would be ADD and attention-deficit/hyperactivity disorder (ADHD; Barkley, 1997; Klorman et al., 1999; Luman, Oosterlaan, Hyde, van Meel, & Sergeant, 2007; Vassileva et al., 2001; Weyandt, Rice, Linterman, Mitzlaff, & Emert, 1998).

Direct Interventions on Attention?

As a final note, we point out that there is considerable and mounting evidence of the ability to intervene directly on attentional function (Tang & Posner, 2009). Success in improving attentional performance through "attention training" has been demonstrated with various types of attention, and with a host of clinical populations, including persons with schizophrenia (Benedict et al., 1994; Medalia, Aluma, Tryon, & Merriam, 1998; Suslow, Schonauer, & Arolt, 2001), individuals recovering from strokes (Rohling, Faust, Beverly, & Demakis, 2009; Sturm et al., 2004; Wilson & Manly, 2003), children with reading impairments (Coelho, 2005; Sinotte & Coelho, 2007), children with ADHD (Dupaul, Guevremont, & Barkley, 1992; Gordon, Thomason, Cooper, & Ivers, 1991; O'Connell et al., 2008; Rabiner, Murray, Skinner, & Malone, 2010; Sohlberg & Mateer, 2001), and autism (Whalen & Schreibman, 2003; Whalen, Schreibman, & Ingersoll, 2006). In our own work, we have been interested in when attention comes under the influence of verbal instruction in early childhood when children are working on tasks in the midst of distraction (Kannass, Colombo, & Wyss, 2010). Children as young as 3 years of age were able to use task instruction to guide their attention. We also found that the effectiveness of the amount of instruction depended on how well children could comprehend or understand the distractor in this procedure. For example, *any* amount of instruction helped children stay on task if the distractor was comprised of, for example, jumbled video clips or video clips presented in a non-native language. However, only frequent instruction helped them when the distractor was more comprehensible (e.g., the video clip followed a coherent story, or was presented in the child's native language). This suggests that parents and caregivers need to consider the nature of environmental distraction and scaffold their interactions appropriately, providing more guidance in challenging contexts.

Our stance in writing this chapter has been that a greater understanding and awareness of the ubiquity, importance, and basic functions of attention would hold promise in various applications within the domain of early childhood research and practice. We hope that this brief introduction to the concept and its relevance is helpful in advancing this point for both early childhood educators and interventionists.

REFERENCES

Anderson, C. J., & Colombo, J. (2009). Larger tonic pupil size in young children with autism spectrum disorder. *Developmental Psychobiology, 51,* 207–211.

Anderson, C. J., Colombo, J., & Shaddy, D. J. (2006). Visual scanning and pupillary responses in young children with autism spectrum disorder. *Journal of Clinical and Experimental Neuropsychology, 28,* 1238–1256.

Aston-Jones, G. (2005). Brain structures and receptors involved in alertness. *Sleep Medicine, 6,* S3–S7.

Aston-Jones, G., Chen, S., Zhu, Y., & Oshinsky, M. L. (2001). A neural circuit for circadian regulation of arousal. *Nature Neuroscience, 4,* 732–738.

Aston-Jones, G., & Cohen, J. D. (2005). An integrative theory of locus coeruleus-norepinephrine function: Adaptive gain and optimal performance. *Annual Review of Neuroscience, 28,* 403–450.

Auerbach, J. G., Landau, R., Berger, A., Arbelle, S., Faroy, M., & Karplus, M. (2005). Neonatal behavior of infants at familial risk for ADHD. *Infant Behavior and Development, 28,* 220–224.

Banich, M. T. (2009). Executive function: The search for an integrated account. *Current Directions in Psychological Science, 18,* 89–94.

Banks, M. S., & Ginsburg, A. P. (1985). Infant visual preferences: A review and new theoretical treatment. *Advances in Child Development and Behavior, 19,* 207–246.

Barkley, R. A. (1997). Behavioral inhibition, sustained attention, and executive functions: Constructing a unifying theory of ADHD. *Psychological Bulletin, 121,* 65–94.

Bell, M., & Wolfe, C. D. (2007). Changes in brain functioning from infancy to early childhood: Evidence from EEG power and coherence during working memory tasks. *Developmental Neuropsychology, 31,* 21–38.

Benedict, R. H. B., Harris, A. E., Markow, T., McCormick, J. A., Nuechterlein, K. H., & Asarnow, R. F. (1994). Effects of attention training on information processing in schizophrenia. *Schizophrenia Bulletin, 20,* 537–546.

Best, T., Kemps, E., & Bryan, J. (2005). Effects of saccharides on brain function and cognitive performance. *Nutrition Reviews, 63,* 409–418.

Bettes, B. A. (1988). Maternal depression and motherese: Temporal and intonational features. *Child Development, 59,* 1089–1096.

Bishop, D. V. M., Aamodt-Leeper, G., Creswell, C., McGurk, R., & Skuse, D. H. (2001). Individual differences in cognitive planning on the tower of Hanoi task: Neuropsychological maturity or measurement error? *Journal of Child Psychology and Psychiatry and Allied Disciplines, 42,* 551–556.

Black, M. M., Sazawal, S., Black, R. E., Khosla, S., Kumar, J., & Menon, V. (2004). Cognitive and motor development among small-for-gestational-age infants: Impact of zinc supplementation, birth weight, and caregiving practices. *Pediatrics, 113,* 1297–1305.

Blaga, O. M., & Colombo, J. (2006). Visual processing and infant ocular latencies in the overlap paradigm. *Developmental Psychology, 42,* 1069–1076.

Blaga, O. M., Shaddy, D. J., Anderson, C. J., Kannass, K. N., Little, T. D., & Colombo, J. (2009). Structure and continuity of intellectual development in early childhood. *Intelligence, 37,* 106–113.

Blaser, E., Sperling, G., & Lu, Z. L. (1999). Measuring the amplification of attention. *Proceedings of the National Academy of Sciences of the United States of America, 96,* 11681–11686.

Booth, A. E., & Waxman, S. R. (2002). Object names and object functions serve as cues to categories for infants. *Developmental Psychology, 38,* 948–957.

Booth, A. E., & Waxman, S. R. (2008). Taking stock as theories of word learning take shape. *Developmental Science, 11,* 185–194.

Bornstein, M. H., & Sigman, M. D. (1986). Continuity in mental development from infancy. *Child Development, 57,* 251–274.

Bradley, R. H., Caldwell, B. M., Rock, S. L., Barnard, K. E., Gray, C., Hammond, M. A., et al. (1989). Home-environment and cognitive-development in the first 3 years of life: A collaborative study involving 6 sites and 3 ethnic-groups in North America. *Developmental Psychology, 25,* 217–235.

Brady, N. C., & Warren, S. F. (2003). Language interventions for children with mental retardation. *International Review of Research in Mental Retardation, 27,* 231–254.

Buzhardt, J., Greenwood, C., Walker, D., Carta, J., Terry, B., & Garrett, M. (2010). A web-based tool to support data-based early intervention decision making. *Topics in Early Childhood Special Education, 29,* 201–213.

Carlson, S. M., Moses, L. J., & Claxton, L. J. (2004). Individual differences in executive functioning and theory of mind: An investigation of inhibitory control and planning ability. *Journal of Experimental Child Psychology, 87,* 299–319.

Carpenter, M., Nagell, K., & Tomasello, M. (1998). Social cognition, joint attention, and communicative competence from 9 to 15 months of age. *Monographs of the Society for Research in Child Development, 63*(4), 176.

Ciesielski, K. T., & Harris, R. J. (1997). Factors related to performance failure on executive tasks in autism. *Child Neuropsychology, 3*, 1–12.

Coelho, C. A. (2005). Direct attention training as a treatment for reading impairment in mild aphasia. *Aphasiology, 19*, 275–283.

Coldren, J. T., & Colombo, J. (1994). On the development of the processes underlying learning across the life span. *Monographs of the Society for Research in Child Development, 59*, 90–92.

Coldren, J. T., & Colombo, J. (2009). Attention as a cueing function during kindergarten children's dimensional change task performance. *Infant and Child Development, 18*, 441–454.

Colombo, J. (1993). *Infant cognition: Predicting later intellectual functioning.* Newbury Park, CA: Sage.

Colombo, J. (1995). On the neural mechanisms underlying developmental and individual differences in visual fixation in infancy: Two hypotheses. *Developmental Review, 15*, 97–135.

Colombo, J. (2001a). The development of visual attention in infancy. *Annual Review of Psychology, 52*, 337–367.

Colombo, J. (2001b). Recent advances in infant cognition: Implications for long-chain polyunsaturated fatty acid supplementation studies. *Lipids, 36*, 919–926.

Colombo, J. (2002). Infant attention grows up: The emergence of a developmental cognitive neuroscience perspective. *Current Directions in Psychological Science, 11*, 196–200.

Colombo, J. (2004). Visual attention in infancy: Process and product in early cognitive development. In M. I. Posner (Ed.), *Cognitive neuroscience of attention* (pp. 329–341). New York: Guilford Press.

Colombo, J., & Bundy, R. S. (1981). A method for the measurement of infant auditory selectivity. *Infant Behavior and Development, 4*, 219–223.

Colombo, J., & Bundy, R. S. (1983). Infant response to auditory familiarity and novelty. *Infant Behavior and Development, 6*, 305–311.

Colombo, J., Carlson, S., Cheatham, C., Kannass, K., Gustafson, K., & Schmeidler, T. (2008). *Dietary supplementation with DHA in infancy lowers heart rate and increases sustained attention.* Paper presented at the International Society for the Study of Fatty Acids and Lipids, Kansas City, MO.

Colombo, J., & Cheatham, C. L. (2006). The emergence and basis of endogenous attention in infancy and early childhood. *Advances in Child Development and Behavior, 34*, 283–322.

Colombo, J., Kannass, K. N., Shaddy, D. J., Kundurthi, S., Maikranz, J. M., Anderson, C. J., et al. (2004). Maternal DHA and the development of attention in infancy and toddlerhood. *Child Development, 75*, 1254–1267.

Colombo, J., & Mitchell, D. W. (1990). Individual differences in early visual attention: Fixation time and information processing. In J. Colombo & J. W. Fagen (Eds.), *Individual differences in infancy: Reliability, stability, prediction* (pp. 193–227). Hillsdale, NJ: Erlbaum.

Colombo, J., & Mitchell, D. W. (2009). Infant visual habituation. *Neurobiology of Learning and Memory, 92*, 225–234.

Colombo, J., Mitchell, D. W., Coldren, J. T., & Atwater, J. D. (1990). Discrimination learning during the first year: Stimulus and positional cues. *Journal of Experimental Psychology: Learning, Memory, and Cognition, 16*, 98–109.

Colombo, J., Mitchell, D. W., & Horowitz, F. D. (1988). Infant visual attention in the paired-comparison paradigm: Test–retest and attention–performance relations. *Child Development, 59,* 1198–1210.

Colombo, J., & Richman, W. A. (2002). Infant timekeeping: Attention and temporal estimation in 4-month-olds. *Psychological Science, 13,* 475–479.

Colombo, J., Richman, W. A., Shaddy, D. J., Greenhoot, A. F., & Maikranz, J. M. (2001). Heart rate-defined phases of attention, look duration, and infant performance in the paired-comparison paradigm. *Child Development, 72,* 1605–1616.

Colombo, J., & Saxon, T. F. (2002). Infant attention and the development of cognition: Does the environment moderate continuity? In H. Fitzgerald, K. Karraker, & T. Luster (Eds.), *Infant development: Ecological perspectives* (pp. 35–60). Washington, DC: Garland Press.

Colombo, J., Shaddy, D. J., Anderson, C. J., Gibson, L. J., Blaga, O. M., & Kannass, K. N. (2010). What habituates in infant visual habituation? A psychophysiological analysis. *Infancy, 15,* 107–124.

Colombo, J., Shaddy, D. J., Blaga, O. M., Anderson, C. J., & Kannass, K. N. (2009). High cognitive ability in infancy and early childhood. In F. D. Horowitz, R. F. Subotnik, & D. J. Matthews (Eds.), *The development of giftedness and talent across the life span* (pp. 23–42). Washington, DC: American Psychological Association.

Colombo, J., Shaddy, D. J., Blaga, O. M., Anderson, C. J., Kannass, K. N., & Richman, W. A. (2009). Early attentional predictors of vocabulary in childhood. In J. Colombo, P. McCardle, & L. Freund (Eds.), *Infant pathways to language: Methods, models, and research directions* (pp. 143–167). New York: Psychology Press.

Colombo, J., Shaddy, D. J., Richman, W. A., Maikranz, J. M., & Blaga, O. M. (2004). The developmental course of habituation in infancy and preschool outcome. *Infancy, 5,* 1–38.

Cooper, R. P., Abraham, J., Berman, S., & Staska, M. (1997). The development of infants' preference for motherese. *Infant Behavior and Development, 20,* 477–488.

Creem, S. H., & Proffitt, D. R. (2001). Defining the cortical visual systems: "What," "Where," and "How." *Acta Psychologica, 107,* 43–68.

Dannemiller, J. L. (1998). A competition model of exogenous orienting in 3.5-month-old infants. *Journal of Experimental Child Psychology, 68,* 169–201.

Desimone, R., & Duncan, J. (1995). Neural mechanisms of selective visual attention. *Annual Review of Neuroscience, 18,* 193–222.

Dosher, B. A., & Lu, Z. L. (2000). Noise exclusion in spatial attention. *Psychological Science, 11,* 139–146.

Dujardin, K., Guerrien, A., & Leconte, P. (1990). Sleep, brain activation, and cognition. *Physiology and Behavior, 47,* 1271–1278.

Dupaul, G. J., Guevremont, D. C., & Barkley, R. A. (1992). Behavioral treatment of attention-deficit hyperactivity disorder in the classroom: The use of the attention training system. *Behavior Modification, 16,* 204–225.

Durston, S., Thomas, K. M., Yang, Y. H., Ulug, A. M., Zimmerman, R. D., & Casey, B. J. (2002). A neural basis for the development of inhibitory control. *Developmental Science, 5,* F9–F16.

Eckhorn, R., Gail, A., Bruns, A., Gabriel, A., Al-Shaikhli, B., & Saam, M. (2004). Neural mechanisms of visual associative processing. *Acta Neurobiologiae Experimentalis, 64*, 239–252.

Elsabbagh, M., Volein, A., Holmboe, K., Tucker, L., Csibra, G., Baron-Cohen, S., et al. (2009). Visual orienting in the early broader autism phenotype: Disengagement and facilitation. *Journal of Child Psychology and Psychiatry, 50*, 637–642.

Engle, R. W. (2002). Working memory capacity as executive attention. *Current Directions in Psychological Science, 11*, 19–23.

Everitt, B. J., & Robbins, T. W. (1997). Central cholinergic systems and cognition. *Annual Review of Psychology, 48*, 649–684.

Fernald, A. (1985). 4-month-old infants prefer to listen to motherese. *Infant Behavior and Development, 8*, 181–195.

Fernald, A., & Kuhl, P. (1987). Acoustic determinants of infant preference for motherese speech. *Infant Behavior and Development, 10*, 279–293.

Fletcher-Watson, S., Leekam, S. R., Turner, M. A., & Moxon, L. (2006). Do people with autistic spectrum disorder show normal selection for attention? Evidence from change blindness. *British Journal of Psychology, 97*, 537–554.

Flom, R., & Bahrick, L. E. (2010). The effects of intersensory redundancy on attention and memory: Infants' long-term memory for orientation in audiovisual events. *Developmental Psychology, 46*, 428–436.

Frick, J. E., Colombo, J., & Saxon, T. F. (1999). Individual and developmental differences in disengagement of fixation in early infancy. *Child Development, 70*, 537–548.

Fuster, J. M. (2002). Frontal lobe and cognitive development. *Journal of Neurocytology, 31*, 373–385.

Gayl, I. E., Roberts, J. O., & Werner, J. S. (1983). Linear systems analysis of infant visual pattern preferences. *Journal of Experimental Child Psychology, 35*, 30–45.

Gordon, M., Thomason, D., Cooper, S., & Ivers, C. L. (1991). Nonmedical treatment of ADHD hyperactivity: The attention training system. *Journal of School Psychology, 29*, 151–159.

Graham, F. K., & Clifton, R. K. (1966). Heart-rate change as a component of orienting response. *Psychological Bulletin, 65*, 305–320.

Greenwood, C. R., Walker, D., Hornbeck, M., Hebbeler, K., & Spiker, D. (2007). Progress developing the Kansas early childhood special education accountability system: Initial findings using ECO and COSF. *Topics in Early Childhood Special Education, 27*, 2–18.

Grossberg, S., & Versace, M. (2008). Spikes, synchrony, and attentive learning by laminar thalamocortical circuits. *Brain Research, 1218*, 278–312.

Gustafson, K. M., Colombo, J., & Carlson, S. E. (2008). Docosahexaenoic acid and cognitive function: Is the link mediated by the autonomic nervous system? *Prostaglandins, Leukotrienes and Essential Fatty Acids, 79*, 135–140.

Hart, S., Boylan, L. M., Border, B., Carroll, S. R., McGunegle, D., & Lampe, R. M. (2004). Breast milk levels of cortisol and secretory immunoglobulin A (SIgA) differ with maternal mood and infant neuro-behavioral functioning. *Infant Behavior and Development, 27*, 101–106.

Hobson, J. A., & Pace-Schott, E. F. (2002). The cognitive neuroscience of sleep:

Neuronal systems, consciousness and learning. *Nature Reviews Neuroscience, 3,* 679–693.

Hockenberger, E. H., Goldstein, H., & Haas, L. S. (1999). Effects of commenting during joint book reading by mothers with low SES. *Topics in Early Childhood Special Education, 19,* 15–27.

Hollich, G., & Prince, C. G. (2009). Comparing infants' preference for correlated audiovisual speech with signal-level computational models. *Developmental Science, 12,* 379–387.

Hughes, C., & Russell, J. (1993). Autistic childrens' difficulty with mental disengagement from an object: Its implications for theories of autism. *Developmental Psychology, 29,* 498–510.

Ibanez, L. V., Messinger, D. S., Newell, L., Lambert, B., & Sheskin, M. (2008). Visual disengagement in the infant siblings of children with an autism spectrum disorder (ASD). *Autism, 12,* 473–485.

Iverson, J. M., Capirci, O., Longobardi, E., & Caselli, M. C. (1999). Gesturing in mother–child interactions. *Cognitive Development, 14,* 57–75.

James, W. (1890). *Principles of psychology.* New York: Holt.

Jankowski, J. J., Rose, S. A., & Feldman, J. E. (2001). Modifying the distribution of attention in infants. *Child Development, 72,* 339–351.

Kaiser, A. P., & Trent, J. A. (2007). Communication interventions for young children with disabilities. In S. L. Odom, R. H. Horner, M. E. Snell, & J. Blacher (Eds.), *Handbook of developmental disabilities* (pp. 234–245). New York: Guilford Press.

Kane, M. J., & Engle, R. W. (2002). The role of prefrontal cortex in working-memory capacity, executive attention, and general fluid intelligence: An individual-differences perspective. *Psychonomic Bulletin and Review, 9,* 637–671.

Kane, M. J., & Engle, R. W. (2003). Working-memory capacity and the control of attention: The contributions of goal neglect, response competition, and task set to Stroop interference. *Journal of Experimental Psychology: General, 132,* 47–70.

Kane, M. J., Poole, B. J., Tuholski, S. W., & Engle, R. W. (2006). Working memory capacity and the top-down control of visual search: Exploring the boundaries of "executive attention." *Journal of Experimental Psychology: Learning, Memory, and Cognition, 32,* 749–777.

Kannass, K. N., Colombo, J., & Carlson, S. E. (2009). Maternal DHA levels and toddler free-play attention. *Developmental Neuropsychology, 34,* 159–174.

Kannass, K. N., Colombo, J., & Wyss, N. (2010). Now, pay attention! The effects of instruction on children's attention. *Journal of Cognition and Development, 11,* 509–532.

Kannass, K. N., & Oakes, L. M. (2008). The development of attention and its relations to language in infancy and toddlerhood. *Journal of Cognition and Development, 9,* 222–246.

Kawakubo, Y., Kasai, K., Okazaki, S., Hosokawa-Kakurai, M., Watanabe, K., Kuwabara, H., et al. (2007). Electrophysiological abnormalities of spatial attention in adults with autism during the gap overlap task. *Clinical Neurophysiology, 118,* 1464–1471.

Klorman, R., Hazel-Fernandez, L. A., Shaywitz, S. E., Fletcher, J. M., Marchione, K. E., Holahan, J. M., et al. (1999). Executive functioning deficits in attention-deficit hyperactivity disorder are independent of oppositional defiant or reading disorder. *Journal of the American Academy of Child and Adolescent Psychiatry, 38,* 1148–1155.

Kopp, C. B., & Vaughn, B. E. (1982). Sustained attention during exploratory manipulation as a predictor of cognitive competence in preterm infants. *Child Development, 53,* 174–182.

Landry, R., & Bryson, S. E. (2004). Impaired disengagement of attention in young children with autism. *Journal of Child Psychology and Psychiatry, 45,* 1115–1122.

Lansink, J. M., & Richards, J. E. (1997). Heart rate and behavioral measures of attention in six-, nine-, and twelve-month-old infants during object exploration. *Child Development, 68,* 610–620.

Lee, H. C., & Seong, P. H. (2009). A computational model for evaluating the effects of attention, memory, and mental models on situation assessment of nuclear power plant operators. *Reliability Engineering and System Safety, 94,* 1796–1805.

Lippert, M., Logothetis, N. K., & Kayser, C. (2007). Improvement of visual contrast detection by a simultaneous sound. *Brain Research, 1173,* 102–109.

Lu, Z. L., & Dosher, B. A. (1998). External noise distinguishes attention mechanisms. *Vision Research, 38,* 1183–1198.

Luman, M., Oosterlaan, J., Hyde, C., van Meel, C. S., & Sergeant, J. A. (2007). Heart rate and reinforcement sensitivity in ADHD. *Journal of Child Psychology and Psychiatry, 48,* 890–898.

Luze, G. J., Linebarger, D. L., Greenwood, C. R., Carta, J. J., Walker, D., Leitschuh, C., et al. (2001). Developing a general outcome measure of growth in the expressive communication of infants and toddlers. *School Psychology Review, 30,* 383–406.

McBride, S. L., & Peterson, C. (1997). Home-based early intervention with families of children with disabilities: Who is doing what? *Topics in Early Childhood Special Education, 17,* 209–233.

Medalia, A., Aluma, M., Tryon, W., & Merriam, A. E. (1998). Effectiveness of attention training in schizophrenia. *Schizophrenia Bulletin, 24,* 147–152.

Ming, X., Julu, P. O. O., Brimacombe, M., Connor, S., & Daniels, M. L. (2005). Reduced cardiac parasympathetic activity in children with autism. *Brain and Development, 27,* 509–516.

Mishra, J., Fellous, J. M., & Sejnowski, T. J. (2006). Selective attention through phase relationship of excitatory and inhibitory input synchrony in a model cortical neuron. *Neural Networks, 19,* 1329–1346.

Morales, M., Mundy, P., Delgado, C. E. F., Yale, M., Messinger, D., Neal, R., et al. (2000). Responding to joint attention across the 6- through 24-month age period and early language acquisition. *Journal of Applied Developmental Psychology, 21,* 283–298.

Mundy, P., Fox, N., & Card, J. (2003). EEG coherence, joint attention and language development in the second year. *Developmental Science, 6,* 48–54.

Murray, L., Kempton, C., Woolgar, M., & Hooper, R. (1993). Depressed mothers' speech to their infants and its relation to infant gender and cognitive development. *Journal of Child Psychology and Psychiatry and Allied Disciplines, 34,* 1083–1101.

Niebur, E. (2002). Electrophysiological correlates of synchronous neural activity and attention: A short review. *BioSystems, 67,* 157–166.

Niebur, E., Hsiao, S. S., & Johnson, K. (2002). Synchrony: A neuronal mechanism for attentional selection? *Current Opinion in Neurobiology, 12,* 190–194.

Oakes, L. M., Kannass, K. N., & Shaddy, D. J. (2002). Developmental changes in endogenous control of attention: The role of target familiarity on infants' distraction latency. *Child Development, 73,* 1644–1655.

Oakes, L. M., & Madole, K. L. (2000). The future of infant categorization research: A process-oriented approach. *Child Development, 71,* 119–126.

O'Connell, R. G., Bellgrove, M. A., Dockree, P. M., Lau, A., Fitzgerald, M., & Robertson, I. H. (2008). Self-alert training: Volitional modulation of autonomic arousal improves sustained attention. *Neuropsychologia, 46,* 1379–1390.

Ohgi, S., Akiyama, T., & Fukuda, M. (2005). Neurobehavioural profile of low-birthweight infants with cystic periventricular leukomalacia. *Developmental Medicine and Child Neurology, 47,* 221–228.

Ohgi, S., Takahashi, T., Nugent, J. K., Arisawa, K., & Akiyama, T. (2003). Neonatal behavioral characteristics and later behavioral problems. *Clinical Pediatrics, 42,* 679–686.

Paller, K. A., & Voss, J. L. (2004). Memory reactivation and consolidation during sleep. *Learning and Memory, 11,* 664–670.

Parasuraman, R., & Wilson, G. F. (2008). Putting the brain to work: Neuroergonomics past, present, and future. *Human Factors, 50,* 468–474.

Posner, M. I., & Dehaene, S. (1994). Attentional networks. *Trends in Neurosciences, 17,* 75–79.

Posner, M. I., & Driver, J. (1992). The neurobiology of selective attention. *Current Opinion in Neurobiology, 2,* 165–169.

Posner, M. I., & Petersen, S. E. (1990). The attention system of the human brain. *Annual Review of Neuroscience, 13,* 25–42.

Pribram, K. H., & McGuinness, D. (1975). Arousal, activation, and effort in control of attention. *Psychological Review, 82,* 116–149.

Rabiner, D. L., Murray, D. W., Skinner, A. T., & Malone, P. S. (2010). A randomized trial of two promising computer-based interventions for students with attention difficulties. *Journal of Abnormal Child Psychology, 38,* 131–142.

Richards, J. E. (1985a). The development of sustained visual-attention in infants from 14 to 26 weeks of age. *Psychophysiology, 22,* 409–416.

Richards, J. E. (1985b). Respiratory sinus arrhythmia predicts heart-rate and visual responses during visual-attention in 14 and 20 week old infants. *Psychophysiology, 22,* 101–109.

Richards, J. E. (1997). Peripheral stimulus localization by infants: Attention, age, and individual differences in heart rate variability. *Journal of Experimental Psychology—Human Perception and Performance, 23,* 667–680.

Richards, J. E., & Cameron, D. (1989). Infant heart-rate-variability and behavioral developmental status. *Infant Behavior and Development, 12,* 45–58.

Richman, W. A., & Colombo, J. (2007). Joint book reading in the second year and vocabulary outcomes. *Journal of Research in Childhood Education, 21,* 242–253.

Rieger, M., Pirke, K. M., Buske-Kirschbaum, A., Wurmser, H., Papousek, M., & Hellhammer, D. H. (2004). Influence of stress during pregnancy on HPA activity and neonatal behavior. In R. Yehuda & B. McEwen (Eds.), *Biobehavioral stress response: Protective and damaging effects* (Vol. 1032, pp. 228–230). New York: New York Academy of Sciences.

Robbins, T. W., & Everitt, B. J. (1995). Arousal systems and attention. In M. Gazzaniga (Ed.), *The cognitive neurosciences* (pp. 703–720). Cambridge: MIT Press.

Robbins, T. W., Granon, S., Muir, J. L., Durantou, F., Harrison, A., & Everitt, B. J. (1998). Neural systems underlying arousal and attention—Implications for drug abuse. *Annals of the New York Academy of Sciences, 846,* 222–237.

Rohling, M. L., Faust, M. E., Beverly, B., & Demakis, G. (2009). Effectiveness of cognitive rehabilitation following acquired brain injury: A meta-analytic re-examination of Cicerone et al.'s (2000, 2005) systematic reviews. *Neuropsychology, 23,* 20–39.

Rose, S. A., & Feldman, J. F. (1997). Memory and speed: Their role in the relation of infant information processing to later IQ. *Child Development, 68,* 630–641.

Roy, A., Steinmetz, P. N., Hsiao, S. S., Johnson, K. O., & Niebur, E. (2007). Synchrony: A neural correlate of somatosensory attention. *Journal of Neurophysiology, 98,* 1645–1661.

Rueda, M. R., Fan, J., McCandliss, B. D., Halparin, J. D., Gruber, D. B., Lercari, L. P., et al. (2004). Development of attentional networks in childhood. *Neuropsychologia, 42,* 1029–1040.

Rueda, M. R., Posner, M. I., & Rothbart, M. K. (2005). The development of executive attention: Contributions to the emergence of self-regulation. *Developmental Neuropsychology, 28,* 573–594.

Ruff, H. A., & Lawson, K. R. (1990). Development of sustained, focused attention in young children during free play. *Developmental Psychology, 26,* 85–93.

Sanes, J. N. (2003). Neocortical mechanisms in motor learning. *Current Opinion in Neurobiology, 13,* 225–231.

Saxon, T. F., Colombo, J., Robinson, E. L., & Frick, J. E. (2000). Dyadic interaction profiles in infancy and preschool intelligence [special issue]. *Journal of School Psychology: Developmental Perspectives in Intelligence, 38,* 9–25.

Saxon, T. F., Frick, J. E., & Colombo, J. (1997). A longitudinal study of maternal interactional styles and infant visual attention. *Merrill-Palmer Quarterly, 43,* 48–66.

Schoen, S. A., Miller, L. J., Brett-Green, B., & Hepburn, S. L. (2008). Psychophysiology of children with autism spectrum disorder. *Research in Autism Spectrum Disorders, 2,* 417–429.

Shinar, D. (2008). Looks are (almost) everything: Where drivers look to get information. *Human Factors, 50,* 380–384.

Sigman, M., Cohen, S. E., Beckwith, L., & Topinka, C. (1987). Task persistence in 2-year-old preterm infants in relation to subsequent attentiveness and intelligence. *Infant Behavior and Development, 10,* 295–305.

Sinotte, M. P., & Coelho, C. A. (2007). Attention training for reading impairment in mild aphasia: A follow-up study. *Neurorehabilitation, 22,* 303–310.

Sohlberg, M. M., & Mateer, C. A. (2001). Improving attention and managing attentional problems—Adapting rehabilitation techniques to adults with ADD. *Adult Attention Deficit Disorder, 931,* 359–375.

Steinmetz, P. N., Roy, A., Fitzgerald, P. J., Hsiao, S. S., Johnson, K. O., & Niebur, E. (2000). Attention modulates synchronized neuronal firing in primate somatosensory cortex. *Nature, 404,* 187–190.

Stone, W. L., Coonrod, E. E., & Ousley, O. Y. (2000). Brief report: Screening tool for autism in two-year-olds (STAT): Development and preliminary data. *Journal of Autism and Developmental Disorders, 30,* 607–612.

Sturm, W., Longoni, F., Weis, S., Specht, K., Herzog, H., Vohn, R., et al. (2004). Functional reorganisation in patients with right hemisphere stroke after training of alertness: A longitudinal PET and fMRI study in eight cases. *Neuropsychologia, 42,* 434–450.

Suslow, T., Schonauer, K., & Arolt, V. (2001). Attention training in the cognitive rehabilitation of schizophrenic patients: A review of efficacy studies. *Acta Psychiatrica Scandinavica, 103,* 15–23.

Sutton, E., Youssef, Y., Meenaghan, N., Godinez, C., Xiao, Y., Lee, T., et al. (2010). Gaze disruptions experienced by the laparoscopic operating surgeon. *Surgical Endoscopy and Other Interventional Techniques, 24,* 1240–1244.

Tang, Y. Y., & Posner, M. I. (2009). Attention training and attention state training. *Trends in Cognitive Sciences, 13,* 222–227.

Thompson, L. A., & Trevathan, W. R. (2008). Cortisol reactivity, maternal sensitivity, and learning in 3-month-old infants. *Infant Behavior and Development, 31,* 92–106.

Toichi, M., & Kamio, Y. (2003). Paradoxical autonomic response to mental tasks in autism. *Journal of Autism and Developmental Disorders, 33,* 417–426.

Toth, K., Munson, J., Meltzoff, A. N., & Dawson, G. (2006). Early predictors of communication development in young children with autism spectrum disorder: Joint attention, imitation, and toy play. *Journal of Autism and Developmental Disorders, 36,* 993–1005.

Treue, S. (2001). Neural correlates of attention in primate visual cortex. *Trends in Neurosciences, 24,* 295–300.

Usher, M., & Donnelly, N. (1998). Visual synchrony affects binding and segmentation in perception. *Nature, 394,* 179–182.

van der Geest, J. N., Kemner, C., Camfferman, G., Verbaten, M. N., & van Engeland, H. (2001). Eye movements, visual attention, and autism: A saccadic reaction time study using the gap and overlap paradigm. *Biological Psychiatry, 50,* 614–619.

Vassileva, J. L., Vongher, J. M., Fischer, M., Conant, L., Risinger, R. C., Salmeron, B. J., et al. (2001). Working memory deficits in adults with ADHD. *Brain and Cognition, 47,* 216–219.

Vertes, R. P. (2004). Memory consolidation in sleep: Dream or reality. *Neuron, 44*, 135–148.

Virsu, V., Oksanen-Hennah, H., Vedenpaa, A., Jaatinen, P., & Lahti-Nuuttila, P. (2008). Simultaneity learning in vision, audition, tactile sense and their cross-modal combinations. *Experimental Brain Research, 186*, 525–537.

Wainwright, J. A., & Brown, S. E. (1996). Visual–spatial orienting in autism. *Journal of Autism and Developmental Disorders, 26*, 423–438.

Wainwright-Sharp, J. A., & Bryson, S. E. (1993). Visual orienting deficits in high-functioning people with autism. *Journal of Autism and Developmental Disorders, 23*, 1–13.

Ward, L. M., Doesburg, S. M., Kitajo, K., MacLean, S. E., & Roggeveen, A. B. (2006). Neural synchrony in stochastic resonance, attention, and consciousness. *Canadian Journal of Experimental Psychology-Revue Canadienne De Psychologie Experimentale, 60*, 319–326.

Watson, J. S. (1966). Development and generalization of contingency awareness in early infancy: Some hypotheses. *Merrill-Palmer Quarterly of Behavior and Development, 12*, 123–135.

Watson, J. S. (2001). Contingency perception and misperception in infancy: Some potential implications for attachment. *Bulletin of the Menninger Clinic, 65*, 296–320.

Waxman, S. R., & Booth, A. E. (2003). The origins and evolution of links between word learning and conceptual organization: New evidence from 11-month-olds. *Developmental Science, 6*, 128–135.

Weyandt, L. L., Rice, J. A., Linterman, I., Mitzlaff, L., & Emert, E. (1998). Neuropsychological performance of a sample of adults with ADHD, developmental reading disorder, and controls. *Developmental Neuropsychology, 14*, 643–656.

Whalen, C., & Schreibman, L. (2003). Joint attention training for children with autism using behavior modification procedures. *Journal of Child Psychology and Psychiatry and Allied Disciplines, 44*, 456–468.

Whalen, C., Schreibman, L., & Ingersoll, B. (2006). The collateral effects of joint attention training on social initiations, positive affect, imitation, and spontaneous speech for young children with autism. *Journal of Autism and Developmental Disorders, 36*, 655–664.

Willatts, P. (1999). Development of means–end behavior in young infants: Pulling a support to retrieve a distant object. *Developmental Psychology, 35*, 651–667.

Wilson, F. C., & Manly, T. (2003). Sustained attention training and errorless learning facilitates self-care functioning in chronic ipsilesional neglect following severe traumatic brain injury. *Neuropsychological Rehabilitation, 13*, 537–548.

Wojciulik, E., & Kanwisher, N. (1998). Implicit but not explicit feature binding in a Balint's patient. *Visual Cognition, 5*, 157–181.

Yerkes, R. M., & Dodson, J. D. (1908). The relation of strength of stimulus to rapidity of habit-formation. *Journal of Comparative Neurology and Psychology, 18*, 459–482.

Yeshurun, Y., & Carrasco, M. (1998). Attention improves or impairs visual performance by enhancing spatial resolution. *Nature, 396,* 72–75.

Yoder, P. J., & Warren, S. F. (2001a). Intentional communication elicits language-facilitating maternal responses in dyads with children who have developmental disabilities. *American Journal on Mental Retardation, 106,* 327–335.

Yoder, P. J., & Warren, S. F. (2001b). Relative treatment effects of two prelinguistic communication interventions on language development in toddlers with developmental delays vary by maternal characteristics. *Journal of Speech Language and Hearing Research, 44,* 224–237.

CHAPTER 3

Facilitating Learning and Memory in Infants and Young Children

Mechanisms and Methods

Patricia J. Bauer

A major goal of early child care providers and educators is to facilitate learning. If we want to facilitate learning, we must facilitate memory. This "formula" is patently obvious. Unless all of a child's knowledge is built in, it must be acquired. The means by which it is acquired is through learning. In turn, learning may come about through observation, study, practice, direct tuition, and so forth, and it may be intentional or unintentional. Regardless of the source and the objective, for the products of learning to be maintained over time, they must be stored in memory. In the course of this chapter, I elaborate on relations between learning and memory with special focus on infancy and very early childhood. A guiding principle of the review is that although learning and memory are intimately related, they are not one in the same, such that equal learning does not result in equal remembering. This observation leads to consideration of memory and related processes that occur after a learning episode and of the developmental status of the neural structures and network that support the processes. Consideration of these factors helps to explain some of the vulnerabilities in young children's learning and memory. It also opens a window on educational practices that may aid students in overcoming—and even capitalizing—on them.

How Learning and Memory Are Related

The literature features a plethora of examples of effects of prior learning on memory and of effects of memory on learning of new information. Research by Chi (1978) provided an early and dramatic example of the effects of domain knowledge on memory. Chi administered to children and adults a task requiring them to remember string of digits of various lengths (e.g., 7-4-3, 8-6-1-9, 3-2-5-4-7, 1-6-8-3-5-2, 7-4-2-5-9-1-8). As expected, the adults remembered more digits than the children. Another of the findings was, at the time, quite unexpected, however. The children in the study had been selected because they were experts in the game of chess; the adults knew how to play chess but were not experts. When the young chess experts and the adult chess novices were required to remember chess positions—rather than strings of digits—the children outperformed the adults. This research provides a now classic demonstration of effects of domain knowledge (or expertise) on memory.

The literature also features demonstrations of the influence of memory on learning and acquisition of new knowledge. An illustrative example comes from the literature on relations between working memory and reading comprehension. From the preschool through the college years, working memory capacity correlates with reading comprehension (e.g., Daneman & Carpenter, 1980). In addition, differences in working memory capacity differentiate reading disabled from nonreading disabled readers (e.g., Siegel & Ryan, 1989). These few illustrations make clear that if we are to understand learning, we must think about memory. Further, if we are to understand how learning processes change over developmental time, we must understand developmental differences in memory.

Developmental Differences in Learning and in Memory in Infancy

It is abundantly clear that learning changes over the course of development and that there are age-related differences in memory. The question is how developmental differences in one domain relate to differences in the other, such that one can facilitate the other. When this question is asked with regard to infants and very young children, address of it is complicated by the fact that we cannot rely on the measures of these processes that we use with older, verbal children. Infants do not play chess. They obviously do not read either, thus making it impossible to test them with reading comprehension tasks. In fact, infants cannot be tested with any of the language-based assessments designed for use with older children and adults. Thus, assessments of learning and memory in infancy require nonverbal tasks.

Measuring Learning and Memory in Pre- and Early-Verbal Children

A commonly used measure of learning and memory in infancy is elicited imitation of multistep sequences. In elicited or deferred imitation, props are used to produce a sequence of actions that the infant is invited to imitate either immediately (elicited imitation), after a delay (deferred imitation), or both. Although the task is nonverbal and depends on behavior, there is ample reason to believe that it taps the same type of memory as assessed through verbal report in language-using children and adults (see Bauer, 2004, 2005b, 2007, for discussions). An example sequence is "make a gong" by (1) folding a bar across a swing-set-shaped base, thus forming a cross piece; (2) hanging a metal disk from the bar; and (3) striking the metal disk with a small mallet, thus causing it to "gong."

Use of this technique with infants as young as 6 months of age (e.g., Barr, Dowden, & Hayne, 1996), and throughout the second year of life (e.g., Bauer, Wenner, Dropik, & Wewerka, 2000), has revealed a number of age-related differences in memory. First, based on a single learning trial, infants learn and remember. For example, relative to an uninstructed baseline (during which we observe spontaneous production of target actions and their order), immediately after seeing sequences demonstrated, 16- and 20-month-old infants produce both more of the actions of sequences such as the gong (i.e., folding the bar, hanging the disk from the bar, striking the disk with the mallet), and more actions in the demonstrated order. This provides strong evidence of learning, based on a single experience of an event. After a delay of 2 weeks, they still remember the sequences, though some forgetting is apparent (e.g., Bauer & Mandler, 1989). Thus, even preverbal infants learn and remember multistep sequences of action.

Second, on the basis of a single experience of an event, older infants remember more than younger infants (e.g., Bauer & Mandler, 1989). Third, with more learning trials, memory is more robust. That is, when they are tested after a 1-month delay, infants who have had three experiences of sequences remember more of the actions and their temporal order relative to infants who have seen the sequences demonstrated twice or only once (Bauer, Wiebe, Waters, & Bangston, 2001). Thus, learning accrues with experience.

Are Differences in Memory Explained by Differences in Learning?

The tight coupling of learning and memory raises the question of whether age-related differences in memory reflect nothing more than age-related differences in learning. If that is the case, then were we to equalize learning, we could also equalize remembering. Since learning accrues over trials, we could give younger children more learning trials, relative to older children, and eliminate age-related differences. Although this is a logical prediction, research reported in Bauer (2005a) makes clear that age-related differences in memory are not explained by differences in learning, at least not as we typically conceive of learning.

Bauer (2005a) involved three groups of infants 16 months of age and three groups of infants 20 months of age. All of the infants learned multistep sequences prior to imposition of 1-, 3-, or 6-month delays (the delay interval was between subjects). To examine age-related differences in remembering, we controlled age-related differences in learning. Specifically, we matched the 16- and 20-month-olds for the amount learned prior to the delay. For example, a younger infant who produced three actions prior to the delay was matched with an older infant who produced three actions, and so forth. Thus, the infants of different ages entered the delay interval with equal learning.

In spite of the fact that the infants learned the same amount about the events, they did not remember the same amount; age differences were especially apparent at the longer delays. When they were retested after 1 month, the older and younger infants had forgotten approximately the same amount about the events: They had lost about one in four of the individual actions they had learned. After both 3 months and 6 months, age-related differences were pronounced. After 3 months, younger and older infants forgot roughly 2.5 and 1.4 actions, respectively; after 6 months, younger and older infants forgot roughly 3.1 and 2.2 actions, respectively (see Bauer, 2005a, for details). Clearly, equal learning does not result in equal forgetting (or its complement, remembering).

One possible explanation for the pattern of findings was that older and younger infants remembered the same amount, but that the older infants were better at retrieving their memories, especially after the long delays. To address this possibility, after the test trial, we demonstrated the sequences once again and then tested the infants' recall. Even with the burden of retrieval lifted (by demonstration of the event), younger infants still performed less well than older infants. Thus, the difference in long-term recall could not be attributed to differences in accessibility at retrieval (see Bauer, 2005a, for details and discussion). With both "bookends" eliminated (initial learning and retrieval), we must look to the middle (the period between learning and test) to find the source of age-related differences.

The Importance of the Postlearning Processes

To understand how equal learning can produce unequal retention, we must look to processes that take place after learning, but before the long-term retrieval test. A likely candidate postlearning process is *consolidation*. Consolidation is the process by which an initially labile memory trace is stabilized and integrated into long-term storage. The process involves a particular neural substrate, one that undergoes substantial postnatal developmental change. This makes it an attractive candidate as a source of age-related differences in retention of newly learned information.

Consolidation originally was hypothesized by Müller and Pilzecker (1900) to account for retroactive interference. In laboratory tests they observed that new material learned shortly after (but not long after) old material produced deficits in memory for the old material. For example, when word List 1 was learned, time was allowed to pass, and then List 2 was learned, both lists were well recalled. In contrast, if List 1 was learned, and then very shortly thereafter List 2 was presented, there was good recall of List 2, but poor recall of List 1. It seemed that in the short-delay situation, List 2 retroactively interfered with List 1. Müller and Pilzecker hypothesized that retroactive interference occurred because at the time List 2 was learned, List 1 had not yet been stabilized or integrated into storage, a process they termed "consolidation."

Müller and Pilzecker's (1900) work illustrate two important principles about learning and memory, namely, that processes that take place after learning influence later remembering, and that those postlearning processes take time. In the years since the introduction of the concept of consolidation, we have learned more about this critical process, including that it involves multiple steps and that it depends upon a network of neural structures. In the next sections, I provide a summary of "how the brain builds a memory," followed by discussion of the implications of these processes for learning and memory in development.

The Neural Substrate of Learning and Memory

Through work with patient populations, animal models of lesion and disease, and with the aid of neuroimaging techniques such as positron emission tomography (PET) and functional magnetic resonance imaging (fMRI), we have learned a great deal about the neural structures and networks involved in the encoding, consolidation, and later retrieval of the products of learning. Briefly, the process depends on a multicomponent neural network involving structures in the medial temporal lobes and the frontal lobes of the brain. The process begins as perceptual experience of an event impinges on and thus produces excitation across multiple brain regions distributed across the cortex (see Figure 3.1). Certain areas of cortex, termed "association areas" (e.g., the front portion of the frontal lobe, known as the anterior or prefrontal cortex), bring the information together (thus the name: "association" areas), giving rise to conscious awareness of the experience. Neural structures on the medial (inside) surface of the

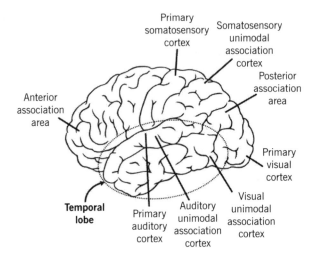

FIGURE 3.1. Lateral view of the association areas of the human brain. Drawing by Ayzit O. Doydum.

temporal lobe are involved in the consolidation of the distributed representation into a durable memory trace. Over the long term, memories are stored in the same cortical areas that participated in initial registration of experience. Prefrontal cortex is implicated in retrieval of memories from long-term stores (e.g., Kandel & Squire, 2000). In the sections to follow, I outline each of these steps in greater detail.

Initial Registration

Information about events and experiences registers in multiple cortical areas across the surface of the brain. Specifically, neurons in primary visual cortex (see Figure 3.1) respond to the form, color, and motion of objects or events. In parallel, neurons in primary somatosensory cortex respond to inputs from the skin (registering information about light touch) and muscles and joints (registering information about the position and movement of our extremities); and neurons in primary auditory cortex respond to various attributes of the sounds made by the object or event. Inputs from these primary sensory areas are sent (projected) to sensory association areas that are dedicated to a single modality (vision, somatic sensation, or audition) where they are integrated into whole percepts of what the object or event looks like, feels like, and sounds like, respectively. These unimodal sensory association areas in turn project to polymodal (also termed "multimodal") posterior-parietal, anterior-prefrontal, and limbic-temporal association areas where inputs from the different sense modalities are integrated.

Research with nonhuman primates has shown that over very brief time intervals (on the order of seconds), information about objects or events is maintained in the cortical association areas. For example, when a visual stimulus is presented, neurons in the prefrontal cortex begin to fire. If the stimulus is hidden from view, the neurons continue to fire during a short delay interval (typically less than 30 seconds). When the delay is over, the animal is able to make a correct reach or look to where the object or cue had been. Thus, the neurons "represented" the object in the brain even after the sensory stimulation was gone. In contrast, if during the delay period the neurons stop firing, the monkey is unable to locate the stimulus (e.g., Fuster & Alexander, 1971; see Eichenbaum & Cohen, 2001, for a review). These and other findings make clear that the association cortices play a role in the initial registration and temporary representation of information.

Consolidation

As just described, cortical association areas are involved in the short-term registration of experience. The association areas also are the ultimate long-term storage sites for memories. Yet between initial registration and commitment to long-term storage there is substantial additional processing. That processing generally is described as involving stabilization and integration of the various inputs from different cortical regions and is thought to be performed by structures within the temporal lobes (i.e., in the medial aspect of the lobe). Stabilization and integration processes begin upon registration of a stimulus, and by some estimates, continue for hours, days, months, and even years. Importantly, throughout the consolidation period, memories are vulnerable to disruption and interference and thus, forgetting.

There are two major types of evidence that imply that for memory traces to endure beyond immediate experience, they must undergo additional processing. The first source comes from patients who suffer from *anterograde amnesia,* or an inability to form new explicit memories. Patients with damage in the medial temporal lobe have normal intelligence (as measured by standardized IQ tests) and normal short-term memory (e.g., over intervals of a few seconds, they can remember a series of digits as well as healthy control subjects can). However, they perform poorly on memory tasks that require new learning, including reproducing a diagram after a 5- to 10-minute delay, recalling and recognizing individual words presented on lists, and recognizing words and faces after a 24-hour delay (Reed & Squire, 1998). The memory deficits cannot be accounted for by problems with retrieval alone because lower levels of performance are apparent on tests of recognition as well as recall, even though tests of recognition make lower retrieval demands. These observations imply that for new memories to be effectively stored, they must undergo additional processing after initial registration.

The second source of evidence that memories undergo postencoding processes is the observation of *temporally graded retrograde amnesia*: Memory for more recent events is impaired, relative to memory for more remote events (see Brown, 2002, for a review). Notice that this pattern is precisely the opposite of normal forgetting. The phenomenon is observed in a variety of patient populations, and can be induced in nonhuman animals (including rabbits, mice, and monkeys; see Eichenbaum & Cohen, 2001; Squire & Alvarez, 1995, for reviews) by creating a lesion in medial temporal structures at different points after learning of a novel association, for example (e.g., association between a tone and an electrical shock). Lesions made shortly after learning produce a large deficit in performance; lesions made well after training produce only mild or no disruption of performance (e.g., Kim & Fanselow, 1992; Takehara, Kawahara, & Kirino, 2003). Together, the data on temporally graded retrograde amnesia and on anterograde amnesia provide strong evidence that for memories to be preserved over the long term, they must undergo additional processing for some time after the experience of an event.

There is general consensus that the additional processing that results in consolidation of a memory actually involves two processes that occur in parallel: (1) stabilization of a memory trace through formation of associations among the individual elements of experience, and (2) integration of the memory trace in cortical association areas (e.g., Zola & Squire, 2000). Stabilization of a memory trace begins as inputs from the association areas are projected to structures in the medial temporal lobes (see Figure 3.2). Whereas at the time of experience, inputs from different sensory modalities

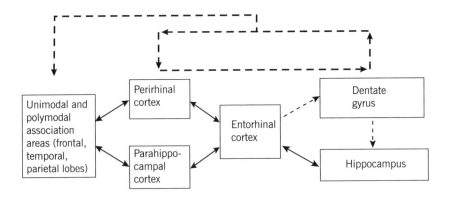

FIGURE 3.2. Schematic representation of the temporal-cortical network implicated in encoding, consolidation, storage, and retrieval of memories. Based on Kandel, Schwartz, and Jessell (2000) and Zola and Squire (2000).

are processed by different association cortices, the inputs come together in the perirhinal and parahippocampal cortices of the medial temporal lobes. These cortices then relay the information to another medial temporal structure—the entorhinal cortex—which in turn relays it into the hippocampus itself (by way of the dentate gyrus). It is in the hippocampus that enduring links between the different elements of experience are forged.

Even as it is being processed in the hippocampus, new information is being associated with old information in cortical storage areas (note in Figure 3.2 the bidirectional nature of information flow into and out of the hippocampal formation). The basis for association is shared elements that are simultaneously activated: neurons that are repeatedly activated together tend to become associated. The result is an entire pattern of interconnection of new information with old. Throughout the period of consolidation, the pattern is regularly "refreshed" by additional neural signaling within the hippocampus and surrounding cortices, and between the medial temporal structures and the association areas (depicted by dashed lines at the top of Figure 3.2). Eventually, the connections between cortical neurons become "cemented," after which medial temporal activity is no longer necessary for the continued existence of the representation (Alvarez & Squire, 1994; McClelland, McNaughton, & O'Reilly, 1995).

We may think of the entire consolidation process as analogous to gelatin setting. At first, gelatin is liquid and the only way to hold it in one place is with a mold. With refrigeration, the gelatin hardens to the point that the mold can be removed and the gelatin will maintain its shape. New memories are like gelatin, the hippocampus is the mold, and the coordinated processing within the medial temporal lobes (to bind the elements together) and between the medial temporal structures and the neocortex (to bind new elements to old) is the refrigeration. Once refrigeration (coordinated processing) has done its work, the mold (hippocampus) is no longer necessary to maintain the integrity of the gelatin (the memory). Unlike gelatin, which sets in a matter of hours, the process of consolidation of new memories may require days, weeks, and even years to complete.

Retrieval

The raison d'être for the formation and consolidation of memories is so that they can be retrieved at some later time. Retrieval is, in essence, a reactivation of the neural network that represents the event (Fuster, 1997). Reactivation occurs because "An internal or external stimulus, whose cortical representation is part of the network by prior association, will reactivate that representation and, again by association, the rest of the network" (Fuster, 1997, p. 455). It is increasingly clear that retrieval of information from long-term stores is accomplished by the same circuits as were involved in initial registration of the experience, namely, the association cortices in general, and prefrontal cortex in particular. Damage to the prefrontal cortex disrupts long-term memory retrieval of both post- and premorbidly experienced facts and episodes (e.g., Janowsky, Shimamura, & Squire, 1989). Prefrontal involvement also is implied by neuroimaging studies (fMRI and PET) that reveal increased activation in prefrontal cortex during memory retrieval. The findings generalize across many kinds of retrieval tasks, including auditory and visual stimuli, and recall and recognition (see Maguire, 2001, for a review).

Consolidation (and Reconsolidation) as a Developmental Challenge

It is apparent that the process of consolidation takes time and that during the period of consolidation, newly learned information is vulnerable to forgetting. The period of consolidation may be especially critical for infants and young children due to relative immaturity of the neural structures and network involved in memory trace construction (see Bauer, 2006, for discussion).

Development of the Temporal–Cortical Network

The period of consolidation may be especially "perilous" for children (Bauer, 2006, 2009) because the structures involved in the process—medial temporal and cortical areas—undergo a protracted course of development. As described in detail elsewhere (e.g., Bauer, 2006, 2007, 2009; Richman & Nelson, 2008), in terms of brain development in general, there are changes in both gray matter (neurons) and white matter (myelinated axons) well into adolescence (e.g., Giedd et al., 1999; Sowell et al., 2004). By 5 years of age, the child's brain is roughly 90% of adult volume (Kennedy, Makris, Herbert, Takahashi, & Caviness, 2002) with an additional 5% increase in volume by the end of the second decade (Caviness, Kennedy, Richelme, Rademacher, & Filipek, 1996). Beyond puberty, gray matter volume actually declines (Gogtay et al., 2004). White matter volume increases linearly with age (Giedd et al., 1999), and is associated with greater connectivity between brain regions and with myelination processes that continue into young adulthood (e.g., Klingberg, Vaidya, Gabrielli, Soseley, & Hedehus, 1999; Schneider, Il'yasov, Hennig, & Martin, 2004).

In terms of the temporal–cortical memory network, in primates, much of the hippocampus matures early, with adult levels of synapses and glucose use by 6 months (Serres & Abraham, 2008). Yet there are gradual increases in hippocampal volume into adolescence (e.g., Gogtay et al., 2004; Pfluger et al., 1999; Utsunomiya, Takano, Okazaki, & Mistudome, 1999). In dentate gyrus (which links the temporal cortices and hippocampal cell fields; see Figure 3.2), as many as 30% of the cells proliferate, migrate, differentiate, and establish connections postnatally. Whereas much of the work is accomplished by the second year of life (e.g., the rise to peak numbers of synapses occurs at 8 to 20 postnatal months), neurogenesis continues throughout childhood and into adulthood (Altman & Das, 1965; see Tanapat, Hastings, & Gould, 2001, for discussion). Functional maturity of the structure is expected to be reached by 16 to 20 months of age, coincident with the rise to peak number of synapses. Full maturity—associated with achievement of the adult number of synapses—is delayed until at least 4 to 5 years (Eckenhoff & Rakic, 1991; see Webb, Monk, & Nelson, 2001, for discussion). Myelination in the hippocampal region continues throughout childhood and adolescence (Arnold & Trojanowski, 1996; Benes, Turtle, Khan, & Farol, 1994; Schneider et al., 2004).

In the prefrontal cortex, the rise to peak number of synapses occurs at 8 to 24 months. Pruning to adult levels does not begin until late childhood and adult levels are not reached until late adolescence or even early adulthood (Huttenlocher, 1979; Huttenlocher & Dabholkar, 1997). As mentioned above, as a result of pruning and other regressive events (i.e., loss of neurons and axonal branches), by adolescence, there are declines in the thickness of the cortical mantle (e.g., Giedd et al., 1999; Gogtay et al., 2004; Sowell, Delis, Stiles, & Jernigan, 2001; see Van Petten, 2004, for discussion). Coincident with decreases in gray matter volume are increases in connectivity between brain regions and with myelination processes that continue well into adolescence or young adulthood (e.g., Klingberg et al., 1999; Schneider et al., 2004).

Implications for Consolidation (and Reconsolidation)

The relative immaturity of the structures and connections of the temporal–cortical network implies that consolidation processes may be less efficient and thus, less effective, in infancy and early childhood, in particular. As a result, even after successful learning, material remains vulnerable to forgetting. The younger the child, the more vulnerable the trace. To further complicate matters, there is increasing evidence that memory traces undergo reconsolidation each time they are reactivated. That is, each time a stored trace is cued—typically by elements of the present situation that overlap with elements that are part of the stored trace (cueing may be either intentional or unintentional)—it is reactivated and undergoes consolidation all over again. The process of reactivation and reconsolidation is a double-edged sword. On the negative side, each time a memory trace is reconsolidated it returns to a state of increased vulnerability. On the positive side, reconsolidation affords opportunity to integrate new learning with old learning. After describing some of the recent data on reconsolidation at the cellular and systems levels, I turn to discussion of the implications of reconsolidation for learning and memory in development.

Cellular Reconsolidation

Long-term storage of information depends on new protein synthesis that supports structural changes that enhance functional connectivity, including changes in the morphology and growth of new dendritic spines on postsynaptic neurons. This process occurs the first time a memory is stored and, as suggested by the results of research by Debiec, LeDoux, and Nader (2002), is repeated when memories are reactivated.

Debiec and colleagues (Debiec et al., 2002) conditioned rats to expect a shock when placed in a distinctive context, a type of learning that is known to be dependent on the hippocampus. Three days after learning, different subgroups of trained rats underwent different treatments. One subgroup had their memories of the contingency reactivated: They were placed back in the distinctive context, though no shocks were administered. The other subgroup did not have their memories reactivated. Rats in both subgroups then were injected with anisomycin, a compound known to block the new protein synthesis necessary for long-term memory. Later the rats were tested for long-term memory of the contingency by placing them back in the conditioning chamber once again. The rats that had not had their memories reactivated showed evidence of retention of the conditioned response. When they were placed in the conditioning chamber they froze, an indication of fear induced by the distinctive environment. In contrast, the rats that had their memories reactivated showed little evidence of memory, as indicated by high mobility and low freezing. These results strongly suggest that memory traces undergo protein synthesis-dependent reconsolidation after reactivation. When reactivation occurs, the processes that originally converted a temporary pattern of activation into an enduring trace must occur once again. If the processes are blocked, the memory is in effect, functionally erased.

Systems Reconsolidation

As evidenced by the work of Takehara et al. (2003; see also Kim & Fanselow, 1992), memories eventually become independent of the hippocampus. Yet the work of Debiec et al. (2002) indicates that hippocampal dependence is reinstated by reactivation of the memory. Evidence of a return to hippocampal dependence at the neural systems level comes from another study of contextual fear conditioning. In this study, Debiec and colleagues conditioned rats to fear a particular context and then waited 45 days, to allow the memory to fully consolidate and become independent of the hippocampus. Half of the rats then had their memories reactivated by being reexposed to the distinctive context. All of the rats then underwent hippocampal surgery. Days later the rats were once again placed in the distinctive context. The rats that had not had their memories reactivated exhibited retention of the contingency (i.e., by freezing). In contrast, the rats that had their memories reactivated before the hippocampal lesion spent very little time freezing, suggesting loss of memory for the contingency. These results indicate that even once memories have been safely tucked away for long-term storage, when they are reactivated, they are vulnerable all over again.

Summary and Implications

Consolidation is the means by which initially labile memory traces become stabilized and integrated into long-term storage. Work with animal models makes clear that memory traces are vulnerable throughout the period of consolidation. In the developing human, consolidation may be especially perilous because the neural structures implicated in it (medial temporal and cortical structures) are relatively immature. As a result, newly learned information may never make it to long-term storage. Further complicating the matter is the apparent fact that even once they have been successfully stored, memory traces may return to a period of lability (and thus, vulnerability) when they are reactivated by exposure to some element that cues the stored trace. Whereas consolidation and reconsolidation represent periods of vulnerability, as outlined in the next section, they also provide an opportunity for growth and cognitive development.

Facilitating Learning and Memory by Capitalizing on Consolidation Processes

The phenomenon of consolidation initially was identified as a result of memory failure associated with retroactive interference. Two different types of memory failure—anterograde and temporally graded retrograde amnesia—provide additional evidence for the process. Disruptions of memory also serve as the source of evidence that memory traces that are reactivated undergo reconsolidation. And most of the discussion of the developmental implications of consolidation and reconsolidation provided in this chapter thus far has emphasized the vulnerability of newly formed memory traces. Fortunately, consolidation and reconsolidation also have positive implications. In fact, consideration of these processes provides a means of understanding a number of well-established phenomena in learning and memory, including findings that (1) memory traces are strengthened with repetition; (2) once established, memory traces can be embellished or elaborated upon; and (3) memory traces become integrated with one another, thereby forming a broader or more general base of knowledge. I discuss each in turn, followed by some suggestions for how we might capitalize on these phenomena to facilitate learning and remembering in child care settings.

Strengthening of Memory Traces

We have long known that additional learning trials can strengthen existing memory traces. In fact, for very young infants, repetition may be necessary to ensure long-term retention. For example, in Bauer et al. (2001), 9-month-olds were exposed to events (like "make a gong") once, twice, or three times prior to imposition of a 1-month delay. The infants in the three-experience condition had higher levels of recall 1 month later, relative to the infants in the one- and two-experience groups (which did not differ from one another). In addition, only the infants in the three-experience condition demonstrated memory for the order in which the events occurred. The process of consolidation provides a neural mechanism for the strengthening of the representation. We can think of each trial as a "pulse" that keeps the material reverberating through the medial-temporal system (see Figure 3.2), increasing the likelihood that it will stabilize and become integrated into long-term storage.

Elaborating Memory Traces

Once established, memory traces can be embellished or elaborated upon by repeated experience. For example, with each additional learning trial, infants recall more actions of a sequence as well as more pairs of actions in temporal order, thus indicating better-organized memory traces with additional learning trials. The processes of consolidation and reconsolidation provide a possible neural means by which this is accomplished. That is, with the experience of an event, the process of stabilization of a memory trace begins. Hours or days later, the event can be reactivated by a cue; there is no better cue than the reexperience of the same event. Once reactivated, the memory trace is open to incorporation of new elements, such as an action that was not adequately encoded on an earlier learning trial, or additional information about the temporal order of actions. Thus, with each reconsolidation, initially "sparse" memory representations can become augmented with additional information. The new elements become part of the reconsolidated trace leaving it "improved" relative to the original.

Integration of Memory Traces

The phenomena of consolidation and reconsolidation also provide possible mechanisms by which separate learning episodes can be integrated with one another. Consider that an initial learning episode sets into motion the process of encoding and consolidation. A subsequent episode of a similar—but not identical—kind sets into motion its own process of encoding and consolidation. Assuming that some elements are shared between the episodes, a demand for retrieval of either will cause both to be reactivated. Once activated simultaneously, the two episodes will "intermingle," and be reconsolidated, each embellished by the other.

At the behavioral level, this process was demonstrated in Bauer and San Souci (2010). Four- and 6-year-old children participated in three interactions with an experimenter. In the first, they learned a novel fact, such as that "Dolphins communicate by clicking and squeaking." In the second episode, they learned that "Dolphins live in groups called pods." Our expectation was that because the two episodes share mention of the feature "dolphin," Learning Episode 2 would reactivate Learning Episode 1 and the two would become integrated. We tested this possibility through a third interaction, in which children were challenged to answer the question "How does a pod communicate?" If the separate learning episodes remained separate, there would be no basis for address of this question, because children were not explicitly taught that pods communicate by clicking and squeaking. However, if the episodes become integrated, through simultaneous activation, then children should be able to provide an answer to the question. As reported in Bauer and San Souci, children were highly successful in the task, implying integration of memory traces between episodes.

Summary

Learning involves storing new facts and experiences and also relating them to old facts and experiences. Each time a memory trace is reactivated it can be strengthened. Each reactivation also provides an opportunity for new information to be added to previously acquired knowledge, leaving it elaborated, relative to the original. Once reactivated, a memory trace also is open to linkage or integration with information already stored in memory based on shared (or similar) elements that result in simultaneous activation of memory traces containing them.

Implications for Child Care Settings

We have much to learn about consolidation and reconsolidation, especially in developmental populations. Yet the need for additional research should not stop us from considering possible educational implications of what we already know about these processes. With the processes of consolidation and reconsolidation in mind, there are two basic principles around which curricula seemingly should be organized, to maximize positive outcomes. As introduced in Bauer (2009), in bumper sticker form, the principles are "Repeat, with variation on the theme," and "Link early, link often."

"Bumper Sticker" Themes

The mandate for repetition comes from what we know about the process of consolidation. To invoke an analogy used earlier in the chapter—the elements of memory traces must remain refrigerated long enough for the gelatin to set. But what if our refrigerator is in a developing country, and electricity to operate it is only available a few hours at a time? In this case, on the basis of a single bout of refrigeration, only a thin layer may form on the surface of the mold. For the gelatin to solidify all the way through, we may need several bouts of refrigeration, distributed over time. So it goes with learning and memory, especially in the developing brain. A learning episode that seems to have "taken" may really be only skin deep, such that it cannot endure without reinforcement (as in Bauer et al., 2001). For the young child, a single learning episode may be sufficient to give the *illusion* that the lesson has been learned, but like the gelatin, it loses its integrity quickly (it does not survive consolidation). Reinforcement in the form of repetition serves to keep the lesson reverberating long enough for consolidation to occur. Variations on a theme serve to ensure that the resulting memory trace has a strong core, with multiple different associates.

The mandate for links comes from what we know about the process of reconsolidation. A single learning episode established a trace comprised of several elements (A, B, and C, for example). A subsequent episode establishes a trace comprised of different elements, some of which overlap with the first (e.g., elements C, D, and E). Establishment of the second trace means the shared element (C) is reinstated, which simultaneously serves to reinstate the other elements as well (A and B). The result is that the links in the original episode are strengthened and linked to the subsequent episode. By "linking early" the new associate serves almost as a separate learning trial for the original trace. By "linking often" the network of associations grows, strengthening and elaborating along the way.

The suggestions that lessons be reinforced through repetition and that links with related material be made both early and often, translate into recommendations regarding means by which learning and memory may be facilitated in infants and very young children. It is relatively clear that for infants and young children to learn new things and retain the information over time, they must be exposed to the new material more than once. The necessary research to determine the number of experiences required to solidify new learning simply has not been done; no doubt the number will vary for different types of experiences and materials. Yet it is apparent that the younger the infant, the more times she or he must experience an event in order to learn and remember it. For example, at 6 months of age, infants remember sequences of actions they have seen modeled six times, but not sequences of actions they have seen modeled only once, twice, or three times (Barr et al., 1996). By the middle of the second year of life, infants retain memory representations of events they have seen modeled only once (Bauer & Dow, 1994). The necessary research to identify the optimal spacing of experiences also has not been done. Again, we may anticipate that the optimal spacing will vary as a function of the type of experience and the materials. We may be relatively confident though that the younger the infant, the closer together the lessons must be in order for experience to accumulate. This principle follows from the fact that the benefits of repetition will accrue only if the repetitions occur within the span of time over which the original lesson is retained, and from the observation that the span of time over which infants and young children remember is shorter for younger relative to older infants (see Bauer, 2007, 2009, for reviews).

The suggestion that lessons be provided with slight "variations on a theme" translates into the recommendation that educators might, for example, vary the materials they use to demonstrate a principle or event. It is clear that infants retain information about the specific features of their experiences. For instance, they reliably remember the specific props used to produce event sequences, even when they are presented among different props that could be used to produce the same sequence of actions with the same outcome (Bauer & Dow, 1994). That is, when they have seen a rattle made of two round nesting cups and a ball (put the ball inside one cup, cover it with the other, shake the combination to make a rattle sound), infants correctly identify the props from among distracters including square nesting cups and a block that fits inside. Memory for the specific features of events is related to memory for the entire sequence of actions (Bauer & Lukowski, 2010. Although they remember the specifics of events, infants and young children also readily extend learning to new materials. For example, after seeing the rattle produced with round cups and a ball, if given square cups and a block rather than the original materials, they will use the new materials to produce the rattle (e.g., Bauer & Dow, 1994; Bauer & Lukowski, 2010). The necessary experiments have not been done, yet application of the principles of consolidation and reconsolidation suggests that memories that have been extended across different sets of props will be more robust over time and to interference, relative to memories that have been encoded using only a single set of stimuli. Thus, a potentially productive means of facilitating learning and memory is to produce the same or similar actions using materials that are similar yet not identical.

The suggestion that links be made both early and often translates into the recommendation that as new material is being presented, educators deliberately remind infants and young children of prior learning episodes. To date, this principle has been demonstrated with preschool-age and older children only, yet there is reason to believe that it would apply to infants and younger children as well. The simple hint to "Think about the stories you heard earlier" is sufficient to increase the likelihood that preschoolers will integrate the facts that "Dolphins communicate by clicking and squeaking" and "Dolphins live in groups called pods," in order to generate the fact that pods communicate by clicking and squeaking (Bauer, King, Larkina, Varga, & White, 2012). Preliminary research suggests that this type of "hint" is better when delivered earlier rather than later in a retention interval. Thus, to facilitate learning, educators might explicitly suggest to children that they link their knowledge of separate yet related episodes of experience. We may reasonably predict that the younger the infant or child, the more explicit the hint to link should be in order to be effective.

Though no doubt there are other elements not captured in the equation, the principles of "Repeat, with variation on the theme," and "Link early, link often," are consistent with Bruner's (1960) conceptualization of a *spiral curriculum*. Bruner suggested that an effective curriculum is one that as it develops, revisits basic ideas repeatedly, "building upon them until the student has grasped the full formal apparatus that goes with them" (p. 13). The curriculum is a spiral (rather than a circle) because although it exposes students to a concept over and over again, it does not stay at the same level of complexity or demand over time. Rather, concepts are introduced and reintroduced, each time in different contexts, with different neighbors, and at different levels of sophistication. Some students may grasp the concept the first time around and use subsequent "passes" to elaborate it. For other students, the first pass (or two) may have little impact, but the concept will be revisited, granting them another opportunity. When activities with similar educational functions are repeated and coordinated with one another, and when the learning experiences in one course or subject matter are coordinated with those in another, the spiral widens. A spiral curriculum seems ideally suited to reveal the "silver lining" in what might otherwise be the dark cloud of consolidation and reconsolidation.

What might a spiral curriculum look like for infants and children in the the first years of life? Dougherty's (1999) lessons for language learning can be used as an illustration. Dougherty outlined five methods for building early language skills, the first four of which can be conceived in a spiral: naming, describing, comparing, and explaining. To get the spiral started, the first language lesson provides a label or name: "It's a ball." When the object is experienced again, it not only is named, but also described: "It's a ball. The ball is round. It's a round ball." The second "pass" thus reinforces the original naming lesson and builds on it with adjectival description. The third exposure might involve the same objects now in a different room, along with other objects. The "old" objects are named and described and also explicitly compared with the new objects: "It's a ball. It's a round ball. Here's a block. It's a square block." A subsequent exposure might involve explanation of how the object can be used or of what it is made, for example. On the way to the explanation, previous lessons of naming and describing are repeated once again: "It's a ball. It's a round ball. Round balls roll." Because encounters involve repetition and elaboration of a basic lesson, children have multiple opportunities to grasp it. Because each encounter involves a new level of complexity and demand, children have multiple opportunities to elaborate the basic lesson. When lessons are repeated, elaborated, and coordinated with one another, the spiral widens.

Challenged Populations

Learning and memory are fundamental processes that occur in all infants and children. Similarly, all infants and children experience a slow course of development of the neural structures and networks involved in learning and memory. As such, we may expect that all infants and children experience challenges to the processes associated with turning new learning into stable memory traces that are integrated with the products of prior learning. The unfortunate reality is that some populations of infants and young children may experience even greater challenges, associated with adverse prenatal experiences, adverse postnatal experiences, or both. Many such experiences stem from poverty and the "omissions" and "commissions" associated with it (Cheatham, Sesma, Bauer, & Georgieff, 2010).

Omission is when a factor important for brain or cognitive development does not occur as expected; omission can occur at any point in the developmental trajectory. A number of potential "errors of omission" (Cheatham, Sesma, et al., 2010) are associated with poverty, including insufficient time between pregnancies, low prepregnancy weight, and poor maternal nutrition. Maternal malnutrition is related to fetal malnutrition, which is a prime cause of intrauterine growth restriction. In addition, factors such as protein or iron deficiencies can result in decreased cell replication and thus, limited brain size and complexity (Cordero, Valenzuela, Rodriquez, & Aboitiz, 2003; King et al., 2004). The proper levels of nutrients (e.g., oxygen, protein, iron, zinc, carbohydrates) are necessary for both neuroanatomic processes (functions of cells and their supporting structures) and neurochemical processes (neurotransmitter and receptor synthesis) in the brain. Thus, the lack of proper placental support to the fetus can result in a profound disruption of brain development. Effects of poverty extend into postnatal life, in the form of decreased perceptual and cognitive stimulation, that may retard postnatal synaptogenesis and pruning.

Commissions are defined as adverse biological conditions to which the brain would not normally have been exposed and which have a noxious effect on brain development (Cheatham, Sesma, et al., 2010). Environmental embryonic commission events include insults from toxins. Maternal alcohol abuse (see West, Chen, & Pantazis, 1994, for a review), intrauterine infections (e.g., Mallard, Welin, Peebles, Hagberg, & Kjellmer, 2003), and environmental toxins (e.g., mercury, lead, ionizing radiation; e.g., Palomo, Beninger, Kostrzewa, & Archer, 2003), can result in restricted brain growth by decreasing cell replication, thereby reducing cell numbers and synaptic connections. These stressors also can affect brain development by altering the metabolism and thus, the function of the cells. The psychopathology associated with these factors includes mental retardation, hyperkinetic disorders, and significant emotional disturbance (see Trask & Kosofsky, 2000, for a review). Postnatally, the conditions of poverty may result in commission events in the form of chronic maternal and infant stress associated with food and shelter insufficiency. Chronic high levels of the stress hormone cortisol are related to cell damage in the hippocampus (Sapolsky, Uno, Rebert, & Finch, 1990).

The omissions and commissions associated with poverty may be expected to negatively impact learning and memory, thus making attention to conditions that foster these processes all the more critical. Consistent with this suggestion, impaired learning and memory has been observed in several populations that experience some of the same risk factors. Infants of mothers with maternal gestational diabetes experience prenatal conditions that can result in iron deficiency, with attendant presumed compromise of hippocampal development. They show impaired performance on tasks that require memory over a brief delay (e.g., Riggins, Bauer, Georgieff, & Nelson, 2010). Infants born prior to term experience both prenatal and postnatal conditions that are outside the range of expected experience. They too show impaired performance on delayed recall tasks (Cheatham, Sesma, et al., 2010; de Haan, Bauer, Georgieff, & Nelson, 2000). Infants who spent the first months of life in the relative deprivation of institutional care (Kroupina, Bauer, Gunnar, & Johnson, 2010) and infants neglected by their caregivers (Cheatham, Larkina, Bauer, Toth, & Cicchetti, 2010) show impairments in learning as well as memory (see Bauer, 2010, for discussion). It is reasonable to expect that factors known to facilitate learning and memory in typically developing infants and children—such as multiple experiences, optimally spaced—would aid infants in overcoming the challenges they experience in learning new material and committing it to memory. The hypothesis awaits empirical test.

Conclusions

Learning and remembering are intimately related to one another. The process of forming a new memory—and thus of acquiring new information—involves several steps beginning with initial registration of the information across distributed cortical regions. For the event or experience to live on beyond the immediate present, the initially labile representation of the experience must be stabilized and the resulting trace must be integrated with information already in storage. Retrieval of a stored memory trace occurs when an internal or external stimulus that shares elements with the trace reactivates it. Every act of retrieval is an opportunity to strengthen and elaborate upon the original trace, and also to create new linkages between it and other traces with elements in common. Thus, every act of retrieval of previously stored information is an opportunity to solidify and expand the knowledge base.

The means by which memory traces are born and develop, and the processes that take place each time they are retrieved or reactivated, have implications for learning and memory in educational settings. In sound-bite terms, they suggest that educators "Repeat, with variation on the theme," and "Link early, link often." These mandates stem from what we know about the process of consolidation and reconsolidation and the developmental status of the neural structures and network that subserves them. Even for the young child, a single lesson or learning episode may be sufficient to support retention over the short term. However, essential elements of the representation likely will be lost as the trace undergoes consolidation. Reinforcement in the form of repetition serves to keep the lesson-related trace alive long enough for it to be successfully consolidated and integrated with existing knowledge. Variations on the lesson theme serve to increase the number of associations to the trace and thus the number of routes to retrieval (and reactivation) of it. The mandate for links stems from the observation that shared elements—and their associates—are strengthened each time they are activated. Thus, a new association that shares elements with an old one strengthens the original trace in much the same way as an additional learning trial. By "linking often" the network of associations grows, strengthening and elaborating along the way.

The principles of "Repeat, with variation on the theme," and "Link early, link often," are consistent with conceptualization of *spiral curricula* (Bruner, 1960). In such curricula, students are introduced and reintroduced to key concepts, in different contexts, and at different levels of sophistication. When learning experiences in one course or subject matter are coordinated with those in another, the spiral widens, providing a firm foundation for continued learning and expansion. Attention to these principles may be especially important—and beneficial—for children in poverty. The conditions of poverty virtually ensure prenatal and postnatal exposure to a number of "errors" of omission and commission that in turn may compromise brain and cognitive development. These events may make it even more difficult for the "gelatin" of learning and memory to set. A concerted research effort to identify the optimal conditions for consolidation and reconsolidation of new memories is called for, in both typically developing infants and young children, and in children coping with the challenges of poverty.

REFERENCES

Altman, J., & Das, G. D. (1965). Autoradiographic and histological evidence of postnatal hippocampal neurogenesis in rats. *Journal of Comparative Neurology, 124,* 319–335.

Alvarez, P., & Squire, L. R. (1994). Memory consolidation and the medial temporal lobe: A simple network model. *Proceedings of the National Academy of Sciences, 91,* 7041–7045.

Arnold, S. E., & Trojanowski, J. Q. (1996). Human fetal hippocampal development: I. Cytoarchitecture, myeloarchitecture, and neuronal morphologic features. *Journal of Comparative Neurology, 367,* 274–292.

Barr, R., Dowden, A., & Hayne, H. (1996). Developmental change in deferred imitation by 6- to 24-month-old infants. *Infant Behavior and Development, 19,* 159–170.

Bauer, P. J. (2004). Getting explicit memory off the ground: Steps toward construction of a neuro-developmental account of changes in the first two years of life. *Developmental Review, 24,* 347–373.

Bauer, P. J. (2005a). Developments in declarative memory: Decreasing susceptibility to storage failure over the second year of life. *Psychological Science, 16,* 41–47.

Bauer, P. J. (2005b). New developments in the study of infant memory. In D. M. Teti (Ed.), *Blackwell handbook of research methods in developmental science* (pp. 467–488). Oxford, UK: Blackwell.

Bauer, P. J. (2006). Constructing a past in infancy: A neuro-developmental account. *Trends in Cognitive Sciences, 10,* 175–181.

Bauer, P. J. (2007). *Remembering the times of our lives: Memory in infancy and beyond.* Mahwah, NJ: Erlbaum.

Bauer, P. J. (2009). Neurodevelopmental changes in infancy and beyond: Implications for learning and memory. In O. A. Barbarin & B. H. Wasik (Eds.), *Handbook of child development and early education: Research to practice* (pp. 78–102). New York: Guilford Press.

Bauer, P. J. (2010). Declarative memory in infancy: An introduction to typical and atypical development. In P. J. Bauer (Ed.), *Advances in child development and behavior: Vol. 38. Varieties of early experience: Implications for the development of declarative memory in infancy* (pp. 3–28). London: Elsevier.

Bauer, P. J., & Dow, G. A. A. (1994). Episodic memory in 16- and 20-month-old children: Specifics are generalized, but not forgotten. *Developmental Psychology, 30,* 403–417.

Bauer, P. J., King, J. E., & Larkina, M., Varga, N., & White, E. (2012). Characters and clues: Factors affecting children's extension of knowledge through integration of separate episodes. *Journal of Experimental Child Psychology, 111,* 681–694.

Bauer, P. J., & Lukowski, A. F. (2010). The memory is in the details: Relations between memory for the specific features of events and long-term recall in infancy. *Journal of Experimental Child Psychology, 107,* 1–14.

Bauer, P. J., & Mandler, J. M. (1989). One thing follows another: Effects of temporal structure on one- to two-year-olds' recall of events. *Developmental Psychology, 25,* 197–206.

Bauer, P. J., & San Souci, P. (2010). Going beyond the facts: Young children extend knowledge by integrating episodes. *Journal of Experimental Child Psychology, 107,* 452–465.

Bauer, P. J., Wenner, J. A., Dropik, P. L., & Wewerka, S. S. (2000). Parameters of remembering and forgetting in the transition from infancy to early childhood. *Monographs of the Society for Research in Child Development, 65*(4, Serial No. 263).

Bauer, P. J., Wiebe, S. A., Waters, J. M., & Bangston, S. K. (2001). Reexposure breeds recall: Effects of experience on 9-month-olds' ordered recall. *Journal of Experimental Child Psychology, 80,* 174–200.

Benes, F. M., Turtle, M., Khan, Y., & Farol, P. (1994). Myelination of a key relay zone in the hippocampal formation occurs in the human brain during childhood, adolescence, and adulthood. *Archives of General Psychiatry, 51,* 477–484.

Brown, A. S. (2002). Consolidation theory and retrograde amnesia in humans. *Psychonomic Bulletin and Review, 9,* 403–425.

Bruner, J. (1960). *The Process of Education.* Cambridge, MA: Harvard University Press.

Caviness, V. S., Kennedy, D. N., Richelme, C., Rademacher, J., & Filipek, P. A. (1996). The human brain age 7–11 years: A volumetric analysis based on magnetic resonance images. *Cerebral Cortex, 6,* 726–736.

Cheatham, C. L., Larkina, M., Bauer, P. J., Toth, S. L., & Cicchetti, D. (2010). Declarative memory in abused and neglected infants. In P. J. Bauer (Ed.), *Advances in child development and behavior: Vol. 38. Varieties of early experience: Implications for the development of declarative memory in infancy* (pp. 161–183). London: Elsevier.

Cheatham, C. L., Sesma, H. W., Bauer, P. J., & Georgieff, M. K. (2010). The development of declarative memory in infants born preterm. In P. J. Bauer (Ed.), *Advances in child development and behavior: Vol. 38. Varieties of early experience: Implications for the development of declarative memory in infancy* (pp. 112–137). London: Elsevier.

Chi, M. T. H. (1978). Knowledge structures and memory development. In R. S. Siegler (Ed.), *Children's thinking: What develops?* (pp. 73–96). Hillsdale, NJ: Erlbaum.

Cordero, M. E., Valenzuela, C. Y., Rodriguez, A., & Aboitiz, F. (2003). Dendritic morphology and orientation of pyramidal cells of the neocortex in two groups of early postnatal undernourished–rehabilitated rats. *Developmental Brain Research, 142,* 37–45.

Daneman, P., & Carpenter, P. (1980). Individual differences in working memory and reading. *Journal of Verbal Learning and Verbal Behavior, 19,* 450–466.

Debiec, J., LeDoux, J. E., & Nader, K. (2002). Cellular and systems reconsolidation in the hippocampus. *Neuron, 36,* 527–538.

de Haan, M., Bauer, P. J., Georgieff, M. K., & Nelson, C. A. (2000). Explicit memory in low-risk infants aged 19 months born between 27 and 42 weeks of gestation. *Developmental Medicine and Child Neurology, 42,* 304–312.

Dougherty, D. P. (1999). *How to talk to your baby.* New York: Penguin Putnam.

Eckenhoff, M., & Rakic, P. (1991). A quantitative analysis of synaptogenesis in the molecular layer of the dentate gyrus in the rhesus monkey. *Developmental Brain Research, 64,* 129–135.

Eichenbaum, H., & Cohen, N. J. (2001). *From conditioning to conscious recollection: Memory systems of the brain.* New York: Oxford University Press.

Fuster, J. M. (1997). Network memory. *Trends in Neuroscience, 20,* 451–459.

Fuster, J. M., & Alexander, G. E. (1971). Neuron activity related to short-term memory. *Science, 173,* 652–654.

Giedd, J. N., Blumenthal, J., Jeffries, N. O., Castellanos, F. X., Liu, H., Zijdenbos, A., et al. (1999). Brain development during childhood and adolescence: A longitudinal MRI study. *Nature Neuroscience, 2,* 861–863.

Gogtay, N., Giedd, J. N., Lusk, L., Hayashi, K. M., Greenstein, D., Vaituzis, A. C., et al. (2004). Dynamic mapping of human cortical development during childhood through early adulthood. *PNAS, 101,* 8174–8179.

Huttenlocher, P. R. (1979). Synaptic density in human frontal cortex: Developmental changes and effects of aging. *Brain Research, 163,* 195–205.

Huttenlocher, P. R., & Dabholkar, A. S. (1997). Regional differences in synaptogenesis in human cerebral cortex. *Journal of Comparative Neurology, 387,* 167–178.

Janowsky, J. S., Shimamura, A. P., & Squire, L. R. (1989). Source memory impairment in patients with frontal lobe lesions. *Neuropsychologia, 27,* 1043–1056.

Kandel, E. R., Schwartz, J. H., & Jessell, T. M. (2000). *Principles of neural science* (4th ed.). New York: McGraw-Hill.

Kandel, E. R., & Squire, L. R. (2000). Neuroscience: Breaking down scientific barriers to the study of brain and mind. *Science, 290,* 1113–1120.

Kennedy, D. N., Makris, N., Herbert, M. R., Takahashi, T., & Caviness, V. S. (2002). Basic principles of MRI and morphometry studies of human brain development. *Developmental Science, 5,* 268–278.

Kim, J. J., & Fanselow, M. S. (1992). Modality-specific retrograde amnesia of fear. *Science, 256,* 675–677.

King, R. S., DeBassio, W. A., Kemper, T. L., Rosene, D. L., Tonkiss, J., Galler, J. R., et al. (2004). Effects of prenatal protein malnutrition and acute postnatal stress on granule cell genesis in the fascia dentata of neonatal and juvenile rats. *Developmental Brain Research, 150,* 9–15.

Klingberg, T., Vaidya, C. J., Gabrielli, J. D., Soseley, M. E., & Hedehus, M. (1999). Myelination and organization of the frontal white matter in children: A diffusion tensor MRI study. *Neuroreport, 10,* 2817–2821.

Kroupina, M. G., Bauer, P. J., Gunnar, M. R., & Johnson, D. E. (2010). Institutional care as a risk for declarative memory development. In P. J. Bauer (Ed.), *Advances in child development and behavior: Vol. 38. Varieties of early experience: Implications for the development of declarative memory in infancy* (pp. 138–160). London: Elsevier.

Maguire, E. A. (2001). Neuroimaging studies of autobiographical event memory. *Philosophical Transactions. Royal Society of London, 356,* 1441–1451.

Mallard, C., Welin, A. K., Peebles, D., Hagberg, J., & Kjellmer, I. (2003). White matter injury following systemic endotoxemia or asphyxia in the fetal sheep. *Neurochemical Research, 28,* 215–223.

McClelland, J. L., McNaughton, B. L., & O'Reilly, R. C. (1995). Why there are complementary learning systems in the hippocampus and neocortex: Insights from the successes and failures of connectionist models of learning and memory. *Psychological Review, 102,* 419–457.

Müller, G. E., & Pilzecker, A. (1900). Experimentalle Beitrage zur Lehre vom Gedachtnis. *Zeitschrift fur Psychologie, 1,* 1–30.

Palomo, T., Beninger, R. J., Kostrzewa, R. M., & Archer, T. (2003). Brain sites of movement disorder: Genetic and environmental agents in neurodevelopmental perturbations. *Neurotoxicity Research, 5,* 1–26.

Pfluger, T., Weil, S., Wies, S., Vollmar, C., Heiss, D., Egger, J., et al. (1999). Normative volumetric data of the developing hippocampus in children based on magnetic resonance imaging. *Epilepsia, 40,* 414–423.

Reed, J. M., & Squire, L. R. (1998). Retrograde amnesia for facts and events: Findings from four new cases. *Journal of Neuroscience, 18,* 3943–3954.

Richman, J., & Nelson, C. A. (2008). Mechanisms of change: A cognitive neuroscience approach to declarative memory development. In C. A. Nelson & M. Luciana (Eds.), *Handbook of developmental cognitive neuroscience* (2nd ed., pp. 541–552). Cambridge, MA: MIT Press.

Riggins, T., Bauer, P. J., Georgieff, M. K., & Nelson, C. A. (2010). Declarative memory performance in infants of diabetic mothers. In P. J. Bauer (Ed.), *Advances in child development and behavior: Vol. 38. Varieties of early experience: Implications for the development of declarative memory in infancy* (pp. 73–111). London: Elsevier.

Sapolsky, R. M., Uno, H., Rebert, C. S., & Finch, C. E. (1990). Hippocampal damage associated with prolonged glucocorticoid exposure in primates. *Journal of Neuroscience, 10,* 2897–2902.

Schneider, J. F. L., Il'yasov, K. A., Hennig, J., & Martin, E. (2004). Fast quantitative difusion-tensor imaging of cerebral white matter from the neonatal period to adolescence. *Neuroradiology, 46,* 258–266.

Seress, L., & Abraham, H. (2008). Pre- and postnatal morphological development of the human hippocampal formation. In C. A. Nelson & M. Luciana (Eds.), *Handbook of developmental cognitive neuroscience* (2nd ed., pp. 187–212). Cambridge, MA: MIT Press.

Siegel, L. S., & Ryan, E. B. (1989). The development of working memory in normally achieving and subtypes of learning disabled children. *Child Development, 60,* 873–908.

Sowell, E. R., Delis, D., Stiles, J., & Jernigan, T. L. (2001). Improved memory functioning and frontal lobe maturation between childhood and adolescence: A structural MRI study. *Journal of International Neuropsychological Society, 7,* 312–322.

Sowell, E. R., Thompson, P. M., Leonard, C. M., Welcome, S. E., Kan, E., & Toga, A. W. (2004). Longitudinal mapping of cortical thickness and brain growth in normal children. *Journal of Neuroscience, 24,* 8223–8231.

Squire, L. R., & Alvarez, P. (1995). Retrograde amnesia and memory consolidation: A neurobiological perspective. *Current Opinion in Neurobiology, 5,* 169–177.

Takehara, K., Kawahara, S., & Kirino, Y. (2003). Time-dependent reorganization of the brain components underlying memory retention in trace eyeblink conditioning. *Journal of Neuroscience, 23,* 9897–9905.

Tanapat, P., Hastings, N. B., & Gould, E. (2001). Adult neurogenesis in the hippocampal formation. In C. A. Nelson & M. Luciana (Eds.), *Handbook of developmental cognitive neuroscience* (2nd ed., pp. 93–105). Cambridge, MA: MIT Press.

Trask, C. L., & Kosofsky, B. E. (2000). Developmental considerations of neurotoxic exposures. *Neurologic Clinics, 18,* 541–562.

Utsunomiya, H., Takano, K., Okazaki, M., & Mistudome, A. (1999). Development of the tempral lobe in infants and children: Analysis by MR-based volumetry. *American Journal of Neuroradiology, 20,* 717–723.

Van Petten, C. (2004). Relationship between hippocampal volume and memory ability in healthy individuals across the lifespan: Review and meta-analysis. *Neuropsychologia, 42,* 1394–1413.

Webb, S. J., Monk, C. S., & Nelson, C. A. (2001). Mechanisms of postnatal neurobiological development: Implications for human development. *Developmental Neuropsychology, 19,* 147–171.

West, J. R., Chen, W. J., & Pantazis, N. J. (1994). Fetal alcohol syndrome: The vulnerability of the developing brain and possible mechanisms. *Metabolic Brain Disease, 9,* 291–322.

Zola, S. M., & Squire, L. R. (2000). The medial temporal lobe and the hippocampus. In E. Tulving & F. I. M. Craik (Eds.), *The Oxford handbook of memory* (pp. 485–500). New York: Oxford University Press.

PART II

LANGUAGE DEVELOPMENT

CHAPTER 4

How Babies Talk

Six Principles of Early Language Development

Kathy Hirsh-Pasek and Roberta Michnick Golinkoff

In 1995, Hart and Risley's (1995) research became headline news. The language experience of children growing up in poverty was distinctly different than that of children growing up in working-class or professional families. On average, the number of words heard per hour in the welfare group was 616 compared to 1,251 in the working-class group and 2,153 in the professional group. These findings are dramatic and consistent with results of recent studies (Hoff, 2006a; Cristofaro & Tamis-LeMonda, 2012). Further, disparities in early cognitive development even as early as 9 months grow larger over time by 24 months (Halle et al., 2009).

These findings have enormous implications. First, Hart and Risley (1995) noted that vocabulary assessed at age 3 significantly predicted scores of language competence at ages 9 and 10. Second, the amount of early language heard in infancy is strongly related to the speed with which children process language at 18 and 25 months of age (Fernald, Perfors, & Marchman, 2006), to vocabulary size at 25 months, and to linguistic and cognitive skills at 8 years of age (Marchman & Fernald, 2008).

Third, not only does early language exposure predict later language ability, but there is also some evidence that it might be related to brain differences in 5-year-olds. Hackman and Farah (2009) suggest that the great disparities in language resulting from socioeconomic status (SES) differences have neurological consequences: "On the basis of our three studies, the effects of poverty were disproportionate for certain neurocognitive systems, including language and executive function" (p. 66). Though SES did not uniformly predict poor performance in all areas of the brain, middle-class kindergarteners did outperform their low-SES counterparts in tests that tapped the left perisylvian/language system.

Finally, it is important to note that early language differences are also related to school readiness and to later school outcomes in both reading and math (NICHD Early Child Care Research Network, 2005). For example, a large literature links early language competence to reading readiness in kindergarten and primary school (National Early Literacy Panel, 2008; Dickinson, Golinkoff, & Hirsh-Pasek, 2010). Indeed, Dickinson and Tabors (2001) report that early language input in kindergarten accounted for over two-thirds of the variance in fourth-grade reading ability. Early language ability relates to improvement in the ability to detect separable sounds that feed phonological awareness (Munson, Kurtz, & Windsor, 2005), to vocabulary acquisition, and to grammatical development (Hoff, 2006b), and each of these language systems is critical to later reading success. Language comprehension difficulties in children are linked to poor oral language comprehension (Clarke, Snowling, Truelove, & Hulme, 2010) such that intervention in oral language training was more positively related to reading outcomes than was training in text comprehension.

The good news that lies beneath these shocking statistics is that the trajectory of language development is malleable. A number of studies find that children's vocabulary and grammar are related to the amount and quality of their language input (e.g., Hoff & Naigles, 2002). Importantly, intervention studies that coached parents of infants in ways to support language development have been successful, and with medium to large effect sizes (National Early Literacy Panel, 2008). Some of these programs achieved higher language outcomes by videotaping parents and offering feedback. The goal was to get parents to offer more language input about what their children were looking at and interested in (Play and Learning Strategies [PALS]; Landry, Smith, & Swank, 2006). These intervention studies give reason to be optimistic. They suggest that with sustained intervention we can change the trajectory of language development!

This chapter begins to tell the backstory of language development in an effort to better understand the mechanisms of language growth and hence, ways in which we can use current scientific data to support strong language skills for all children. The story is told in two parts. First, we explore what we know about language development—reviewing what is obvious to the naked eye and importantly what we are learning that is often hidden from view. Second, we suggest six principles of language learning gleaned from the last two decades of research. We conclude with suggestions on how these principles can be directly translated for classroom use with very young children and how they might particularly profit low-income children.

A Selective Review of the Evidence on Language Learning

Charting Language Development

What You See

The trajectory of language production has been documented. Diary studies dating to the late 1800s from scientists the likes of Darwin (1877) among many others relate the momentous climb from the first coos and gurgles of the 3-month-old to the first words at around 1 year of age to multiword speech at around 2 years of age. Figure 4.1 presents an overview of these productive milestones.

What You Don't See

The real story of language development, however, comes not merely from what children say, but also from what they understand well before they can

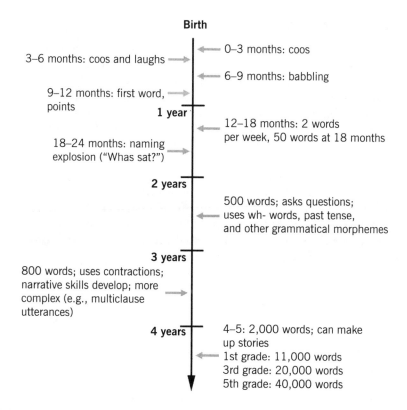

FIGURE 4.1. Milestones of productive language development. Figure developed by Russell Richie.

speak. New methodologies have allowed the field to see beneath production—or the lack thereof—and to better understand *how* children learn,
not just *what* they learn.

These methodologies enable us to assemble the puzzle of language
development. To learn a language, for example, children must be able to
segment the continuous flow of speech or the "melodies" of speech into sentences, phrases, words, and sounds (or hand shapes in the case of children
learning sign language). They must also parse continuous events into the
objects and actions referenced in language. Finally they must map the units
of sound onto the objects, actions, and events using words and grammar.
What might infants know in each of these areas? Here we describe just a
few of these methods to give a flavor of the tools that allow us entrée into
the emerging language system. These new methodologies are shaping the
landscape of early language development and offering clues to what types
of early intervention might prove most profitable (Golinkoff & Hirsh-
Pasek, 2012).

A Methodological Sampler

High-amplitude sucking (Eimas, Siqueland, Jusczyk, & Vigorito, 1971)
indicated that infants just a few weeks old heard the sounds of language
as falling into the same categories possessed by adults. The *habituation
paradigm* (Bornstein, 1985) that presents infants with a repeated visual,
or auditory, stimulus (or both) indicated that infants can detect relational
components in the events they witness (e.g., Pulverman, Golinkoff, Hirsh-
Pasek, & Buresh, 2008). The *head-turn preference procedure* (Fernald,
1985; Hirsh-Pasek et al., 1987) moved beyond asking whether infants
could discriminate *individual* sounds to asking how they segment fluent
speech into units like clauses, phrases, and words. The *intermodal preferential looking paradigm* (IPLP; Golinkoff, Hirsh-Pasek, Cauley, & Gordon, 1987; Hirsh-Pasek & Golinkoff, 1996) enabled us to complete the last
part of the puzzle—asking how preverbal infants might map words and
grammar onto objects, actions, and events.

A host of other popular methodologies populate infant and toddler
language research (e.g., the switch paradigm; Werker, Cohen, Lloyd, Casasola, & Stager, 1998) as well as various new neurological techniques (e.g.,
Kuhl & Rivera-Gaxiola, 2008). Collectively, these methods opened the
vistas of language learning that now allow us to paint a new portrait of
what children know well before they can speak. We review selective findings using these methods in the context of the emergentist coalition model
of language (ECM; Hollich, Hirsh-Pasek, & Golinkoff, 2000), a framework developed as a comprehensive and integrative look at the earliest
language growth.

The ECM

Introduced by Hirsh-Pasek and Golinkoff (1996), the ECM was designed to organize findings in language acquisition and to ask how the perceptual, social, and linguistic input available to children might be integrated to promote both vocabulary and grammatical growth. The model makes three assumptions. First, children are sensitive to multiple language inputs at any given time. Second, these inputs are differentially weighted over development such that children first use perceptual information to parse the incoming flow of sounds and the visual information in events; later attend to social cues in the service of language learning; and finally, to grammatical information. Third, these principles emerge as children weigh the different sources of information over time although none disappear.

The ECM answered a call from a number of theorists looking for a more holistic approach to language development (Bloom, 1993; Thelen & Smith, 1994; Woodward & Markman, 1998). In fact, Nelson (1996) wrote, "There are no single effective pushes to the developing system but rather a combination of influences that lead to observable change" (p. 85). However, most studies of language growth focused on one aspect of language development—the sounds, the words, or the grammar—rather than on a broader approach. The ECM invites us to look beyond milestones at particular ages and toward the processes that enable language development. Sternberg (1984) put it best when he wrote:

> There are two fundamental questions in developmental psychology. First, what are the psychological states individuals pass through at different points in their development? Second, what are the mechanisms of development by which individuals pass from one state to another? A strong case could be made that the second question is the more basic one. . . . (p. vii)

Here we use the ECM as a guide to organize research in various areas of language development. We next turn to a set of principles that can be derived from these findings. A visual representation of the model can be seen in Figure 4.2.

Perception

Detecting the Sounds of Language

A now classic study by DeCasper and Spence (1986) showed that, even in the womb, infants begin to listen to and remember speech such as stories like *The Cat in the Hat* (Seuss, 1957). Others report that newborns prefer listening to human language over an artificial "language" that mimics some of its properties (Vouloumanos & Werker, 2007). Eimas et al. (1971) using a high

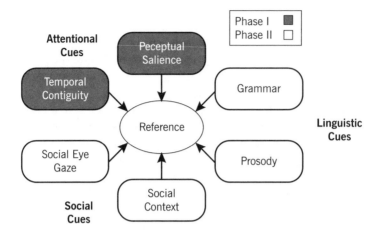

FIGURE 4.2. The emergentist coalition model. The coalition of cues available for establishing word reference are utilized differently across developmental time. Children shift from Phase I, a reliance on attentional cues such as how compelling an object is (perceptual salience) and the coincident appearance of an object and a label (temporal contiguity), to Phase II, a greater dependency on social and linguistic cues like eye gaze and grammar. By 12 months, dependence on Phase I cues has begun to wane and shift to the social cues in Phase II. From Hollich, Hirsh-Pasek, and Golinkoff (2000). Copyright 2000 by the Society for Research in Child Development. Reprinted with permission from John Wiley & Sons, Inc.

amplitude sucking task, demonstrated that shortly after birth infants can discriminate between sounds in all the world's languages—until approximately 8 months when they become less sensitive to sounds not used in the home language and morph into language specialists (Kuhl et al., 2006).

For bilingual children, the ability to discriminate between sounds in non-native languages lasts for a longer time than for monolingual children—a quality that may be adaptive as children sort out which sounds matter for meaning in their languages (Fennell, Byers-Heinlein, & Werker, 2007). At around 4.5 months, Mandel, Jusczyk, and Pisoni (1995) reported that infants recognize the sound pattern of their own name compared to a name with the same number of syllables and stress pattern (e.g., LAUren vs. HARRy). By 6 months, infants use their own name as a *wedge* into the speech stream, recognizing a new word that appears after their name but not after an unfamiliar name (Bortfeld, Morgan, Golinkoff, & Rathbun, 2005).

Perhaps the most celebrated of the perception studies launched a new and critical field relevant to later intervention. Conducted by Saffran, Aslin and Newport (1996), infants listened to 2 minutes of artificial speech created out of nonsense syllables that were strung together and presented in monotone with no temporal breaks between the syllables. Within the string were embedded three-syllable nonsense "words" (e.g., *pidago*) that always appeared together. Thus, Saffran et al. manipulated the transitional probabilities between syllables such that some syllables were more likely to occur together. With only 2 minutes of exposure to the artificial syllable string, infants showed a preference for syllable pairs that had been part of "words" (e.g., *dago*) over syllables that were not part of "words" (e.g., *lapi*).

This study made clear that infants bring computational abilities to the language-learning task and act as statisticians on the input *before* it has meaning to them. One consequence of this finding is that infants need to hear enough input on which to perform the statistics. Marcus, Vijayan, Rao, and Vishton (1999) found that 7-month-olds not only calculate statistics over particular elements in a sequence, but also abstract algebraic-like patterns in the language data they hear, mimicking how grammar works.

A final note on the perceptual properties of language is that infants tend to pay more attention to *infant-directed* speech rather than to *adult-directed* speech. Characteristically, when adults are speaking to infants rather than to adults, they often modify word order (Narasimhan & Dimroth, 2008), exaggerate semantically meaningful tones (Liu, Tsao, & Kuhl, 2007), speak more slowly, use simpler words with fewer syllables per phrase, use higher than average frequency, and exaggerate intonation contours by stretching vowels (e.g., Fernald & Simon, 1984; Grieser & Kuhl, 1988). This change in register improves word recognition (Singh, 2008), word segmentation (Thiessen, Hill, & Saffran, 2005), and even word learning (Ma, Golinkoff, Houston, & Hirsh-Pasek, 2011).

Detecting Objects and Actions in Events

In the first year, infants are not only statisticians, but physicists. A rich literature reviews their attention to properties of objects as early as 4 months of age (Carey, 2009). Learning about objects and their properties, and being able to categorize them, is critically related to word learning (Gopnik & Meltzoff, 1987). More recently, researchers are also asking about how infants might parse the events that they witness to prepare them for learning action words and relational terms like prepositions and verbs (Song, Golinkoff, & Hirsh-Pasek, 2011). To learn a verb like "march," for example, English-reared infants must differentiate the act of "marching" from, say, "hopping." They must recognize that how the person moves (e.g., marching vs. hopping) is distinct even if they travel along the same *path*. These *manners* of motion are carried out by an agent who serves as the *figure* of the action, and they always occur against a *ground* (e.g., running on the beach vs. the street).

What is interesting is that learning verbs is not only contingent upon dissecting events in ways that will be labeled by language but also in packaging the components together in language-ready ways. For example, "marching" is encoded as a verb in English, "*march into* the class," whereas in Turkish "sınıfa *yürüyerek girdi*—means *go into* the class *marchingly*" surfacing as an adverb—if at all. Spanish patterns in the same way as does Turkish with the path information conflated in the verb and the manner (how the action is performed) in an adverb. Notice that bilingual children and children learning English as a second language (ESL) might have to learn that the packaging of event components required in their two languages is different. This might pose a particular problem in the learning of relational terms versus nouns especially for ESL children.

As a backdrop to asking how children might master relational terms like verbs, some are now investigating when children zoom in on the foundational semantic properties of events like manner and path and how attention to these event components might wane or wax when the processing of events meets up against the native language (Göksun, Hirsh-Pasek, & Golinkoff, 2010). The findings suggest that 7-month-olds can discriminate between different paths (over/under) and manners (e.g., spinning vs. toe touching; Pulverman et al., 2008; Song et al., 2011) and can categorize these properties of events by the beginning of the second year of life (Pruden, Göksun, Roseberry, Hirsh-Pasek, & Golinkoff, 2012; Pruden, Roseberry, Göksun, Hirsh-Pasek, & Golinkoff, in press) whether they are learning English, Spanish, or Mandarin (Pulverman, Chen, Chan, Tardif, & Meng, 2007; Pulverman et al., 2008).

Infants viewing events are also sensitive to properties like containment (English "in") and support relationships (English "on"; Hespos & Spelke, 2007), figures and grounds (Göksun et al., 2010), and the source and goal of the same action (e.g., the bird flew from the tree [source] to the bush [goal]; Lakusta & Carey, 2008). Infants also seem to tell the difference between agents and patients of action in events (Golinkoff, 1975).

What is particularly exciting about these findings is that infants are not only processing language-relevant information in the continuous events that they witness but they seem to start with a set of universal divisions in events. As children learn their native language they "reframe" the event in ways that conform to their native language (Golinkoff & Hirsh-Pasek, 2008; Göksun et al., 2010). In some ways this shift is analogous, though not homologous, to the shift from a universal set of sounds discriminated by all infants that becomes refined and tailored to the native language with language experience (Hespos & Spelke, 2004).

In sum, then, infants in the first year of life already have important analytic tools that allow them to perceive the sounds of speech and the elements in events that will prepare them for language learning. These perceptual beginnings might predict later language competence as the following examples suggest. Speech segmentation ability measured in children younger than 1 year of age is related to language ability and cognitive abilities 3 to 5 years later (Newman, Ratner, Jusczyk, Jusczyk, & Dow, 2006). For monolingual children, detecting phonemes in one's *native* language at 7.5 months is predictive of later language abilities, but the ability to detect phonemes from *other* languages is negatively correlated with language outcome (Kuhl, 2009); bilingual children "stay open" to phoneme variation longer (Fennell et al., 2007).

The study of individual differences in language factors during infancy and how these predict later language learning is a new research focus. Longitudinal studies like Marchman and Fernald's (2008) suggest that the *amount* of language directed to infants and the ability to segment the language stream is predictive of later differences in processing speed and word learning in an IPLP-type task.

Mapping Sounds and Events onto Words and Grammar

As many have noted, the task of mapping words to world is deceptively simple. A child who sees Quine's (1960) proverbial rabbit hopping by while a linguist utters *gavagai* might think the word refers to the whole rabbit, the rabbit's ears, or color of the rabbit's ears, or the rabbit's hopping. How is a child to know? Researchers have proposed a number of answers to this question ranging from those who argue for perceptual salience or attentional cues as the link between word and meaning (Imai & Gentner, 1997; Smith, 2003) to those who hold that infants have certain cognitive constraints that guide them to one interpretation for a word over another (e.g., children assume the word maps to the entire rabbit; Markman, 1994; Hollich, Golinkoff, & Hirsh-Pasek, 2007) to those who suggest that children attend to social cues in the environment that supports word mapping (Adamson & Bakeman, 1991; Tomasello, 1995).

The ECM, however, suggests that rather than endorse one theory to the exclusion of the others, this research can be unified in a developmental model of word learning. Hollich et al. (2000), for example, presented infants with two toys in a live adaptation of the IPLP. The experimenter looked at and trained children on either the name of the interesting toy (coincident condition) or looked at and labeled the boring toy (conflict condition). While hiding behind a barrier that displayed both toys side by side, the experimenter then asked the child: "Where is the modi? Can you find the modi?" At 10 months of age, infants formed associations between the object they preferred (the interesting toy) and the word that they heard— regardless of whether the interesting or the boring toy was labeled by the experimenter (Pruden, Hirsh-Pasek, Golinkoff, & Hennon, 2006). By 12 months of age, infants learned the label in the coincident condition but not in the conflict condition. That is, they started to notice the social cues but could not recruit them in the service of word learning. By 24 months of age, toddlers could override their interest in the perceptually interesting object to map the label onto the boring object designated by the experimenter. They used social cues like eye gaze to interpret the speaker's intent. A reliance on social over perceptual cues in word learning is critical as we do not necessarily label the most interesting objects in our immediate environment.

The role that social cues play in word mapping has been extensively studied. Research on communicative intentions suggests that children figure out the referent of a word by attending to what a person *means to convey* by word or action (e.g., Baldwin & Moses, 2001; Liszkowski, Carpenter, & Tomasello, 2008) and that attention to social cues like eye gaze direction predicts later language outcomes (Brooks & Meltzoff, 2008). Children also learn words best when the adult looks at the object that the child is focused on rather than trying to draw the child to the object he or she finds interesting (Dunham, Dunham & Curwin, 1993; Tomasello, 1995). Tomasello, Carpenter, Call, Behne, and Moll (2005) argue that these moments of joint *attention* are also episodes of joint *intention* where the child tunes into the intentional goals of the speaker. With this window into the other person's mind (what Bloom [2001] called the "principle of relevance"), children move from apprentice word learners to seasoned speakers.

Evidence from both typical and atypical populations suggests that early access to and experience with social cues is crucial to long-term language outcome, and that certain measurable social behaviors in the first year of life are predictive of later language ability (Morales, Mundy, & Rojas, 1998). For example, Morales et al. (1998) found that 6-month-olds' ability to follow a person's gaze to an object (considered an early indicator of joint attentional skills) correlated positively with receptive and expressive vocabulary size at 12, 18, 21, and 24 months. Further studies revealed that infants' responses to various parental and experimenter bids for joint attention (e.g., pointing, looking, touching) are related to later language ability (Morales et al., 2000). In fact, populations that have less access to social cues tend to have poorer language abilities. Parish-Morris, Hennon, Hirsh-Pasek, Golinkoff, and Tager-Flusberg (2007) engaged children diagnosed on the autistic spectrum in a series of tasks designed to measure their access to social intent. Attention to social intent predicted 68% of the variability in their vocabulary outcomes.

Finally, mapping comes not only from attention to perceptual salience and social intent, but also through sensitivity to the grammatical structure of the language. By the second year of life, children use tense agreement and morphology (e.g., a word ending with *-ing* is probably a verb and therefore labeling an action or event; Fisher & Song, 2006). Brown (1957) offers a classic example of the way in which young children employ their knowledge of syntax to determine word meaning. Three- to 5-year-old children were shown a picture of an action, a substance, and an object (e.g., person kneading a confetti-like mass in a bowl) and given a novel word ("sib") in one of three syntactic contexts: as a noun (a "sib"), a verb ("sibbing"), or as a quantifier (*some* "sib"). Depending upon the syntactic context in which children heard the novel word, they interpreted it to mean either the bowl (noun), the process of kneading (verb), or the confetti-like mass (substance/ material). Recently, Song et al. (2010) showed that 3-year-olds (English- and French-reared) used the morphology of a novel adjective or verb to detect the meaning and part of speech of a new word.

The use of these grammatical cues in the service of word learning is referred to as *syntactic bootstrapping* (Gleitman, 1990; Naigles, Gleitman, & Gleitman, 1993). The term refers to when children use their knowledge of abstract linguistic structure (such as the fact that transitive verbs may be causal; Fisher & Snedeker, 2002) to guide their interpretation of novel words. Some argue that given the ephemeral nature of verbs and the fact that verbs are generally harder to learn than nouns (Gentner, 1982; Imai et al., 2008), syntactic bootstrapping might be even more critical for verb learning than for noun learning. Studies suggest that even toddlers as young as 21 months of age can use syntactic cues such as the arrangement and number of a verb's noun arguments to determine something of the meaning of a novel verb (Fisher & Song, 2006; Lee & Naigles, 2008).

In a stunning demonstration of the role grammar can play in verb learning, Gillette, Gleitman, Gleitman, and Lederer (1999) conducted their "human simulation" study. Researchers asked adults to guess the words used by mothers captured on videotape interacting with their 18-to 24-month-old children. With the sound turned off, adults correctly guessed the missing nouns in 45% of the cases; their score for verbs was only 15%, and for mental verbs, 0%. When syntax was systematically added verb identification improved substantially (see Snedeker, Li, & Yuan, 2003, for a replication with Mandarin).

The findings on mapping from word to world have several important lessons for those interested in supporting strong language growth. First, children will notice perceptually interesting objects and actions and will attempt to attach labels to these first. Second, if we are sensitive to what children find interesting and label those objects and actions, children will engage in joint attention and master more vocabulary. Toddlers (Akhtar, Dunham, & Dunham, 1991) who follow our gaze to new objects more effectively become better word learners. Conversations are the grist for learning words and sentence structures. Third and critically, this research suggests that exposing children to full sentences (rather than one word at a time) best promotes word learning. *Vocabulary and grammar acquisition are reciprocal processes.*

Implications for the Classroom and for Intervention

The new findings we have reviewed give us direction on how we can intervene to ensure positive language trajectories for young children. We have seen that language learning can be distilled into three main tasks: (1) finding the units of speech (segmentation) that will become the sounds, words, phrases, and sentences; (2) finding the units in the world (objects, actions, and events) that will be labeled by language; and (3) forming mappings between elements of the world and words. With these basics and the research as the backdrop, we offer six principles of language learning that might guide practice in the home and the classroom.

Principle 1: Children Learn the Words That They Hear Most

As Neuman and Dwyer (2009) suggested, "Talk may be cheap but it is priceless for young developing minds" (p. 384). Support for this principle comes from the Hart and Risley (1995) study, many correlational studies (e.g., Hoff, 2006a; Hoff & Naigles, 2002), and the fact that the amount of language exposure has long-range consequences for later language and reading levels (Clarke et al., 2010; Marchman & Fernald, 2008). Saffran et al.'s (1996) findings begin to shed light on *why* the amount of language input is critical for young learners. Language must be heard in sufficient quantity for the computational brain to do the calculations necessary to derive the units of language.

This relationship between adult input and child output not only appears in home environments but also in studies of child care and early schooling (Hoff, 2006b; NICHD Early Child Care Research Network, 2000, 2002, 2005). Research also finds that children learn not only language that is directed to them, but from overheard speech (Akhtar, 2005). In short, providing environments filled with opportunities to hear and respond to language supports children's growing vocabulary and grammar.

Principle 2: Social Interaction Matters:
Interactive and Responsive Contexts Favor Language Learning

Language input is important, but input alone does not support language competencies. For example, it is not enough to just hear language or words spewing forth from a television. Findings by Kuhl, Tsao, and Liu (2003) and Roseberry, Hirsh-Pasek, Parish-Morris, and Golinkoff (2009) suggest that children under the age of 3 are unlikely to learn language from mere exposure to television (DeLoache et al., 2010). Language learning requires sensitive and responsive conversations with children where language input is *tailored* to the interest and timing of the child's attention. Adults who take turns in interactions with young children, share periods of joint focus, and express positive affect provide children with the scaffolding needed to facilitate language and cognitive growth (e.g., Bronfenbrenner & Morris, 1998; Landry, Smith, Swank, Assel, & Vellet, 2001). This link has been observed in child care homes and relative care as well as in center care (Kontos, Howes, Shinn, & Galinsky, 1997; NICHD Early Child Care Research Network, 1998; Hirsh-Pasek & Burchinal, 2006. A longitudinal study that examined teacher–child conversations when children were 4, controlling for children's language ability at age 3 (i.e., the mean length of their utterances), parental income, education, and home support for literacy (e.g., reading), found that higher-quality conversations and richer vocabulary exposure during free play and group book reading were related to children's language, comprehension, and print skills at the end of kindergarten (Dickinson, 2001b; Tabors, Snow, & Dickinson, 2001) and fourth grade (Dickinson, 2001b; Dickinson & Porche, 2011). Parental sensitivity across time also fostered change in child outcomes (Bornstein & Tamis-LeMonda, 1989; NICHD Early Child Care Research Network & Duncan, 2003). The moral of this story is that language competencies grow when we remain conversational and attuned to children's focus of attention and interests during the course of the infant, toddler, and preschool years.

Why might social interactive settings be critical for language growth? Contingent interaction not only facilitates advanced babbling in infants (Goldstein, King, & West, 2003) but also helps older children come to discern adults' intentions (Baldwin & Moses, 2001). Contingent responsivity is crucial for language growth (Roseberry, 2010), possibly because it engages the child and mirrors the child's responses. Perhaps this explains why children under 3 have trouble learning language from television (Roseberry et al., 2009) but not from video chats (Roseberry, 2010).

Principle 3: Children Learn Words for Things and Events That Interest Them

Bloom (2000) wrote that "Language learning is enhanced when the words a child hears bear upon and are pertinent to the objects of engagement, interest and feelings . . . " (p. 19). In fact, the evidence suggests that younger children readily assume that words map onto objects they find interesting (Hollich et al., 2000). The joint attention literature attests to the fact that parents who talk about what children are looking at have more advanced vocabularies. The corollary is also true: Parents who try to redirect children's attention and label objects not of interest have children who learn fewer words (e.g., Dunham et al., 1993; Hollich et al., 2000).

When children are interested and actively engaged in activities they also learn language from their peers. Dickinson (2001a) noted that the amount of time 3-year-olds spent talking with peers while pretending was positively associated with the size of their vocabularies 2 years later. Bergen and Mauer (2000) found that 4-year-olds' play, in the form of making shopping lists and "reading" storybooks to stuffed animals, predicted both language and reading readiness after the children had entered kindergarten (Nicolopoulou, McDowell, & Brockmeyer, 2006).

Principle 4: Children Learn Words Best in Meaningful Contexts

Sparking interest is often a first step in meaning making. People learn best when information is presented in integrated contexts rather than as a set of isolated facts (Bartlett, 1932; Bruner, 1972). Words connected in a grocery list are better remembered than the same list of words presented without context.

Meaningful connections between words develop in conversations and in studies that use thematic play as a prop for language development. Christie and Roskos (2006), for example, find that children who learn connected vocabulary for the category of building (words like "hammers," "hard hats," "screw drivers," and "tool belts") better remember and use these words than do children who do not learn in this more integrative way.

Meaning comes not only by connecting words with experiences, but also by hearing them used in sentences within narratives. Play can often provide a rich context for those narratives. New research by Han, Moore, Vukelich, and Buell (2010) finds that children who are given an opportunity to use vocabulary in a playful context learn it better than those who learn only under explicit instruction. As Neuman and Dwyer (2009) pointed out, experimental research on comparing vocabulary learning in meaningful versus less meaningful contexts is scant. Yet, correlational studies in language, play, and memory research converge to suggest that teaching vocabulary in integrated and real-world contexts enriches and deepens children's background knowledge and hence their mental lexicons (Hirsh-Pasek, Golinkoff, Berk, & Singer, 2009).

Principle 5: Vocabulary Learning and Grammatical Development Are Reciprocal Processes

The amount and diversity of verbal stimulation fosters earlier and richer language outcomes in terms of both vocabulary and grammar (Hart & Risley, 1995, 1999; Tamis-LeMonda, Bornstein, & Baumwell, 2001). Vocabulary and grammar are not divorced; they feed one another. Dixon and Marchman (2007), for example, argue from a large sample of children ages 16 to 30 months ($N = 1461$) that words and grammar are "developing in synchrony across the first few years of life" (p. 209). This relationship between grammar and vocabulary learning is also found in research with bilingual children. Conboy and Thal (2006) find, for example, that toddlers'

English vocabulary predicted their English grammar and the reverse, and their Spanish vocabulary predicted their Spanish grammar.

Why might language environments that offer more sophisticated language support learning? First, syntactic bootstrapping, which assists children in narrowing word meaning, can only be useful if children hear many sentences. Upon hearing "John is blicking Mary," for example, the child may assume that John did something to Mary—an assumption not licensed by the sentence "John and Mary are blicking." Second, observing the diverse linguistic contexts in which words are used helps children detect nuances in word meaning (Gillette et al., 1999; Naigles, 1990). Finally, it is worth noting that oral language measured as *both* vocabulary and grammar (NICHD Early Child Care Research Network, 2005) is crucial for early literacy (Clarke et al., 2010).

Principle 6: Keep It Positive

One of Hart and Risley's (1995) startling findings was that lower-income children are more likely to hear prohibitions (e.g., "Don't touch that!") than to hear what they called "affirmations" (e.g., "That's an interesting toy"). Prohibitions are not only more negative in tone, but they serve as conversation closers. In a lovely illustration, Chase-Lansdale and Takanishi (2009) opened a recent report entitled *How Do Families Matter?* with a vignette they called "Three Mothers and an Eggplant."

> The first mother wheels her shopping cart down the produce aisle, where her kindergartner spots an eggplant and asks what it is. The mother shushes her child, ignoring the question. A second mother, faced with the same question, responds curtly, "Oh, that's an eggplant, but we don't eat it." The third mother coos, "Oh, that's an eggplant. It's one of the few purple vegetables." She picks it up, hands it to her son, and encourages him to put it on the scale. "Oh, look, it's about two pounds!" she says. "And it's $1.99 a pound, so that would cost just about $4. That's a bit pricey, but you like veal parmesan, and eggplant parmesan is delicious too. You'll love it. Let's buy one, take it home, cut it open. We'll make a dish together."

Rather than closing off the conversation, the third mother affirms the child's interest, speaks in full sentences, and continues the conversation in a way that builds vocabulary and grammar. When we expand on our children's language and ask questions rather than simply giving directives, we talk more and we create a climate that spurs language growth. Continuing the conversation increases the amount of talk, uses language in a social context, builds on children's interest, makes language meaningful, and generates more complex language samples.

Taken collectively, the six research-derived principles of language development offer a way to alter the trajectory of a child's language development. The principles dictate a kind of pedagogical approach that yields optimal language growth regardless of language or culture. Teachers and parents can confidently give children a rich language base by applying the principles in areas that are of interest to them and their children. The trick is to start the conversation and keep it going. As David K. Dickinson said (personal communication, 2010), "Strive for five," meaning five back-and-forth turns with the child. When conversations are only one-side prohibitions or one-word answers, children are not hearing the language they need to fuel their language-learning engine. Nor are they being sufficiently exposed to the concepts language encodes.

Final Thoughts

Language is a core mental ability that serves as the foundation for communication, academic learning, and social navigation. Children growing up in poverty are at a significant disadvantage for developing these language competencies (e.g., Hart & Risley, 1995). Given the centrality of language and communication for school readiness and academic success, this research has sent ripples to the highest levels of government. In the last 15 years, researchers have not only replicated these findings, but also expanded them, suggesting that the lack of positive language input might have lasting effects on children's mental processing speed (e.g., Marchman & Fernald, 2008), their later reading abilities (e.g., Clarke et al., 2010), and possibly in brain functioning (e.g., Hackman & Farah, 2009).

Research in the last decade, however, also offers an antidote. Language learning is malleable and we can change young children's trajectories. We now know enough about the course of language learning to make the leap from the pages of scientific journals into application. Using a smorgasbord of the latest research, we offered six principles that distill the science into a road map for practitioners who work with young children and their families. If we are to narrow the achievement gap between rich and poor, it is imperative that we build strong language competencies in all children and that we put our science to work.

ACKNOWLEDGMENTS

This research was funded by joint grants to the authors from the National Science Foundation, Grant No. SBR9615391, and from the National Institutes of Health, Grant No. RO1HD050199. Thanks to Russell Richie for his help in preparing the chapter.

REFERENCES

Adamson, L., & Bakeman, R. (1991). The development of shared attention during infancy. In R. Vasta (Ed.), *Annals of child development* (Vol. 8, pp. 1–41). London: Kingsley.

Akhtar, N. (2005). The robustness of learning through overhearing. *Developmental Science, 8,* 199–209.

Akhtar, N., Dunham, F., & Dunham, P. (1991). Directive interactions and early vocabulary development: The role of joint attentional focus. *Journal of Child Language, 18,* 41–49.

Baldwin, D. A., & Moses, L. J. (2001). Links between social understanding and early word learning: Challenges to current accounts. *Social Development, 10,* 309–329.

Bartlett, F. (1932). *Remembering: A study in experimental and social psychology.* New York: Cambridge University Press.

Bergen, D., & Mauer, D. (2000). Symbolic play, phonological awareness, and literacy skills at three age levels. In K. Roskos & J. F. Christie (Eds.), *Play and literacy in early childhood: Research from multiple perspectives* (pp. 45–62). Mahwah, NJ: Erlbaum.

Bloom, L. (1993). *The transition from infancy to language: Acquiring the power of expression.* New York: Cambridge University Press.

Bloom, L. (2000). The intentionality model of word learning: How to learn a word, any word. In R. Golinkoff, K. Hirsh-Pasek, L. Bloom, L. Smith, A. Woodward, N. Akhtar, et al. (2000), *Becoming a word learner: A debate on lexical acquisition* (pp. 19–50). New York: Oxford University Press.

Bloom, L. (2001). Language acquisition and the child: Developmental and theoretical tensions [Keynote address]. In A. Do, L. Domínguez, & A. Johansen (Eds.), *BUCLD 25: Proceedings of the 25th Annual Boston University Conference on Language Development* (pp. 16–33). Medford, MA: Cascadilla Press.

Bornstein, M. (1985). Habituation of attention as a measure of visual information processing in human infants: Summary, systematization, and synthesis. In G. Gottlieb & N. Krasnegor (Eds.), *Measurement of audition and vision in the first year of postnatal life: A methodological overview* (pp. 253–300). Westport, CT: Ablex.

Bornstein, M. H., & Tamis-LeMonda, C. S. (1989). Maternal responsiveness and cognitive development in children. *New Directions for Child Development, 43,* 49–61.

Bortfeld, H., Morgan, J., Golinkoff, R., & Rathbun, K. (2005). Mommy and me: Familiar names help launch babies into speech stream segmentation. *Psychological Science, 16,* 298–304.

Bronfenbrenner, U., & Morris, P. A. (1998). The ecology of developmental processes. In W. Damon & R. M. Lerner (Eds.), *Handbook of child psychology: Vol. 1. Theoretical models of human development* (5th ed., pp. 993–1028). Hoboken, NJ: Wiley.

Brooks, R., & Meltzoff, A. (2008). Infant gaze following and pointing predict accelerated vocabulary growth through two years of age: A longitudinal, growth curve modeling study. *Journal of Child Language, 35,* 207–220.

Brown, R. (1957). Linguistic determinism and the part of speech. *Journal of Abnormal and Social Psychology, 55*(1), 1–5.

Bruner, J. (1972). Nature and uses of immaturity. *American Psychologist, 27,* 687–708.

Carey, S. (2009). *The origin of concepts.* New York: Oxford University Press.

Chase-Lansdale, P. L., & Takanishi, E. (2009). *How do families matter? Understanding how families strengthen their children's educational achievement.* New York: Foundation for Child Development.

Christie, J., & Roskos, K. (2006). Standards, science, and the role of play in early literacy education. In D. Singer, R. M. Golinkoff, & K. Hirsh-Pasek (Eds.), *Play = learning: How play motivates and enhances children's cognitive and social–emotional growth* (pp. 57–73). New York: Oxford University Press.

Clarke, P., Snowling, M. J., Truelove, E., & Hulme, C. (2010). Ameliorating children's reading-comprehension difficulties: A randomized controlled trial. *Psychological Science, 21,* 1106–1116.

Conboy, B. T., & Thal, D. J. (2006). Ties between the lexicon and grammar: Cross-sectional and longitudinal studies of bilingual toddlers. *Child Development, 77,* 712–735.

Cristofaro, T., & Tamis-LeMonda, C. S. (2012). Mother–child conversations at 36 months and at pre-kindergarten: Relations to children's school readiness. *Journal of Early Childhood Literacy, 12,* 68–97.

Darwin, C. (1877). A bibliographical sketch of an infant. *Mind, 2,* 285–294.

DeCasper, A., & Spence, M. (1986). Prenatal maternal speech influences newborns' perception of speech sounds. *Infant Behavior and Development, 9,* 133–150.

DeLoache, J. S., Chiong, C., Sherman, K., Islam, N., Vanderborght, M., Troseth, G. L., et al. (2010). Do babies learn from baby media? *Psychological Science, 21,* 1570–1574.

Dickinson, D. K. (2001a). Large-group and free-play times: Conversational settings supporting language and literacy development. In D. K. Dickinson & P. O. Tabors (Eds.), *Beginning literacy with language: Young children learning at home and school* (pp. 223–255). Baltimore: Brookes.

Dickinson, D. K. (2001b). Putting the pieces together: The impact of preschool on children's language and literacy development in kindergarten. In D. K. Dickinson & P. O. Tabors (Eds.), *Beginning literacy with language: Young children learning at home and school* (pp. 257–287). Baltimore: Brookes.

Dickinson, D., Golinkoff, R., & Hirsh-Pasek, K. (2010). Speaking out for language: Why language is central to reading development. *Educational Researcher, 39,* 305–310.

Dickinson, D. K., & Porche, M. (2011). Relation between language experiences in preschool classroom and children's kindergarten and fourth-grade language reading abilities. *Child Development, 82,* 870–886.

Dickinson, D. K., & Tabors, P. O. (Eds.). (2001). *Beginning literacy with language: Young children learning at home and school.* Baltimore: Brookes.

Dixon, J. A., & Marchman, V. A. (2007). Grammar and the lexicon: Developmental ordering in language acquisition. *Child Development, 78,* 190–212.

Dunham, P., Dunham, F., & Curwin, A. (1993). Joint-attentional states and lexical acquisition at 18 months. *Developmental Psychology, 29,* 827–831.

Eimas, P. D., Siqueland, E. R., Jusczyk, P. W., & Vigorito, J. (1971). Speech perception in infants. *Science, 171,* 303–306.

Fennell, C., Byers-Heinlein, K., & Werker, J. (2007). Using speech sounds to guide word learning: The case of bilingual infants. *Child Development, 78,* 1510–1525.

Fernald, A. (1985). Four-month-old infants prefer to listen to motherese. *Infant Behavior and Development, 8*(2), 181–195.

Fernald, A., Perfors, A., & Marchman, V. A. (2006). Picking up speed in understanding: Speech processing efficiency and vocabulary growth across the second year. *Developmental Psychology, 42,* 98–116.

Fernald, A., & Simon, T. (1984). Expanded intonation contours in mothers' speech to newborns. *Developmental Psychology, 20,* 104–113.

Fisher, C., & Snedeker, J. (2002, November). *Counting the nouns: Simple sentence-structure cues guide verb learning in 21-month-olds.* Paper presented at the 27th Boston University Conference on Language Development, Boston, MA.

Fisher, C., & Song, H. (2006). Who's the subject? Sentence structures as analogs of verb meaning. In K. Hirsh-Pasek & R. M. Golinkoff (Eds.), *Action meets word: How children learn the meanings of verbs* (pp. 392–425). New York: Oxford University Press.

Gentner, D. (1982). Why nouns are learned before verbs: Linguistic relativity versus natural partitioning. In S. A. Kuczaj (Ed.), *Language development: Vol. 2. Language, thought, and culture* (pp. 301–334). Hillsdale, NJ: Erlbaum.

Gillette, J., Gleitman, H., Gleitman, L., & Lederer, A. (1999). Human simulations of vocabulary learning. *Cognition, 73,* 135–176.

Gleitman, L. (1990). The structural sources of verb meanings. *Language Acquisition: A Journal of Developmental Linguistics, 1,* 3–55.

Göksun, T., Hirsh-Pasek, K., & Golinkoff, R. (2010). Trading spaces: Carving up events for learning language. *Perspectives on Psychological Science, 5,* 33–42.

Goldstein, M. H., King, A. P., & West, M. J. (2003). Social interaction shapes babbling: Testing parallels between birdsong and speech. *Proceedings of the National Academy of Sciences, 100,* 8030–8035.

Golinkoff, R. (1975). Semantic development in infants: The concepts of agent and recipient. *Merrill-Palmer Quarterly: Journal of Developmental Psychology, 21,* 181–193.

Golinkoff, R. M., & Hirsh-Pasek, K. (2008). How toddlers begin to learn verbs. *Trends in Cognitive Science, 12,* 397–403.

Golinkoff, R. M., & Hirsh-Pasek, K. (2012). Methods for studying language in infants: Back to the future. In E. Hoff (Ed.), *Guide to research methods in child language* (pp. 60–77). New York: Wiley-Blackwell.

Golinkoff, R. M., Hirsh-Pasek, K., Cauley, K. M., & Gordon, L. (1987). The eyes have it: Lexical and syntactic comprehension in a new paradigm. *Journal of Child Language, 14,* 23–45.

Gopnik, A., & Meltzoff, A. N. (1987). The development of categorization in the second year and its relation to other cognitive and linguistic developments. *Child Development, 58,* 1523–1531.

Grieser, D. L., & Kuhl, P. K. (1988). Maternal speech to infants in a tonal language:

Support for universal prosodic features in motherese. *Developmental Psychology, 24,* 14–20.

Hackman, D., & Farah, M. (2009). Socioeconomic status and the developing brain. *Trends in Cognitive Sciences, 13,* 65–73.

Halle, T., Forry, N., Hair, E., Perper, K., Wandner, L., Wessel, J., et al. (2009). *Disparities in early learning and development: Lessons from the Early Childhood Longitudinal Study–Birth Cohort (ECLS-B).* Washington, DC: Child Trends.

Han, M., Moore, N., Vukelich, C., & Buell, M. (2010). Does play make a difference?: Effects of play intervention on at-risk preschoolers' vocabulary learning. *American Journal of Play, 3,* 82–105.

Hart, B., & Risley, T. (1995). *Meaningful differences in the everyday lives of American children.* Baltimore: Brookes.

Hart, B., & Risley, T. R. (1999). *The social world of children learning to talk.* Baltimore: Brookes.

Hespos, S. J., & Spelke, E. S. (2004). Conceptual precursors to language. *Nature, 430,* 453–456.

Hespos, S., & Spelke, E. (2007). Precursors to spatial language: The case of containment. In A. Michel, M. Hickmann, & L. Vieu (Eds.), *The categorization of spatial entities in language and cognition* (pp. 233–245). Amsterdam, Netherlands: Benjamins.

Hirsh-Pasek, K., & Burchinal, M. (2006). Putting language learning in context: How change at home and in school affects language growth across time. *Merrill Palmer Quarterly, 52,* 449–485.

Hirsh-Pasek, K., & Golinkoff, R. M. (1996). *The origins of grammar: Evidence from early language comprehension.* Cambridge, MA: MIT Press.

Hirsh-Pasek, K., Golinkoff, R. M., Berk, L. E., & Singer, D. G. (2009). *A mandate for playful learning in preschool: Presenting the evidence.* New York: Oxford University Press.

Hirsh-Pasek, K., Kemler Nelson, D., Jusczyk, P., Cassidy, K., Druss, B., & Kennedy, L. (1987). Clauses are perceptual units for young infants. *Cognition, 26,* 269–286.

Hoff, E. (2006a). Environmental supports for language acquisition. In D. K. Dickinson & S. B. Neuman (Eds.), *Handbook of early literacy research* (Vol. 2, pp. 163–172). New York: Guilford Press.

Hoff, E. (2006b). How social contexts support and shape language development. *Developmental Review, 26,* 55–88.

Hoff, E., & Naigles, L. (2002). How children use input to acquire a lexicon. *Child Development, 73,* 418–433.

Hollich, G., Golinkoff, R. M., & Hirsh-Pasek, K. (2007). Young children associate novel words with complex objects rather than salient parts. *Developmental Psychology, 43,* 1051–1061.

Hollich, G., Hirsh-Pasek, K., & Golinkoff, R. (2000). Breaking the language barrier: An emergentist coalition model for the origins of word learning. *Monographs of the Society for Research in Child Development, 65*(3, Serial No. 262).

Imai, M., & Gentner, D. (1997). A cross-linguistic study of early word meaning: Universal ontology and linguistic influence. *Cognition, 62,* 169–200.

Imai, M., Li, L., Haryu, E., Okada, H., Hirsh-Pasek, K., Golinkoff, R. M., et al. (2008). Novel noun and verb learning in Chinese-, English-, and Japanese-speaking children. *Child Development, 79,* 979–1000.

Kontos, S., Howes, C., Shinn, M., & Galinsky, E. (1997). Children's experiences in family child care and relative care as a function of family income and ethnicity. *Merrill-Palmer Quarterly, 43,* 386–403.

Kuhl, P. K. (2009). Linking infant speech perception to language acquisition: Phonetic learning predicts language growth. In P. McCardle, J. Colombo, & L. Freund (Eds.), *Infant pathways to language: Methods, models, and research directions* (pp. 213–243). Mahwah, NJ: Erlbaum.

Kuhl, P. K., & Rivera-Gaxiola, M. (2008). Neural substrates of early language acquisition. *Annual Review of Neuroscience, 31,* 511–534.

Kuhl, P. K., Stevens, E., Hayashi, A., Deguchi, T., Kiritani, S., & Iverson, P. (2006). Infants show facilitation for native language phonetic perception between 6 and 12 months. *Developmental Science, 9,* 13–21.

Kuhl, P. K., Tsao, F.-M., & Liu, H.-M. (2003). Foreign-language experience in infancy: Effects of short-term exposure and social interaction on phonetic learning. *Proceedings of the National Academy of Sciences, 100,* 9096–9101.

Lakusta, L., & Carey, S. (2008, March). Infants' categorization of sources and goals in motion events. In S. Pruden & T. Göksun (Chairs), *Conceptual primitives for processing events and learning relational terms.* Symposium at the 16th International Conference on Infant Studies, Vancouver, Canada.

Landry, S. H., Smith, K. E., & Swank, P. R. (2006). Responsive parenting: Establishing early foundations for social, communication, and independent problem-solving skills. *Developmental Psychology, 42,* 627–642.

Landry, S. H., Smith, K. E., Swank, P. R., Assel, M. A., & Vellet, S. (2001). Does early responsive parenting have a special importance for children's development or is consistency across early childhood necessary? *Developmental Psychology, 37,* 387–403.

Lee, J., & Naigles, L. (2008). Mandarin learners use syntactic bootstrapping in verb acquisition. *Cognition, 106,* 1028–1037.

Liszkowski, U., Carpenter, M., & Tomasello, M. (2008). Twelve-month-olds communicate helpfully and appropriately for knowledgeable and ignorant partners. *Cognition, 108,* 732–739.

Liu, H.-M., Tsao, F.-M., & Kuhl, P. K. (2007). Acoustic analysis of lexical tone in Mandarin infant-directed speech. *Developmental Psychology, 43,* 912–917.

Ma, W., Golinkoff, R. M., Houston, D., & Hirsh-Pasek, K. (2011). Word learning in infant- and adult-directed speech. *Language Learning and Language Development, 7,* 209–225.

Mandel, D. R., Jusczyk, P. W., & Pisoni, D. B. (1995). Infants' recognition of the sound patterns of their own names. *Psychological Science, 6,* 314–317.

Marchman, V. A., & Fernald, A. (2008). Speed of word recognition and vocabulary knowledge in infancy predict cognitive and language outcomes in later childhood. *Developmental Science, 11,* F9–F16.

Marcus, G. F., Vijayan, S., Rao, S. B., & Vishton, P. M. (1999). Rule learning by seven-month-old infants. *Science, 283*(5398), 77–80.

Markman, E. (1994). Constraints on word meaning in early language acquisition. *Lingua, 92*, 199–227.

Morales, M., Mundy, P., Delgado, C., Yale, M., Messinger, D., Neal, R., et al. (2000). Responding to joint attention across the 6- to 24-month age period and early language acquisition. *Journal of Applied Developmental Psychology, 21*, 283–298.

Morales, M., Mundy, P., & Rojas, J. (1998). Following the direction of gaze and language development in 6-month-olds. *Infant Behavior and Development, 21*, 373–377.

Munson, B., Kurtz, B., & Windsor, J. (2005). The influence of vocabulary size, phonotactic probability, and wordlikeness on nonword repetitions of children with and without specific language impairment. *Journal of Speech, Language, and Hearing Research, 48*(5), 1033–1047.

Naigles, L. (1990). Children use syntax to learn verb meanings. *Journal of Child Language, 17*, 357–374.

Naigles, L., Gleitman, L. R., & Gleitman, H. (1993). Children acquire word meaning components from syntactic evidence. In E. Dromi (Ed.), *Language and cognition: A developmental perspective* (pp. 104–140). Norwood, NJ: Ablex.

Narasimhan, B., & Dimroth, C. (2008). Word order and information status in child language. *Cognition, 107*, 317–329.

National Early Literacy Panel. (2008). *Developing early literacy: Report of the National Early Literacy Panel.* Jessup, MD: National Institute for Literacy.

Nelson, K. (1996). *Language in cognitive development.* New York: Cambridge University Press.

Neuman, S. B., & Dwyer, J. (2009). Missing in action: Vocabulary instruction in Pre-K. *The Reading Teacher, 62*, 384–392.

Newman, R. S., Ratner, N. B., Jusczyk, A. M., Jusczyk, P. W., & Dow, K. A. (2006). Infants' early ability to segment the conversational speech signal predicts later language development: A retrospective analysis. *Developmental Psychology, 42*, 643–655.

NICHD Early Child Care Research Network. (1998). Early child care and self-control, compliance, and problem behavior at 24 and 36 months. *Child Development, 69*, 1145–1170.

NICHD Early Child Care Research Network. (2000). The relation of child care to cognitive and language development. *Child Development, 71*, 960–980.

NICHD Early Child Care Research Network. (2002). Early child care and children's development prior to school entry: Results from the NICHD Study of Early Child Care. *American Educational Research Journal, 39*, 133–164.

NICHD Early Child Care Research Network. (2005). Pathways to reading: The role of oral language in the transition to reading. *Developmental Psychology, 41*, 428–442.

NICHD Early Child Care Research Network, & Duncan, G. (2003). Modeling the impacts of child care quality on children's preschool cognitive development. *Child Development, 74*, 1454–1475.

Nicolopoulou, A., McDowell, J., & Brockmeyer, C. (2006). Narrative play and emergent literacy: Storytelling and story-acting meet journal writing. In D. G. Singer, R. M. Golinkoff, & K. Hirsh-Pasek (Eds.), *Play = learning: How play motivates and enhances children's cognitive and social-emotional growth* (pp. 124–144). New York: Oxford University Press.

Parish-Morris, J., Hennon, E., Hirsh-Pasek, K., Golinkoff, R., & Tager-Flusberg, H. (2007). Children with autism illuminate the role of social intention in word learning. *Child Development, 78,* 1265–1287.

Pruden, S. M., Goksün, T., Roseberry, S., Hirsh-Pasek, K., & Golinkoff, R. M. (2012). Find your manners: How do infants detect the invariant manner of motion in dynamic events? *Child Development, 83,* 977–991.

Pruden, S., Hirsh-Pasek, K., Golinkoff, R., & Hennon, E. (2006). The birth of words: Ten-month-olds learn words through perceptual salience. *Child Development, 77,* 266–280.

Pruden, S. M., Roseberry, S., Goksün, T., Hirsh-Pasek, K., & Golinkoff, R. M. (in press). Infant categorization of path relations during dynamic events. *Child Development.*

Pulverman, R., Chen, J., Chan, C., Tardif, T., & Meng, X. (2007, March). *Cross-cultural comparisons of attention to manner and path: Insights from Chinese infants.* Poster presented at the meeting of the Society for Research on Child Development, Boston, MA.

Pulverman, R., Golinkoff, R., Hirsh-Pasek, K., & Buresh, J. (2008). Infants discriminate manners and paths in non-linguistic dynamic events. *Cognition, 108,* 825–830.

Quine, W. V. O. (1960). *Word and object: An inquiry into the linguistic mechanisms of objective reference.* Oxford, UK: Wiley.

Roseberry, S. (2010). *Blicking through video chats: The role of contingency in toddlers' ability to learn novel verbs.* Unpublished doctoral dissertation, Temple University, Pennsylvania.

Roseberry, S., Hirsh-Pasek, K., Parish-Morris, J., & Golinkoff, R. M. (2009). Live action: Can young children learn verbs from video? *Child Development, 80,* 1360–1375.

Saffran, J., Aslin, R., & Newport, E. (1996). Statistical learning by 8-month-old infants. *Science, 274,* 1926–1928.

Singh, L. (2008). Influences of high and low variability on infant word recognition. *Cognition, 106,* 833–870.

Smith, L. (2003). Learning to recognize objects. *Psychological Science, 14,* 244–250.

Snedeker, J., Li, P., & Yuan, S. (2003). Cross-cultural differences in the input to early word learning. *Proceedings of the Twenty-Fifth Annual Conference of the Cognitive Science Society.* Mahwah, NJ: Erlbaum.

Song, L., Golinkoff, R. M., & Hirsh-Pasek, K. (2011). *Infants' categorization of intransitive human actions.* Manuscript submitted for publication.

Song, L., Nazzi, T., Moukawane, S., Golinkoff, R. M., Stahl, A., Ma, W., et al. (2010). Sleepy vs. sleeping: Preschoolers' sensitivity to morphological cues for adjectives and verbs in English and French. In K. Franich, K. M. Iserman, & L. L. Keil (Eds.), *Proceedings of the 34th Annual Boston University Conference on Language Development* (Vol. 2, pp. 409–420). Somerville, MA: Cascadilla Press.

Sternberg, R. J. (1984) Introduction. In R. J. Sternberg (Ed.), *Mechanisms of cognitive development.* New York: Freeman.

Dr. Seuss. (1957). *The cat in the hat*. New York: Random House Books for Young Readers.

Tabors, P. O., Snow, C. E., & Dickinson, D. K. (2001). Homes and schools together: Supporting language and literacy development. In D. K. Dickinson & P. O. Tabors (Eds.), *Beginning literacy with language: Young children learning at home and school* (pp. 313–334). Baltimore: Brookes.

Tamis-LeMonda, C. S., Bornstein, M. H., & Baumwell, L. (2001). Maternal responsiveness and children's achievement of language milestones. *Child Development, 72*(3), 748–767.

Thelen, E., & Smith, L. (1994). *A dynamic systems approach to the development of cognition and action*. Cambridge, MA: MIT Press.

Thiessen, E., Hill, E., & Saffran, J. (2005). Infant-directed speech facilitates word segmentation. *Infancy, 7,* 53–71.

Tomasello, M. (1995). Pragmatic contexts for early verb learning. In M. Tomasello & W. E. Merriman (Eds.), *Beyond the names for things: Young children's acquisition of verbs* (pp. 115–146). Hillsdale, NJ: Erlbaum.

Tomasello, M., Carpenter, M., Call, J., Behne, T., & Moll, H. (2005). Understanding and sharing intentions: The origins of cultural cognition. *Behavioral and Brain Sciences, 28,* 675–735.

Vouloumanos, A., & Werker, J. F. (2007). Listening to language at birth: Evidence for a bias for speech in neonates. *Developmental Science, 10,* 159–164.

Werker, J., Cohen, L., Lloyd, V., Casasola, M., & Stager, C. (1998). Acquisition of word–object associations by 14-month-old infants. *Developmental Psychology, 34,* 1289–1309.

Woodward, A., & Markman, E. (1998). Early word learning. In W. Damon, D. Kuhn, & R. Siegler (Eds.), *Handbook of child psychology: Volume 2. Cognition, perception, and language* (pp. 371–420). Hoboken, NJ: Wiley.

CHAPTER 5

Bilingual Language Learners

Erika Hoff and Silvia Place

Who Are Bilingual Language Learners?

Throughout the world children grow up exposed to two or more languages as a result of multiple factors including immigration, official or unofficial community bilingualism, and exogamous marriage between speakers of different languages. Although exact figures are hard to come by, it has been estimated that half the world's children live in bilingual environments (Grosjean, 1982, 2010). A particular subset of these bilingual language learners is of concern to U.S. policymakers. In the United States, one-fourth of children under the age of 5 years live in households in which a language other than English is spoken (U.S. Census Bureau, 2006), and their numbers are projected to grow in the coming decades (Garcia & Jensen, 2009). These children are of concern because, on average, they fall below norms for monolingual children on measures of English skills when they begin school (Oller & Eilers, 2002), and they underachieve throughout their school years (Garcia, McCardle, & Nixon, 2007).

In the United States, children who are bilingual language learners are, for the most part, children who have one or two immigrant parents. This fact is sometimes surprising to members of the English-speaking majority in the United States to whom the large and continued presence of linguistic minorities in many communities projects the appearance of a linguistically isolated group that speaks the heritage language and passes it on to succeeding generations. To the contrary, however, heritage language maintenance in the United States has been described as following the "three-generation rule." The first generation of immigrants maintains the heritage language—and may learn little English, their children born in the United States become bilingual, and the third generation is typically monolingual in English. Where minority language use persists in the United States, it is supported by continuing immigration (see Eilers, Pearson, & Cobo-Lewis, 2006).

These children of immigrant parents who constitute the population of bilingual language learners in the United States are disproportionately poor. The poverty rate for children in immigrant families is 21%, compared to 14% in native-born families (Haskins, Greenberg, & Fremstad, 2004). Thus, while poverty is not an inherent property of bilingual populations, it is statistically the case that many bilingual language learners in the United States suffer some degree of economic hardship and, conversely, that dual language exposure is a frequent characteristic of children from families that are poor.

Many of these children who are poor and come from homes in which a language other than English is spoken reach school age with low levels of skill in English. In the United States, poor English skills at school entry are not easy to overcome. For example, among fourth-grade children in Florida, 92% of those categorized as English language learners (ELLs) fall below the grade-level standards for reading and language arts (Lesaux, Koda, Siegel, & Shanahan, 2006). Some of the children in the ELL category have low levels of skill in English because they are recent immigrants themselves. However, some are U.S.-born children of immigrants (Shatz & Wilkinson, 2010).

In order to support the development of English language skills among children in poverty who are bilingual language learners, it is necessary to understand what is causing those skills to be low. Low English skill levels are not surprising in children who hear very little English at home, but the reason for low English skills among children who do hear English, in addition to another language, is not clear. Many scholars have claimed that the human language acquisition capacity can handle two languages as easily as one and that bilingual children acquire both their languages on the same timetable as monolingual children acquire one (Kovács & Mehler, 2009; Petitto & Kovelman, 2003; Petitto et al., 2001). It could be that what appear to be effects of dual language exposure among children of immigrants are actually effects of the low income and low parental education levels that are confounded with dual language exposure. Socioeconomic status (SES) has a well-established relation to language development (Hart & Risley, 1995; Hoff, 2003, 2006). Or, it could be that even in the immigrant families where the children do hear English, something about the amount or nature of their English language exposure results in low levels of language skill. There is little research addressing these questions, despite the fact that low academic achievement among children of immigrant households is a problem in many places in the world (see Scheele, Leseman, & Mayo, 2010).

The present chapter presents evidence addressing two basic questions about young bilingual language learners in the United States:

1. What are their early language development trajectories?
2. What are the factors that create variability among bilingual language learners in those trajectories?

The answer to the first question should provide policymakers, program designers, and classroom teachers with guidance as to what to expect in the bilingual language learners they are trying to serve. The answer to the second question will inform expectations, and, in addition, will suggest what features of supportive environments might be included in program design.

This chapter focuses on the findings of a recent research program studying children from Spanish–English bilingual homes in South Florida. We focus on children who have been exposed to both languages from birth, in order to investigate the normal course of bilingual development. Thus, the children we study are not like many of the bilingual language learners in school whose first sustained exposure to English comes with school entry. The bilingual language learners we study are also not typical of the bilingual population in that they come from high-SES homes. The Spanish–English bilingual population in South Florida is unlike most bilingual populations in the United States. The Spanish speakers are immigrants primarily from South America and the Caribbean. Many are highly educated, with middle-class occupations and incomes and, relatedly, they have some degree of proficiency in English. Their children are exposed to Spanish at home because the parents have chosen to do so. This population thus provides a natural experiment in which language development under conditions of dual language exposure can be compared to language development under conditions of monolingual exposure, unconfounded by the SES of the families. The results of studying this population should help to untangle the effects of dual language exposure from the effects of SES on language development in the population of low-SES, bilingual children whose poor academic outcomes are a public policy concern.

Current Views of How Language Development Is Affected by Bilingualism

Two contradictory views of what normative bilingual development should look like can be found in academic, educational, and lay circles. The dominant view in academic circles until the 1960s was that children who hear and acquire two languages from an early age may be confused by their language experience and may experience delays in cognitive and linguistic development as a result (Genesee & Nicoladis, 2007; Hakuta, 1986). That view still circulates in advice to parents from well-intentioned educators and pediatricians (as described in Baker, 2007; King & Fogle, 2006; Pearson, 2008). It is a source of concern and distress to many immigrant parents who would like their children to learn their heritage language but worry about whether they are doing the right thing in speaking a language other than English to their child.

In many academic circles that older view has been supplanted by the view from the discipline of generative linguistics, which was first articulated and made famous by Noam Chomsky beginning in the 1960s (Chomsky, 1965, 1991). The newer view is that children are biologically prepared to acquire language, that language development is paced by a genetic blueprint, and that the process of language acquisition is only minimally dependent on language exposure. While their capacity lasts, children can acquire two languages as easily as one (Gleitman & Newport, 1995). This view can also cause concern and distress to parents because they observe (and our findings confirm) that their bilingually developing children are not acquiring English as rapidly as the children of their monolingual neighbors—and then they worry that there is something wrong with their children.

The scientific literature dispels the view that children are confused by dual language input. To the contrary, children exposed to two languages can distinguish those languages from infancy, and they can learn two phonological systems, two vocabularies, and two grammars (Kovács & Mehler, 2009; Petitto & Kovelman, 2003; Petitto et al., 2001; Werker & Byers-Heinlein, 2008). On the other hand, the literature does not unequivocally support the claim that children exposed to two languages typically acquire them at the same rate as monolingual children learn one. The evidence cited in support of this claim, when it is made, consists of two sorts of findings: (1) that bilingually developing children reach major milestones of language development on a timetable that is within the normal range of variation for monolingual children (Petitto et al., 2001), and (2) findings of no statistically significant difference between very small samples of monolingual and bilingual children (Pearson, Fernández, & Oller, 1993).

The normal range of variation in the timing of language development, and accordingly, in the language skills that are displayed by children at the same age, is large. The finding that bilingually developing children proceed at a pace in each language that is within the normal range is not the same as finding no difference (Bialystok & Feng, 2011). Recent, larger-scale studies have found that young bilingual children score below monolingual norms on a standardized instrument in both vocabulary and grammar (Marchman, Fernald, & Hurtado, 2010; Vagh, Pan, & Mancilla-Martinez, 2009), but it is perilous to draw conclusions from much of this research because the bilingual samples tend to be lower SES than the reference groups on which the norms are based. Here we present data from our study of bilingually developing children that suggest a third possibility: that children can simultaneously acquire two languages without confusion or impediment to the process of learning, but that learning two languages takes longer than learning one.

Effects of Dual Language Exposure on Language Development

Method

We describe trajectories of bilingual development based on longitudinal data from 47 children (25 boys and 22 girls) exposed to both Spanish and English from birth and 56 children (30 boys and 26 girls) exposed only to English. All families resided in South Florida. All children were born in the United States. All children were full term and healthy at birth, had normal hearing, and were screened for evidence of communicative delay at 22 months. The bilingual children were required to hear at least 10% of their total input in the less frequently heard language. All the bilingually developing children were producing at least some words in both languages at 22 months. On average these families were highly educated, and there was no difference between the bilingual and monolingual households in the parents' levels of education. Among parents in bilingual households, 87% of mothers and 60% of fathers had at least a college (4-year) degree; among parents in monolingual households, 75% of mothers and 61% of fathers had at least a college (4-year) degree.

The measures of the children's English and Spanish development came from the widely used MacArthur-Bates communicative development inventories (Fenson et al., 1993; Jackson-Maldonado et al., 2003). These are caregiver report instruments, with parallel forms available for English and Spanish (and many other languages). The English and Spanish forms, although parallel in structure, were independently developed and normed on monolingual samples. Here we report outcomes on two measures: the raw vocabulary score, which is based on caregivers' reporting on a checklist the words their children were heard to produce, and the mean length of the longest three utterances (MLU3), also reported by caregivers. These analyses are drawn from those reported in Hoff et al. (2012).

Results

The first finding we present is that these bilingually developing children were acquiring language knowledge at the same rate as SES-matched monolingual children. Figure 5.1 plots the development of the monolingual children's English vocabulary scores and the bilingual children's total (English

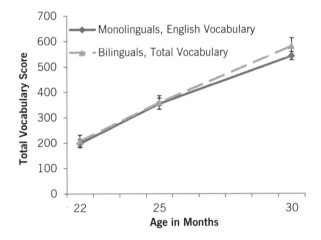

FIGURE 5.1. Total vocabulary growth in monolingual and bilingual language learners from 22 to 30 months. (Total for monolinguals = raw English CDI score; total for bilinguals = raw English CDI score + raw Spanish IDHC score.)

+ Spanish) vocabulary scores from 22 to 30 months. Statistical analysis confirmed what is apparent in the figure: There is no difference between the two groups of children. This is consistent with findings from other studies of bilingual children using total vocabulary measures (e.g., Junker & Stockman, 2002; Pearson et al., 1993). To reiterate, when we count all the words on the Spanish and English checklists combined that the bilingual children use in their speech, it is not different from the number of different English words that the monolingual children use in their speech.

The bilingual children's word knowledge, however, was distributed across two languages. Figure 5.2a repeats the same plot of English vocabulary for the monolingual children and plots the bilingual children's English and Spanish vocabulary scores separately. Again, statistical analysis confirmed what is apparent: a three (Age) × two (Language Group) ANOVA revealed significant main effects of age and language group and a significant Age × Language Group interaction. The monolingual children had larger English vocabularies than the bilingually developing children, and those vocabularies grew at a faster rate during this period. Although the measures in English and Spanish are not directly comparable, it is apparent that on average, English was the stronger language among the bilingually developing children. Thus, the effect of bilingualism seen in this sample is not the result of comparing monolingual English-speaking children to bilingual children who were Spanish dominant.

The next question we asked was whether the same pattern held for grammatical development. The Chomskyan view of language acquisition would predict that grammatical development should not be affected by bilingualism, even where vocabulary development is. Figure 5.2b presents data on the children's grammatical development, using the mean length of their longest three utterances as the outcome measure. (There is no obvious way to calculate a total measure across languages, although see Thordardot-tir, 2005, for one suggestion.) The apparent similarity between the pattern of vocabulary development in Figure 5.2a and grammatical development in Figure 5.2b was confirmed by statistical analysis. There were significant main effects of age and language group and a significant Age × Language Group interaction.

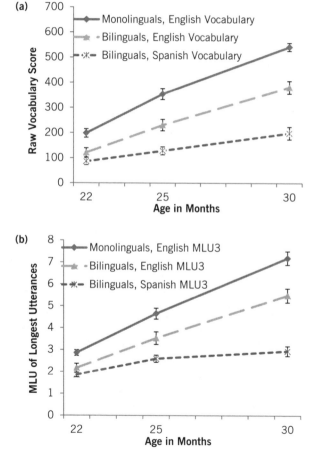

FIGURE 5.2. Growth in single language measures of (a) vocabulary and (b) grammatical development for monolingual and bilingual language learners from 22 to 30 months.

Discussion

These findings provide a clear answer to the question of whether bilingualism affects the rate at which each language is acquired: it does. These findings do not contradict the findings from earlier studies that bilingual children acquire each language within the normal range of variation for monolingual children (Genesee, 2006; Paradis & Genesee, 1996; Petitto & Kovelman, 2003; Petitto et al., 2001); the normal range of variation in the rate of language development is large (Bialystok, 2001), and the distributions of single language skill levels in monolingual and bilingual groups overlap. However, these findings contradict the assertion that the simultaneous acquisition of two languages has no effect on the pace at which each is acquired.

Because these monolingual and bilingual samples were equivalent in terms of parental education levels, the size of the difference between the groups says something about the size of the effect of bilingualism independent of the effect of low SES, which frequently characterizes bilingual samples. Effect sizes were calculated on the data averaged across the three measurement points. Measured in standard deviation units (Cohen's d), the size of the effects were 0.90 for vocabulary and 0.75 for grammar, which are considered to be moderate to large effects. In terms of percentile scores, the monolinguals and bilinguals as groups differed 21 percentile points on the vocabulary measure and 17 percentile points on the length of their longest utterances. Because these children were, on average, more advanced in English than in Spanish the size of the effect of bilingualism on their English language skills provides a conservative estimate of the size of the effect on the acquisition of one language associated with the simultaneous acquisition of another.

Visual inspection of the figures provides another way to gauge the size of the effect of bilingualism. In terms of English vocabulary size, the bilingually developing children at 25 months were at essentially the same level as the monolingual children at 22 months. In terms of MLU of the longest utterances, the bilingual children at 25 months were more advanced than the monolingual children at 22 months. Thus, one could describe these data as showing that the lag associated with bilingualism at this very early stage is less than 3 months. Thus, although these data show that it takes longer to acquire two languages than one, these data also show that it does not take twice as long—at least to reach the level of monolingual children at 2 years. The size of the lag increases with age, however, because the rate of English language development in the monolingual group is faster than the rate of development in the bilingual group.

What causes this lag in the single language development of bilingual language learners? The finding that the trajectories of total language development were virtually identical suggests that the bilingual children did not suffer in their ability to learn language. The fact that both groups of children came from equivalently high-SES homes suggests that the bilingual children did not suffer from inadequate environments. We propose that the lag is caused by the reduced input in each language that must be characteristic of children whose language exposure is divided between two languages. That is, unless children in bilingual environments hear twice as much speech in total as children in monolingual environments, they must hear less of each language. A large body of evidence from the study of monolingual children demonstrates that the rate of language development depends on access to language input (see Hoff, 2006). In addition, previous research on bilingual populations has established that the relative amount of exposure in each language is a strong predictor of children's rates of development (De Houwer, 2009; Gathercole & Thomas, 2009; Hoff et al., 2012; Oller & Eilers, 2002; Pearson, Fernández, Lewedeg, & Oller, 1997; Scheele et al., 2010).

Effects of the Balance of Dual Language Exposure on Language Development

Using the present sample, we tested the hypothesis that access to input influences the rate of language development in bilingual language learners by subdividing the group of bilingual children according to the relative amount of English and Spanish they heard and looking for corresponding differences in their rates of English and Spanish development.

Method

We used the estimates of the percent of English and Spanish in children's experience that were provided by their caregivers in an interview at the first visit to divide the bilingually developing children into three groups: a Spanish-dominant exposure group for whom the percent of English addressed to them at home was 30% or less ($n = 15$), a balanced exposure group for whom the percent of English addressed to them at home was between 50 and 60% ($n = 14$), and an English-dominant exposure group for whom English was 70% or more of their home input ($n = 18$).

Results

Figures 5.3a and 5.3b present the English vocabulary and MLU3 data for the monolingual children and the three groups of bilingually developing children. Both vocabulary and grammatical development showed the same pattern of effects: The monolingual children were the most advanced in English, the bilingual learners with English-dominant exposure were next,

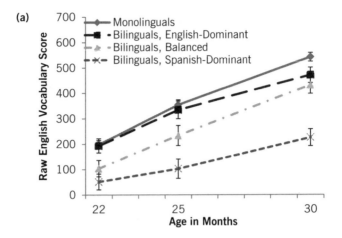

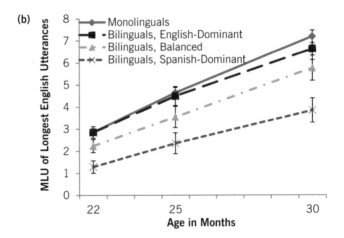

FIGURE 5.3. Growth in English (a) vocabulary and (b) grammar for monolingual and bilingual language learners from 22 to 30 months, with bilingual language learners categorized according to language dominance in input. (English-dominant = English input greater than or equal to 70%, balanced = English input between 50 and 60%, Spanish-dominant = English input less than or equal to 30%.)

followed by the children with balanced exposure and Spanish-dominant exposure, in that order. Not surprisingly—given that the size of the groups and the size of the between-group differences were reduced by subcategorizing the children according to balance—not all the between-group comparisons were significant. On both the vocabulary and grammatical measures, the Spanish-dominant group and the balanced input group differed significantly from the monolingual children; the English-dominant input group was not significantly different from the monolingual children. Although the Spanish-dominant input group had the lowest levels of English skill, they were learning some English. We also found, although we do not report these data here, that the English-dominant children were learning some Spanish. Furthermore, correlations calculated between amount of input in each language and the measures of language development showed a significant linear relation (Hoff et al., 2012).

Discussion

When we divided the bilingual language learners in our study according to the balance of English and Spanish in their experience, we found differences in their English and Spanish development associated with balance. The nature of these differences was entirely consistent with the argument that the average difference between monolingual and bilingual children reflected differences in their exposure to English, and, more generally, that the rate of language acquisition is paced by access to language input (Hoff, 2006). The effects of language balance were not consistent with two other views sometimes argued: our data did not support the view that balanced input allows children to acquire two languages at the same pace as monolingual children acquire one, nor did our data support the view that a minimum threshold of input is required for language acquisition to occur. At this early point in language development, there was evidence that even small amounts of language exposure result in language learning. It may well be, however, that in the long run a minority language that is acquired at such a slow rate becomes not very useful, thus little used and little heard. As English becomes increasingly dominant, Spanish may stop developing and may even decline. Other studies of older children are suggestive of such a process (Jia & Aaronson, 2003; Kohnert, 2004).

Effects of Properties of Dual Language Exposure on Language Development

Bilingual environments vary not only in the relative amount of exposure to each language they provide children but also in the properties of that language exposure. Some of these variable properties are the same as in monolingual experience: Children differ in how much speech they hear in each language, in the contingency of that speech on their own actions or utterances, in the richness of the vocabulary used, and in the complexity and variety of the syntactic structures used. There are other variable properties more relevant to bilingual experience. For some children in bilingual environments, the two languages they hear are quite separated in their experience; other children frequently experience both languages from the same people and even within the same conversation (De Houwer, 2009; Pearson, 2008). Some, but not all children exposed to two languages may hear one or both of their languages from a restricted number of different people, and children in bilingual environments may hear their languages from both native and non-native speakers to varying degrees (Fernald, 2006). These differences in children's bilingual environments are all potential sources of variability in the rate at which children exposed to two languages acquire those languages. We examined the relation of three of these properties of bilingual language experience to the children's bilingual development. We focus here on the findings of the effects on English, employing the same two outcome measures: vocabulary scores and MLU3; other analyses are reported in Place and Hoff (2012).

Method

These analyses made use of language diary data recorded by 29 of the caregivers of bilingually developing children (12 boys and 17 girls) when their children were 25 months old. Following a protocol developed by De Houwer and Bornstein (2003), the caregivers kept a log of their children's language exposure for each day of the week, recorded 1 day for each of 7 weeks. The caregivers recorded for each 30-minute period that the child was awake, the language(s) used during that time period, the person or persons who interacted with the child, and the ongoing activity (e.g., meal-time, bedtime). From these detailed records we calculated measures of the children's relative exposure to English and Spanish (measured as the percent of 30-minute periods in which the child heard only English or only Spanish), and the children's exposure to mixed input (measured as the number of 30-minute periods in which both English and Spanish were addressed to the child). We also counted for each child, the number of different speakers who addressed the child in each language and the percent of input in each language that was provided by native speakers of that language.

Results

We replicated our finding that the relative amount of exposure to each language predicted development in each language, which we had also obtained on the full sample using caregiver-report estimates of language exposure. Using the language diary data we found that the percent of 30-minute time periods in which the children were exposed to English alone accounted for 39% of the variance in English vocabulary scores and 27% of the variance in MLU3. We also found that the separation of the two languages in children's experience was unrelated to their development of either English or Spanish. The number of different speakers who were sources of English exposure and the percent of English exposure that was provided by native

English speakers were also both positive predictors of children's English vocabulary, over and above the effects of the amount of English input. Together these measures of the amount and properties of English exposure accounted for 54% of the variance in English vocabulary. There were no significant effects of the properties of input on the measure of grammatical development. The null effects with respect to grammar may reflect a lesser sensitivity of grammatical development to properties of input—as other findings suggest (Hoff, 2006). They may also reflect a lack of sensitivity in the measure we employed.

Discussion

Our more detailed look at properties of dual language exposure and their effects on bilingual development revealed that English vocabulary development is supported when children have access to multiple speakers of English and when their English exposure is provided by native speakers of English. We found no evidence that separation of the languages in input benefited acquisition.

Effects of Family Constellation on Dual Language Exposure and Language Development

Most of the bilingually developing children in our sample had at least one parent who was a native speaker of Spanish, but for some it was the mother who was the native Spanish speaker and for others it was the father. And for many children, both parents were native Spanish speakers. We asked how these family constellation variables were related to the balance of English to Spanish in the children's language exposure and to the children's English and Spanish language development. There is some evidence in previous studies that when both parents are native speakers of the heritage language, children hear it more and acquire it better than when only one parent is a native speaker (Alba, Logan, Lutz, & Stults, 2002; De Houwer, 2007).

Method

We compared three family types: those with a native Spanish-speaking mother and native English-speaking father, a native Spanish-speaking father and native English-speaking mother, and two native Spanish-speaking parents. These three constellations accounted for 25 of 29 families that provided diary data. (In three of the other households the Spanish-speaking parent described him- or herself as a native bilingual, and in one household both parents were native speakers of English who spoke some Spanish and they employed a Spanish-speaking nanny.) The outcomes were the measures of language exposure calculated from the diary data and the raw vocabulary and MLU3 measures of the children's vocabulary and grammatical development based on the MacArthur-Bates inventories.

Results

Figure 5.4 plots the percent of the children's language exposure that was in English-only, Spanish-only, or English and Spanish blocks. English was the more frequently heard language for the children with one native English-speaking parent—either the mother or the father, and Spanish was the more frequently heard language for the children with two native Spanish-speaking parents. Another difference among these different types of families is in where and from whom the children received their exposure to English. Children with a native English-speaking mother heard 66% of their English from native speakers. Children with a native Spanish-speaking mother and native English-speaking father heard only 28% of their English from native speakers. For children with two native Spanish-speaking parents, only 12% of the speech addressed to them in English that could be coded for native speaker status came from native English speakers.

Figures 5.5a and 5.5b plot the children's raw vocabulary scores and their MLU3 in English and Spanish by family constellation. There was a significant effect of family constellation on both measures of English;

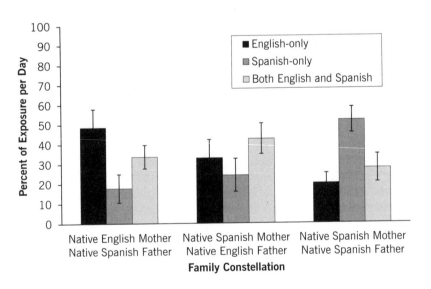

FIGURE 5.4. Percent of 30-minute time periods in which 25-month-old bilingual language learners heard only English, only Spanish, or both English and Spanish within the same period, by constellation of parents' native languages.

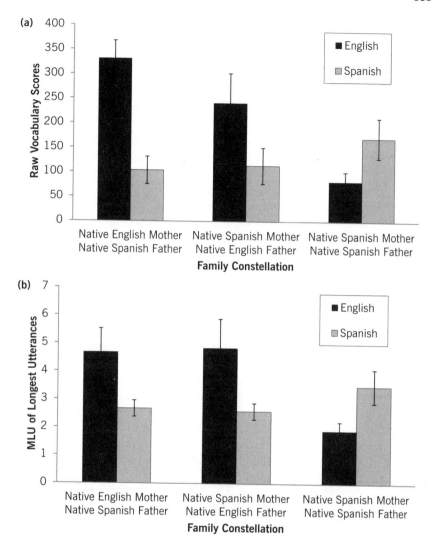

FIGURE 5.5. Twenty-five-month-old bilingual language learners' (a) vocabulary and (b) grammatical development in English and Spanish, by constellation of parents' native languages.

there was no significant effect on Spanish. The bilingual language learners who had a native English-speaking mother were more advanced in English vocabulary and grammar than the bilingual language learners who had two native Spanish-speaking parents.

Discussion

Our data say something about the heterogeneity that characterizes bilingual environments and the language skills of children who are bilingual language learners. The constellation of native languages in children's homes affects how much each language is used in the home and also affects how much of the English that children hear is provided by native English speakers. Both of these factors influence language development (Place & Hoff, 2011). Other family structure variables that we did not consider also may affect young children's dual language exposure and bilingual development. In our sample, there were very few grandparents living in the homes, but where it occurs the presence of a grandparent who is a native—and often more nearly monolingual—speaker of the heritage language will affect use of that language. In other analyses, we also have looked at the effect of older siblings in bilingual households (Bridges & Hoff, in press). We have found that the presence of other children who attend English-language schools results in more English being used in the home, and in more rapid English development and less rapid Spanish language development, as have Duursma et al. (2007). Interestingly, toddlers' exposure to English is increased by the presence of an older sibling both because the older sibling speaks English to the toddler and also because mothers who have older, school-age children in addition to a toddler use English more—even with the toddler. The older child's school attendance moves the household to a more English-dominant pattern of language use (Bridges & Hoff, in press).

What Do Bilingual Language Learners Need from Infant/Toddler Programs?

Infants and toddlers who are bilingual language learners have the same need for developmentally appropriate, cognitively stimulating experiences as other infants and toddlers. Gauging what is developmentally appropriate may be particularly challenging in the case of bilingual language learners. Adults who are used to interacting with monolingual children may unconsciously estimate children's conceptual understandings and intellectual abilities on the basis of their expressive language skills. However, when children are learning two languages simultaneously, their skill level in each one of those languages are not the same indicator of their cognitive level and ability as they would be in monolingual children. Bilingual language learners will have smaller vocabularies and less complex grammar in their languages than monolingual children of the same age, but they are not different on nonverbal cognitive measures, nor do they differ in their conceptual repertoires (see Scheele et al., 2010). It is a challenge to program providers to gear programs to the set of cognitive and linguistics skills that bilingual language learners present.

Like other children from families that are poor, bilingual language learners from low-SES households are likely to need extra support for the development of oral language and literacy skills. The literature on the relation of language experience to language development in monolingual children provides guidance with respect to what properties of language exposure are supportive, and there is every reason to think that these equally apply to bilingual language learners (Scheele et al., 2010). Children benefit from input that is used in one-to-one conversation with an adult who engages their attention, uses a wide range of vocabulary—including rare words, uses complex grammatical structures, and uses a variety of grammatical structures (Hoff, 2006; Huttenlocher, Waterfall, Vasilyeva, Vevea, & Hedges, 2010). There is also a literature on teachers' language use in classrooms and its relation to children's language development (Dickinson, McCabe, & Essex, 2006; Hoff, 2006; Huttenlocher, Vasilyeva, Cymerman, & Levine, 2002). The evidence here is consistent with findings on home language use: lexically rich and syntactically complex speech used in meaningful contexts supports language acquisition.

One finding from our studies that also may be relevant to infant/toddler programs is the value of language input from native speakers. We do not know what makes input from native speakers more supportive of language development than non-native input. Research in progress is addressing that question. We do know that it is often the case that native Spanish speakers talk to their children in English because they have been told by well-intentioned teachers, pediatricians, and others that they should—so that their children will learn English. As a result, some parents who are not highly proficient in English are nonetheless addressing their children in English. Although it may seem that high levels of proficiency ought not to be necessary for talking to small children, it may well be that the richness of vocabulary and the complexity and variety of syntax that support language acquisition in young children are affected when adults use a language in which they have modest proficiency. Pending the results of future research, it seems warranted to suggest that it is important for children's English language development that they hear English produced by speakers who are proficient English speakers. Just what level of proficiency is required to provide children with input as rich and supportive of language development as that provided by native speakers is a question for future research.

A last question for infant/toddler programs is whether they should try to support children's development in their heritage language. In many cases, this is simply not feasible. Children may come from many different heritage language backgrounds, and it may be impossible to provide input in those languages in the classroom. For Spanish it is not impossible. Spanish is the highest-frequency heritage language in the United States, and the low rates of academic success among Hispanic children are a cause for serious concern (Garcia & Jensen, 2009; Haskins et al., 2004). There are reasons to think that supporting bilingual children's Spanish skills in infant/toddler programs might benefit their English literacy and academic skills in the long run. Literacy skills acquired in one language transfer to another language—particularly if both languages share the same alphabet, as English and Spanish do (Oller & Jarmulowicz, 2007). Further, children in immigrant homes who are able to speak the heritage language enjoy better family relationships and their attendant socioemotional and academic benefits (Tseng & Fuligni, 2000). Finally, there is the argument that bilingualism itself is a desired developmental outcome. There are cognitive benefits associated with bilingualism at the individual level (e.g., Bialystok & Feng, 2011), and a bilingual workforce is an economic asset to the nation. When a second language is learned after early childhood and learned through classroom instruction, it is not learned as well as when it is acquired earlier (e.g., Abrahamsson & Hyltenstam, 2009). Children who come from homes in which a language other than English is spoken have the opportunity to become proficient bilinguals. It needs to be recognized, however, that acquiring two languages is more demanding—even for children—than acquiring one.

Summary and Conclusions

A substantial number of children from families that are poor are bilingual language learners. These children have the same need for enriching infant/toddler programs as other children from families that are poor, and, in addition, they need programs that will support their English language development. Research on the course of early bilingual development can inform the design of such programs. Our research on Spanish–English bilingual toddlers in South Florida has begun to provide a description of bilingual development that should help program providers understand the unique profile of competencies that bilingual language learners present. Our research has also identified factors that can be incorporated into program design in order to promote the development of English language proficiency in bilingual language learners.

Our findings clearly indicate that learning two languages takes longer than learning one. As a result, bilingual language learners typically lag behind monolingual children in their acquisition of vocabulary and grammar when only one language is considered. This does not mean there is anything amiss with the children who are bilingual language learners or that bilingual development causes harm. The bilingual language learners who have lower language skills than their monolingual agemates are not less advanced in their conceptual knowledge or cognitive abilities. It is a simple fact that children who are learning two things at the same time make slightly slower progress at each, compared to children who are learning only one. Program providers need to be cognizant of the different pattern of language and cognitive skills that they can expect from children who are bilingual language learners.

The results of our research also identify three factors associated with more rapid English language development among children who are bilingual language learners. The first is the quantity of their English language exposure. The more English children hear, the more rapidly they acquire English. We saw no evidence in our data of thresholds. Even 10% of exposure in English produced some learning, and the benefit of greater exposure did not asymptote at any point. Additional English exposure provided in the setting of infant/toddler programs that does not reduce the children's heritage language exposure should benefit bilingual language learners' English development without impeding their heritage language development. That is, children can learn more if they are provided more input. There are, no doubt, limits on how much children can process and how fast they can learn, but few children are likely to be pushing those limits.

The English exposure that programs provide to bilingual language learners can also be designed to be maximally supportive. Our results indicate that not all English exposure is equally useful. The second factor we found to influence English language development, over and above the quantity of English exposure, is the number of different speakers from whom the children hear English. Children who hear English from several different people learn English more rapidly than children who have fewer sources. The third factor that was positively associated with English language skill was the percent of children's English exposure that was provided by native speakers of English. We are currently investigating the differences between native and non-native child-directed speech, and we do not currently know what is more supportive about language interactions with native speakers. We do conclude from our findings, however, that programs designed to provide language-advancing input to children should include speakers with at least native-like proficiency. We also conclude that the common advice of telling parents with limited English proficiency that they should speak English to their children is probably bad advice (see Hammer, Davison, Lawrence, & Miccio, 2009, for a similar conclusion).

Although the study of bilingual language learners is a new field and much is still unknown, decades of research on monolingual children have made it clear that the amount and properties of children's language exposure affect their rates of language development. It should not be surprising that the same is true for bilingual language learners. Research on monolingual children has also made it clear that children's language development can be supported by their language experiences in preschool (e.g., Dickinson et al., 2006). For bilingual language learners who may not have sources of native-English language exposure at home, infant/toddler programs have an especially important role to play in supporting the development of the language skills they will need to succeed in school.

ACKNOWLEDGMENT

Preparation of this chapter was supported by Grant No. R21HD060718 to Erika Hoff from the National Institute of Child Health and Human Development.

REFERENCES

Abrahamsson, N., & Hyltenstam, K. (2009). Age of onset and native likeness in a second language: Listener perception versus linguistic scrutiny. *Language Learning, 59,* 249–306.

Alba, R., Logan, J., Lutz, A., & Stults, B. (2002). Only English by the third generation? Loss and preservation of the mother tongue among the grandchildren of contemporary immigrants. *Demography, 39,* 467–484.

Baker, C. (2007). *A parents' and teachers' guide to bilingualism.* Clevedon, UK: Multilingual Matters.

Bialystok, E. (2001). *Bilingualism in development: Language, literacy, and cognition.* Cambridge: Cambridge University Press.

Bialystok, E., & Feng, X. (2011). Language proficiency and its implications for monolingual and bilingual children. In A. Y. Durgunoglu & C. Goldenberg (Eds.), *Dual-language learners: The development and assessment of oral and written language* (pp. 121–138). New York: Guilford Press.

Bridges, K., & Hoff, E. (in press). Older sibling influences on the language environment and language development of toddlers in bilingual homes. *Applied Psycholinguistics.*

Chomsky, N. (1965). *Aspects of the theory of syntax.* Cambridge, MA: MIT Press.

Chomsky, N. (1991). Linguistics and cognitive science: Problems and mysteries. In A. Kasher (Ed.), *The Chomskyan turn* (pp. 26–53). Cambridge, MA: Blackwell.

De Houwer, A. (2007). Parental language input patterns and children's bilingual use. *Applied Psycholinguistics, 28,* 411–424.

De Houwer, A. (2009). *Bilingual first language acquisition.* Bristol, UK: Multilingual Matters.

De Houwer, A., & Bornstein, M. (2003, April 30–May 3). *Balancing on the tightrope: Language use patterns in bilingual families with young children.* Paper presented at the meeting of the Fourth International Symposium on Bilingualism, Tempe, Arizona.

Dickinson, D. K., McCabe, A., & Essex, M. J. (2006). A window of opportunity we must open to all: The case for preschool with high-quality support for language and literacy. In D. K. Dickinson & S. B. Neuman (Eds.), *Handbook of early literacy research* (Vol. 2, pp. 11–28). New York: Guilford Press.

Duursma, E., Romero-Contreraa, S., Szuber, A., Proctor, P., Snow, C., August, D., et al. (2007). The role of home literacy and language environment on bilinguals' English and Spanish vocabulary development. *Applied Psycholinguistcs, 28,* 171–190.

Eilers, R. E., Pearson, B. Z., & Cobo-Lewis, A. B. (2006). Social factors in bilingual development: The Miami experience. In P. McCardle & E. Hoff (Eds.), *Childhood bilingualism: Research on infancy through school age* (pp. 68–90). Clevedon, UK: Multilingual Matters.

Fenson, L., Dale, P. S., Reznick, J. S., Thal, D., Bates, E., Hartung, J. P., et al. (1993). *MacArthur communicative development inventories: User's guide and technical manual.* San Diego, CA: Singular.

Fernald, A. (2006). When infants hear two languages: Interpreting research on early speech perception by bilingual children. In P. McCardle & E. Hoff (Eds.), *Childhood bilingualism: Research on infancy through school age* (pp. 30–44). Clevedon, UK: Multilingual Matters.

Garcia, E., & Jensen, B. (2009). Early educational opportunities for children of Hispanic origins. *Social Policy Report, 23*(2), 3–19.

Garcia, G. N., McCardle, P., & Nixon, S. M. (2007). Development of English literacy in Spanish-speaking children: Transforming research into practice. *Language, Speech, and Hearing Services in Schools, 38,* 213–215.

Gathercole, V. C. M., & Thomas, E. M. (2009). Bilingual first-language development: Dominant language takeover, threatened minority language take-up. *Bilingualism: Language and Cognition, 12*(2), 213–237.

Genesee, F. (2006). Bilingual first language acquisition in perspective. In P. McCardle & E. Hoff (Eds.), *Childhood bilingualism: Research on infancy through school age* (pp. 45–67). Clevedon, UK: Multilingual Matters.

Genesee, F., & Nicoladis, E. (2007). Bilingual first language acquisition. In E. Hoff & M. Shatz (Eds.), *Blackwell handbook of language development* (pp. 324–342). West Sussex, UK: Wiley-Blackwell.

Gleitman, L. R., & Newport, E. L. (1995). The invention of language by children: Environmental and biological influences on the acquisition of language. In D. N. Osherson (Ed.), *An invitation to cognitive science: Volume 1. Language* (2nd ed., pp. 1–24). Cambridge, MA: MIT Press.

Grosjean, F. (1982). *Life with two languages: An introduction to bilingualism.* Cambridge, MA: Harvard University Press.

Grosjean, F. (2010). *Studying bilinguals.* Oxford: Oxford University Press.

Hakuta, K. (1986). *Mirror of language: The debate on bilingualism.* New York: Basic Books.

Hammer, C. S., Davison, M. D., Lawrence, F. R., & Miccio, A. W. (2009). The effect of maternal language on bilingual children's vocabulary and emergent literacy development during Head Start and kindergarten. *Scientific Studies of Reading, 13,* 99–121.

Hart, B., & Risley, T. R. (1995). *Meaningful differences in the everyday experience of young American children.* Baltimore: Brookes.

Haskins, R., Greenberg, M., & Fremstad, S. (2004). Federal policy for immigrant children: Room for common ground? *The Future of Children, 14,* 1–5. Retrieved from *http://futureofchildren.org/futureofchildren/publications/ docs/14_02_PolicyBrief.pdf.*

Hoff, E. (2003). Causes and consequences of SES-related differences in parent-to-child speech. In M. H. Bornstein & R. H. Bradley (Eds.), *Socioeconomic status, parenting, and child development* (pp. 147–160). Mahwah, NJ: Erlbaum.

Hoff, E. (2006). How social contexts support and shape language development. *Developmental Review, 26,* 55–88.

Hoff, E., Core, C., Place, S., Rumiche, R., Senor, M., & Parra, M. (2012). Dual language exposure and early bilingual development. *Journal of Child Language, 39,* 1–27.

Huttenlocher, J., Vasilyeva, M., Cymerman, E., & Levine, S. (2002). Language input at home and at school: Relation to child syntax. *Cognitive Psychology, 45,* 337–374.

Huttenlocher, J., Waterfall, H., Vasilyeva, M., Vevea, J., & Hedges, L. V. (2010). Sources of variability in children's language growth. *Cognitive Psychology, 61,* 343–365.

Jackson-Maldonado, D., Thal, D. J., Fenson, L., Marchman, V., Newton, T., & Conboy, B. (2003). *Inventarios del desarrollo de habilidades comunicativas: User's guide and technical manual.* Baltimore: Brookes.

Jia, G., & Aaronson, D. (2003). A longitudinal study of Chinese children and adolescents learning English in the United States. *Applied Psycholinguistics, 24,* 131–161.

Junker, D. A., & Stockman, I. J. (2002). Expressive vocabulary of German–English bilingual toddlers. *American Journal of Speech–Language Pathology, 11,* 381–394.

King, K., & Fogle, L. (2006). Raising bilingual children: Common parental concerns and current research. *Center for Applied Linguistics Digest.* Retrieved from *www.Cal.org /resources/digest/RaiseBilingChild.Html.*

Kohnert, K. (2004). Processing skills in early sequential bilinguals. In B. A. Goldstein (Ed.), *Bilingual language development and disorders in Spanish–English speakers* (pp. 53–76). Baltimore: Brookes.

Kovács, Á. M., & Mehler, J. (2009). Flexible learning of multiple speech structures in bilingual infants. *Science, 325*(5940), 611–612.

Lesaux, N. K., Koda, K., Siegel, L. S., & Shanahan, T. (2006). Development of literacy of language minority learners. In D. L. August & T. Shanahan (Eds.), *Developing literacy in a second language: Report of the national literacy panel* (pp. 75–122). Mahwah, NJ: Erlbaum.

Marchman, V. A., Fernald, A., & Hurtado, N. (2010). How vocabulary size in two languages relates to efficiency in spoken word recognition by young Spanish–English bilinguals. *Journal of Child Language, 37,* 817–840.

Oller, D. K., & Eilers, R. (Eds.). (2002). *Language and literacy in bilingual children.* Clevedon, UK: Multilingual Matters.

Oller, D. K., & Jarmulowicz, L. (2007). Language and literacy in bilingual children in the early school years. In E. Hoff & M. Shatz (Eds.), *Blackwell handbook of language development* (pp. 368–386). Oxford, UK: Blackwell.

Paradis, J., & Genesee, F. (1996). Syntactic acquisition in bilingual children: Autonomous or interdependent? *Studies in Second Language Acquisition, 18,* 1–25.

Pearson, B. Z. (2008). *Raising a bilingual child.* New York: Living Language/Random House.

Pearson, B. Z., Fernández, S. C., Lewedeg, V., & Oller, D. K. (1997). The relation of input factors to lexical learning by bilingual infants. *Applied Psycholinguistics, 18,* 41–58.

Pearson, B. Z., Fernández, S. C., & Oller, D. K. (1993). Lexical development in bilingual infants and toddlers: Comparison to monolingual norms. *Language Learning, 43,* 93–120.

Petitto, L. A., Katerelos, M., Levy, B. G., Gauna, K., Tétreault, K., & Ferraro, V. (2001). Bilingual signed and spoken language acquisition from birth: Implications for the mechanisms underlying early bilingual language acquisition. *Journal of Child Language, 28,* 453–496.

Petitto, L. A., & Kovelman, I. (2003). The bilingual paradox: How signing–speaking bilingual children help us resolve bilingual issues and teach us about the brain's mechanisms underlying all language acquisition. *Learning Languages, 8,* 5–18.

Place, S., & Hoff, E. (2011). Properties of dual language exposure that influence two-year-olds' bilingual proficiency. *Child Development, 82,* 1834–1849.

Scheele, A. F., Leseman, P. P. M., & Mayo, A. Y. (2010). The home language environment of monolingual and bilingual children and their language proficiency. *Applied Psycholinguistics, 31,* 117–140.

Shatz, M., & Wilkinson, L. C. (Eds.). (2010). *The education of English language learners.* New York: Guilford Press.

Thordardottir, E. T. (2005). Early lexical and syntactic development in Québec French and English: Implications for cross-linguistic and bilingual assessment. *International Journal of Language and Communication Disorders, 40,* 243–278.

Tseng, V., & Fuligni, A. J. (2000). Parent–adolescent language use and relationships among immigrant families with East Asian, Filipino, and Latin American backgrounds. *Journal of Marriage and the Family, 62,* 465–476.

U.S. Census Bureau. (2006). *American community survey.* Retrieved April 30, 2008, from *http://factfinder.census.gov.*

Vagh, S. B., Pan, B. A., & Mancilla-Martinez, J. (2009). Measuring growth in bilingual and monolingual children's English productive vocabulary development: The utility of combining parent and teacher report. *Child Development, 80,* 1545–1563.

Werker, J. F., & Byers-Heinlein, K. (2008). Bilingualism in infancy: First steps in perception and comprehension. *Trends in Cognitive Sciences, 12,* 144–151.

PART III

SOCIAL–EMOTIONAL DEVELOPMENT

CHAPTER 6

The Development of Self-Regulation in Infancy and Early Childhood

An Organizing Framework for the Design and Evaluation of Early Care and Education Programs for Children in Poverty

Clancy Blair, Daniel Berry, and Allison H. Friedman

High-quality early care and education for children in poverty remains a centerpiece of social policy in the United States. It represents one potentially viable strategy to redress the extremes of inequality stemming from subsistence-level poverty in a free-market system and helps to ensure the educated populace required to maintain social and economic well-being in a democratic society. There has been great interest in the potential benefits of high-quality early care and education for children in poverty for several decades (e.g., Consortium for Longitudinal Studies, 1983). This interest was initially bolstered by early findings indicating meaningful benefits to IQ, school achievement, and educational attainment for recipients across the triumvirate of carefully studied and extensively evaluated model programs: the Perry Preschool Project (Schweinhart & Weikert, 1984), the Abecedarian Project (Ramey & Campbell, 1984), and the Chicago Parent–Child Center program (Reynolds, 1992). Long-term follow-up of these programs has largely solidified the assumption that high-quality early care and education represents the best and most viable strategy for ensuring the health and well-being of children in poverty (Heckman, 2006). This is particularly the case given that findings of follow-up studies into early and middle adulthood have indicated substantial benefits to program recipients on several meaningful life outcomes, despite the fact that initial cognitive benefits tended to fade over time. Specifically, findings from Perry (Schweinhart, Barnes, & Weikart, 1993), Abecedarian (Campbell, Pungello, Miller-Johnson, Burchinal, & Ramey, 2001), and the Chicago Parent–Child program (Reynolds, Temple, Robertson, & Mann, 2001) indicate increased school completion, reduced special education placements, increased college attendance and, in some of the programs, increased employment, increased earnings, and reduced rates of arrest and incarceration (see Reynolds & Temple, 2008, for review).

Long-term benefits to meaningful life outcomes associated with high-quality early education and care for children in poverty provide the rationale for ongoing comprehensive and methodologically sound investigation of mechanisms through which such program effects occurred. Interrelated areas of inquiry concern questions about the specific content of the programs and, particularly for present purposes, questions about key aspects of psychological development that might have been impacted by children's experiences in the programs. In this chapter we focus on self-regulation as a primary indicator of program effects and discuss approaches and strategies for assessing self-regulation as an outcome of early intervention. To this end, we describe key aspects of the construct in infancy and early childhood, propose approaches to the assessment of self-regulation in infancy and early childhood, and discuss the application of these approaches in newly implemented intervention programs to promote child development.

Self-Regulation: Definition and Relation to High-Quality Early Care and Education

When examining early intervention for children in poverty there are several aspects of child psychological development that need to be considered as key indicators of program effects. One, for example, is language development. A rich and varied language environment provided by caregivers in high-quality programs would be expected to lead to language growth in children that could be associated with increases in IQ and with benefits to school achievement (e.g., Hart & Risely, 1995). A second relates to the quality of social–emotional relationships with caregivers and expected benefits to children's emotional development associated with the presence of a close and secure relationship with a caring adult (e.g., Sroufe, 1996). A third concerns self-efficacy and the idea that the programs provided children with the opportunity to interact with and have an effect on their environments in ways that promoted a strong sense of agency (e.g., Elliott & Dweck, 1988).

A fourth area of development that we see as integral to the preceding three is self-regulation. Self-regulation is in many ways necessary for, as well as dependent on, growth in language ability, social–emotional well-being, and self-efficacy (e.g., Calkins & Leerkes, 2011; Ursache, Blair, & Raver, 2012). Therefore, when considering areas of psychological development that are important for the design and evaluation of future and ongoing high-quality care and education efforts, we suggest that self-regulation serves as an overarching organizing construct, growth in which can be expected to lead to the variety of long-term impacts on academic and life success noted above.

As an overarching construct, self-regulation refers to the primarily volitional control of emotional and cognitive responses to stimulation for the purposes of goal-directed action. For example, individuals exhibit self-regulation when inhibiting impulsive responding, when opting for a larger beneficial long-term gain, rather than smaller short-term gains (Mischel & Ayduk, 2011), when fostering motivation and interests and structuring activities and routines in ways that lead to a desired positive end state (Papies & Aarts, 2011), and when modulating emotional and cognitive responses to stimulation in ways that promote positive social exchanges and sustained engagement (Kochanska, Murray, & Harlan, 2000). Individuals also exhibit self-regulation when deliberately or automatically monitoring and modulating arousal levels (whether increasing them when bored or decreasing them when agitated) in order to effectively engage with the environment (Blair & Ursache, 2011).

Self-regulation has been operationalized in a number of ways across research literatures in personality psychology, cognitive psychology, and cognitive and social neuroscience, each with a greater or lesser emphasis on either the predominantly cognitive or predominantly social–emotional aspects of the construct. In the study of self-regulation in early childhood, for example, research on an aspect of temperament referred to as effortful control can be viewed as an amalgam of social–emotional and cognitive aspects of self-regulation. Behaviorally, effortful control refers to the ability to engage in a given activity for sustained periods to time, to smoothly transition between activities, and to plan and to wait before entering into new activities or situations (Rothbart, Ellis, Rueda, & Posner, 2003). From a cognitive perspective, however, effortful control is also associated with the ability to volitionally monitor and control attention in the context of conflicting information in order to regulate emotion (Posner & Rothbart, 2000). As such, effortful control combines aspects of more automatic, bottom-up processes of behavioral and social–emotional regulation as well as volitional regulation through the top-down control of attention.

The interrelated yet distinct social–emotional and cognitive aspects of self-regulation have been emphasized in different ways in various programs of research. For example, the behavioral and social–emotional aspects of self-regulation development in early childhood have been emphasized in research on the development of conscience and committed compliance (Kochanska et al., 2000) and on the development of emotion regulation (Eisenberg, Valiente, & Eggum, 2010), as well as the ways in which these more automatic aspects of self-regulation relate to the development of social–emotional competence and psychological well-being. Other work has concentrated more on the cognitive aspects of self-regulation, primarily as seen in research on executive functions (Blair & Ursache, 2011; Zelazo, Muller, Frye, & Marcovitch, 2003), defined as working memory, inhibitory control, and attention-shifting cognitive abilities important for children's social and academic development (Carlson, Mandell, & Williams, 2004; Espy et al., 2004; Hughes & Ensor, 2007).

Self-Regulation as a Basis for the Evaluation of Early Care and Education

From both social–emotional and cognitive perspectives, viewing self-regulation development as a central indicator of the effects of high-quality early care and education helps to address key questions concerning how and why such programs can lead to long-term benefits for children in poverty. Although the study of self-regulation in early intervention has been limited, there is some preliminary evidence to support the idea that the long-term impact for programs, such as the Perry Preschool and Abecedarian programs, may be partially mediated by effects on children's self-regulation skills. Recent reevaluation of the Perry program indicates that, for males, many of the long-term beneficial effects of the program on criminal behavior were due to early program impacts on children's social and personal behavior in middle childhood. For example, the beneficial program effects on arrest rates at the ages of 27 and 40 were explained partially by the effect of the program on children's "externalizing" problems (e.g., lying/cheating, stealing, truancy, obscenity) at the ages of 7 through 9. Similarly, for females, early program impacts on externalizing problems in middle childhood had secondary beneficial impacts on criminal behavior and marriage (Heckman, Malofeeva, Pinto, & Savelyev, 2008). Using data from the Abecedarian and Carolina Approach to Responsive Care programs, Burchinal, Campbell, Bryant, Wasik, and Ramey (1997) reported similar indirect effects of high-quality early child care. By the time infants were approximately 1 year old, those receiving high-quality early care tended to engage more responsively with independent observers during testing procedures, referred to as "task orientation." In turn, program effects on task orientation were shown to explain part of the programs' effects on children's cognitive growth trajectories across middle childhood.

As the analyses of these "gold-standard" programs makes clear, consideration of self-regulation as a central focus for the study of program effects provides a valuable organizing construct for program evaluation. Further, this focus on self-regulation is in marked contrast to prior emphases on intelligence (IQ) as a potential central mechanism underlying long-term program impacts. For instance, the positive long-term impacts of the Perry program were notable despite the fact that the program impacts on IQ faded with age. For the Perry program, the diminution over time of program effects on IQ in the face of substantial program effects on life outcomes such as academic achievement and attainment suggest that specific expectations concerning IQ as a central outcome were not as meaningful as once might have been thought. In contrast, follow-up of the Abecedarian sample has indicated that IQ gains have tended to remain over time (Campbell et al., 2001), suggesting that program effects on mental ability are also a likely contributor to long-term program effects. However, rather than juxtapose a focus on a cognitive mechanism, IQ, with a presumed social–emotional or so-called "noncognitive" mechanism referred to under the rubric of self-regulation, it is more appropriate to consider self-regulation in its combined cognitive and social–emotional manifestations as a framework for the evaluation of high-quality early care and education effects on human development. Research on cognitive aspects of self-regulation, including the regulation of attention and the development of executive functions, as well as social manifestations of self-regulation, such as the regulation of emotion and the exercise of self-control, provides testable hypotheses concerning the how and why of the broad impacts of high-quality early care and education on children's development.

One of the tangible benefits of viewing self-regulation as a central focus for the evaluation of early care and education is that self-regulation, including executive functions, emotion regulation, and effortful control, have large and varied research literatures that link them to multiple positive life outcomes. For example, executive functions have been related to school achievement in a number of studies with young children (Blair & Razza, 2007; Bull & Scerif, 2001; Espy et al., 2004). Although correlational, certain of these studies have indicated that the relation of executive functions to later achievement is robust even when controlling for prior levels of achievement and executive function abilities (e.g., McClelland et al., 2007; Welsh, Nix, Blair, Bierman, & Nelson, 2010). As such, these studies suggest that short- or long-term program effects on executive functions would likely serve as one mechanism through which high-quality early education and care would result in benefits to academic achievement and educational attainment.

Similarly, studies have indicated that emotion regulation is also an important contributor to school achievement (Raver, Garner, & Smith-Donald, 2007) and social competence (Denham, 2006). Young children who can appropriately regulate positive and negative emotion have higher levels of social competence (Denham et al., 2003) and reading and math achievement in the early elementary grades (Howse, Calkins, Anastopoulos, Keane, & Shelton, 2003; Trentacosta & Izard, 2007). Reflecting the integrated and interrelated nature of emotional and cognitive influences on self-regulation, these relations are likely partly explained by transactional processes among emotion regualtion, effortful control, and executive functions. Children who can appropriately modulate emotion and stress arousal in response to stimulation are better at focusing attention, holding information in working memory, and inhibiting prepotent responses to stimulation, all key aspects of executive functioning (Blair, Granger, & Razza, 2005; Howse et al., 2003; Raver, 2002).

As well, the relation between emotion regulation and academic achievement may be partially explained by the effect of emotion regulation on social competence. Emotional competence enables children to engage in positive interactions with teachers and peers that promote school engagement, school liking, and early learning and achievement (Hamre & Pianta, 2001; Ladd, Birch, & Buhs, 1999). Children who experience difficulty with social–emotional skills, friendship formation, and relationships with teachers early in school are more likely to experience peer rejection and declining enjoyment and engagement in school and poor academic outcomes (Buhs, Ladd, & Herald, 2006; Hamre & Pianta, 2005). Problems with social–emotional skills and interpersonal relationships are substantial risk factors for poor school outcomes as well as an essential aspect of school readiness and early school adjustment (Ladd, Herald, & Kochdal, 2006).

A focus on self-regulation in the evaluation of early intervention can also serve as a valuable indicator of the potential effects of early care and education programs on longer-term outcomes relating to psychopathology, substance misuse, and criminality. Both emotion regulation and executive function deficits are characteristic of risk for early developing psychopathology and substance dependency. A substantial literature has shown that executive function deficits may be a critical factor underlying the development of attention-deficit/hyperactivity disorder (ADHD; Barkley, 1997; Friedman et al., 2007; Willcutt, Doyle, Nigg, Faraone, & Pennington, 2005). Less effective executive function (Seguin & Zelazo, 2005) and effortful control (Eisenberg et al., 2010) have also been linked with the development of aggression problems in childhood, and some work suggests that executive function deficits may play a notable role in antisocial behavior and criminality (Morgan & Lilienfeld, 2000). Low levels of inhibitory control in middle childhood and early adolescence have also been shown to be a risk factor for later drug and alcohol use in adolescence (Nigg et al., 2006). Similarly, neurobehavioral disinhibition in middle childhood—a construct reflecting emotion regulation, executive functions, and behavior control—is predictive of clinical-level substance abuse problems in late adolescence (Tarter et al., 2003).

Neurobiology of Self-Regulation Development

In sum, there is accumulating evidence indicating that many of the positive life outcomes shown for children receiving high-quality early care intervention are associated with individual differences in self-regulation. Beyond behavioral associations, however, a growing understanding of the neurobiological substrates of self-regulation suggests that high-quality early care and education in infancy and early childhood may have meaningful effects on the developing structure and function of brain areas that underlie self-regulation. This research provides an increasingly clear picture of the neural circuitry, neurotransmitters, and neuromodulators upon which experience, for good or for ill, likely acts to influence behavior and to shape brain morphology and function.

The neurobiological substrates of self-regulation linking brain areas associated with executive functions and the control of attention to brain areas associated with emotional and stress reactivity and regulation are the focus of sustained interest in neuroscience research (Barbas & Zikopoulos, 2007; Holmes & Wellman, 2009). The application of methods in neuroanatomy, neuroimaging, and neuroendocrinology to the study of self-regulation has indicated that neural circuitry of the frontal cortex, striatum, and limbic system underlies the ability to regulate emotion and cognition in the service of goal-directed behavior (Robbins & Arnsten, 2009). Specifically, neural pathways between limbic and prefrontal cortical areas are largely reciprocal and allow for both bottom-up signaling from limbic centers to direct attention and engage executive functions of prefrontal cortex as well as for top-down control and inhibition or excitation from prefrontal cortex to limbic areas (Barbas & Zikopoulos, 2007). The process of signaling occurs in part through levels of neuromodulators associated with synaptic activity in prefrontal cortex, such as dopamine, norepinephrine, and serotonin. Notably, the relation of neuromodulator levels to synaptic activity is nonlinear, in the shape of an inverted U, in which moderate levels of neuromodulators are associated with high levels of neural activity, whereas very low or very high levels are associated with low levels of neural activity (Arnsten, 2000; Ramos & Arnsten, 2007). In this way, the relation between emotional and cognitive regulation at the neural level can be described as a balance between emotional arousal and cognitive control and in which one of the tasks of early development is to manage this balance through the give and take between emotional and cognitive engagement with stimulation (Blair & Dennis, 2010).

Given principles of experience-dependent neural plasticity early in development and the idea that the strength of connectivity in neural circuitry is established in response to experience (i.e., cells that fire together wire together), it is highly likely that high-quality care and education may have meaningful effects on the development of neural systems that underlie self-regulation. Such effects may be particularly evident in the development of the physiological response to stress in children. Stress response systems, such as the limbic hypothalamic–pituitary–adrenal (HPA) axis, influence levels of neuromodulator; in the case of the HPA axis the glucocorticoid hormone cortisol. Importantly, poverty is physiologically as well as psychologically stressful for children (Evans, 2003; Evans & English, 2002), and as such, affects steroid hormone levels that in turn influence activity in prefrontal–limbic cortical circuitry that underlies self-regulation (Liston, McEwen, & Casey, 2009; Liston et al., 2006). For example, correlational research suggests that exposure to poverty and to low-quality physical and psychosocial environments in infancy and early childhood are predictive of heightened levels of resting salivary cortisol, reduced cortisol reactivity, and to a number of indicators of increased burden on stress physiology, referred to as allostatic load (Blair et al., 2008; Blair, Raver, et al., 2011; Evans, 2003). As expected, heightened levels of cortisol are, in turn, predictive of less effective executive functioning skills in early childhood (Blair et al., 2005; Blair, Granger, et al., 2011). As such, one of the ways in which poverty is thought to "get under the skin" to affect children's self-regulation development is by affecting the neural circuitry of developing physiological stress response systems. Providing infants and young children from low-income contexts with high-quality early care likely supports the normative development of these stress systems by providing structured, predictable, and emotionally positive experiences. Indeed, this would be consistent with a number of animal models that have illustrated the beneficial effects of enriched early care on stress physiology (e.g., Bredy, Humpartzoomian, Cain, & Meaney, 2003; Francis, Diorio, Plotsky, & Meaney, 2002). As such, in addition to measures of emotion and cognitive regulation, biological markers of young children's stress physiology may be an informative marker of program impacts.

Taken together, there is clear evidence that children's developing executive function and emotion regulation abilities—self-regulation, broadly conceived—in early childhood are predictive of their social and academic development. As such, the long-term impacts of high-quality early care and education thought to be due to "noncognitive" skills may be better represented as positive impacts on children's self-regulation development. Growing understanding of the neurocognitive underpinnings of self-regulation suggests that high-quality care and education in infancy and early childhood may be particularly important for children growing up in poverty.

Application of Research on Self-Regulation to the Evaluation of Early Care and Education Beginning in Infancy

As the preceding sections emphasize, a focus on self-regulation opens the door to a variety of well-established but generally untested and underutilized approaches to the evaluation of the effects of early care and education. Additionally, a focus on self-regulation allows for the examination of an array of neurobiological variables, including stress hormones such as cortisol, as well as indicators of neural physiology and brain morphology that should prove to be valuable indicators of effective high-quality care and education and that can serve to strengthen inference regarding the extent of program effects on child development. Knowledge of the neurobiology of relations between emotion regulation and executive functions can increasingly provide the basis for specific recommendations as to innovative ways in which to demonstrate the potential short- and long-term benefits of high-quality care.

Growing interest in self-regulation as an indicator of the effects of high-quality care and education programs for children is seen in recent evaluations of innovative center-based care for preschool-age children. These include the Chicago School Readiness Project (CSRP; Raver et al., 2009), the Research-Based Developmentally Informed (REDI) Head Start program (Bierman, Domitrovich, et al., 2008; Bierman, Nix, Greenberg, Blair, & Domitrovich, 2008), and the experimental evaluation of the Tools of the Mind curriculum (Bodrova & Leong, 2007) reported by Barnett et al. (2008) and by Diamond, Barnett, Thomas, and Munro (2007). Each of these programs included content designed to foster academic achievement by building self-regulation skills. For example, CSRP focused on teacher training and coaching by a mental health consultant to improve the emotional climate of the classroom, lower children's level of conflict with peers, and lower teacher stress. Evaluation of CSRP indicated that the program had notable positive impacts on multiple aspects of children's self-regulation skills, such as their attention and executive functioning abilities, as well as on children's behavior problems and preacademic skills. Further, there was some evidence that the program impacts on children's preacademic skills were partially explained by the program effects on children's self-regulation skills (Raver et al., 2008, 2009; Zhai, Raver, & Li-Grining, 2011).

The REDI program included a preschool version of the Promoting Alternative Thinking Strategies (PATHS) curriculum to promote children's emotion knowledge and emotion regulation (Domitrovich, Cortes, & Greenberg, 2007) while also supporting literacy development through the promotion of verbal language (Bierman, Nix, et al., 2008). Similar to CSRP, evaluations of the REDI program indicated positive impacts on children's self-regulation skills, such as task orientation and persistence, as well as children's abilities to effectively shift their attention. The program also showed positive effects on children's academic and social–emotional development, with some evidence suggesting that, as above, these effects were partially explained by children's self-regulation skills.

The Tools of the Mind curriculum (Bodrova & Leong, 2007) provides numerous teacher-scaffolded, child-directed classroom activities that are designed to foster executive functions. With careful scaffolding by teachers, children engage in a number of activities that build skills in turn taking and perspective taking through social interactions related to learning. For example, children take alternate roles as reader or listener in Buddy Reading; or as doer and checker in a math activity to build understanding of one-to-one correspondence, Making Collections. The primary activity to build self-regulation in Tools of the Mind, however, is structured sociodramatic play, in which children plan and engage in extended play scenarios around a given theme, such as a restaurant or a doctor's office. By planning and engaging in well-structured play, children develop abilities related to future-oriented thinking, to planning and problem solving, and to the fulfillment of a defined role upon which one can elaborate and build self-regulation. A prior evaluation of the curriculum indicated that children randomly assigned to receive Tools of the Mind in preschool were more proficient at complex executive function tasks than were children assigned to receive a high-quality literacy-focused curriculum (Diamond et al., 2007). Although academic outcome data are not available for this prior evaluation, large to moderate correlations between executive function abilities and academic measures for children receiving Tools of the Mind suggest that the program is effective in promoting school achievement and school adjustment (Diamond et al., 2007). Future trials of this promising program can help to establish its potential impact on academic and social outcomes and the extent to which program-related improvements in self-regulation are key mediators of such effects.

Notably, the programs described above varied in the degree to which each focused relatively more on emotional or cognitive aspects of self-regulation. The REDI program focuses most explicitly on emotion through the PATHS curriculum, with the goal of supporting emotional development and thereby executive functioning and academic achievement, in combination with enhanced literacy instruction. In contrast, the Tools of the Mind curriculum focuses most specifically on activities designed to build executive functions with the expectation, supported by additional classroom activities, that advances in executive function will translate into advances in emotion regulation, social competence, and academic achievement. And CSRP represents an integrated model, highlighting emotional competence and classroom structure as a prerequisite for effective learning to occur. Yet, each program showed some impacts on children's self-regulation development, suggesting that the effects of high-quality early care and education on self-regulation may be due to supporting either end of the emotion–cognition continuum of self-regulation.

Although there are, to our knowledge, no evaluations of early education and care programs that apply neuroscience methods, there are some promising directions for this research that consider self-regulation in terms of an emotion–cognition balance. In ongoing evaluations of the Tools of the Mind curriculum that we and our collaborators are conducting, saliva samples are being collected from children to determine whether receipt of the curriculum is affecting stress physiology as indicated by cortisol, as well as alpha amylase, a marker of activity in the sympathetic adrenal medullary system. In this aspect of our research, we are interested in the extent to which participation in the program might be associated with reduced burden on stress response systems and greater reactivity and regulation in these indicators of stress physiology.

Similarly, in this evaluation of the program we are also interested in the extent to which participation might be affecting brain morphology and patterns of neural activity. In particular, our hypothesis is that as children develop executive function abilities in response to participation in the program, this will be evident in brain activity and perhaps brain structure in prefrontal cortical regions. Specifically, we expect that patterns of neural activity in response to tasks requiring executive functions will be more efficient in children participating in Tools of the Mind, exhibiting lower levels of activity on moderately difficult executive function tasks but higher levels of activity on more difficult executive function tasks when compared to children participating in the control group. As well, we are also interested in the extent to which treatment-related group differences in behavior and in patterns of neural activity might be associated with differences in gray and white matter volumes in ventral medial and orbital frontal regions of frontal cortex that play a central role in modulating levels of activity in limbic and brainstem structures that initiate stress responses.

Evaluating Self-Regulation through the Measurement of Attention in Programs Beginning in Infancy

Although an interest in self-regulation is emerging in the evaluation of center-based care for 3- to 5-year-olds, an age at which executive functions and effortful control can begin to be effectively measured and at which point an increasing array of neurobiological methods can begin to be employed, it is also important to consider earlier indicators of self-regulation development that can be applied to the evaluation of programs beginning in infancy. This is particularly the case, given the "earlier is better" developmental logic underlying intervention research. Attention in infancy is a potentially valuable early indicator of self-regulation development, and likely a meaningful marker of successful intervention in infancy and toddlerhood. The volitional control of attention shows rapid development across infancy (Johnson, Posner, & Rothbart, 1991) with the emergence of the ability to disengage attention from points of fixation and engage environments broadly over the course of the first 4 months of life (Bahrick, Walker, & Neisser, 1981; Butcher, Kalverboer, & Geuze, 2000; Posner & Rothbart,

2007). In particular, development of the ability to volitionally orient attention over the child's first 18 months has been proposed to play a substantial role in the regulation of emotion and development of temperamental effortful control (Posner & Rothbart, 1998, 2007). Correlational research has shown that infants who are better at orienting attention (e.g., attending to mom, toy, or object), as well as those who use self-comforting strategies (e.g., finger sucking, rocking, gentle rubbing) to distract themselves during times of distress tend to show declines in their displayed levels of negative emotion (Crockenberg & Leerkes, 2004; Stifter & Braungart, 1995). Given the emergence of attention skills in infancy, of course, a good deal of this regulation occurs in the context of the give-and-take of interactions with meaningful adults, or "coregulation" (Tronick, 1982). For example, maternal behaviors in which mothers engage in their infant's attention-orienting process, by either following the infant's self-directed attentional shift or by actively scaffolding these shifts have been found to be associated with reductions in infant negative emotion during times of distress. Some evidence suggests that this may be particularly the case, when these maternal behaviors are contingent on infant behavior (Crockenberg & Leerkes, 2004).

By virtue of early self- and coregulated attention-orienting strategies in infancy, children increasingly gain volitional control of attention, and, in turn, more effective emotional and cognitive self-regulation skills into early childhood and beyond (Posner & Rothbart, 2007). Use of attention-orienting strategies such as distraction in response to distress in toddlerhood is predictive of the ability to effectively delay gratification in early childhood (Sethi, Mischel, Aber, Shoda, & Rodriguez, 2000). Similarly, orienting attention to a novel object at 9 months has been shown to be predictive of higher levels of effortful control at 22 months, and greater regulation of anger at 33 months (Kochanska et al., 2000). Further, individual differences in the degree to which 6-month-old infants orient attention away from distressing events are predictive of lower levels of aggressive behavior in toddlerhood (Crockenberg, Leerkes, & Bárrig Jó, 2008). Infant attention shifting has also been shown to moderate the relation between temperamental distress to novelty in infancy and later anxiety in toddlerhood. Specifically, higher levels of infant distress to novelty were predictive of more anxious behavior, only to the extent that the toddlers rarely adopted attention-orienting strategies to avoid stress as infants. For infants who did tend to adopt more attention-shifting strategies—that is, by inference, those evincing better early self-regulation skills early in life— higher levels of distress to novelty were predictive of *lower* levels of anxious behavior (Crockenberg & Leerkes, 2006). In sum, there is some indication that infants' emerging abilities to orient attention may be a meaningful indicator of later self-regulation abilities.

A growing body of work indicates that other measures of attentional ability in infancy, namely, visual recognition memory and habituation–dishabituation, are predictive of higher-order cognitive processes related to self-regulation. In fact, these measures of infant attentional abilities are stronger predictors of later IQ than traditional measures of infant development (Kavšek, 2004). Infant visual recognition memory concerns an infant's preference to look at a novel stimuli compared to a previously viewed one (Rose, Feldman, & Jankowski, 2004). Habituation is defined as a decrease in attention to a repeatedly presented stimulus, presumably as the infant constructs a memory of the stimulus. Dishabituation is defined as an increase in or recovery of attention to a novel stimulus following habituation. Typically, when presented with two stimuli, an infant will exhibit preferential looking to the stimulus that he or she has not previously seen, suggesting that the infant has encoded the stimulus. Additionally, when continuously presented with the same stimulus, the infant will decrease his or her looking time, suggesting that he or she has encoded the information. Looking time will rebound or increase when a novel stimulus is then shown.

In terms of individual differences, infants who spend less time looking at a stimulus are thought to process visual information more rapidly and efficiently, and to retain the information for a longer period of time. These shorter-looking infants may be developing more efficient inhibitory control mechanisms that enable them to disengage attention once they have fully processed the stimulus rather than become "stuck" (Rose et al., 2004). The ability to inhibit a response to a familiar stimulus may be adaptive in that it prevents the infant from spending time attending to a stimulus he or she has already processed at the cost of exploring new stimuli. As well, this inhibition may be an early precursor of executive function development in that it foreshadows the ability to exercise voluntary control and to more readily direct and engage attention as needed.

There are a number of studies that identify relations between infant attention as assessed in habituation–dishabituation and visual recognition memory paradigms and later cognitive abilities including IQ, vocabulary, and expressive and receptive language (Kavšek 2004; McCall & Carriger, 1993; Rose & Feldman, 1997; Rose et al., 2004). However, there are no studies that we know of that examine the relationship between measures of infant attention and childhood self-regulation abilities. Rose and Feldman found an association between infant visual recognition memory as measured by a novelty preference at 7 months and IQ at 11 years. However, this relationship was significantly mediated by measures of memory and processing speed at age 11, suggesting that these aspects of cognitive ability may be a mechanism underlying the longitudinal relation between early attention and higher-order cognitive processes many years later. Additional studies have found associations between infants' length of fixation and composite visual recognition memory at the ages of 5 and 7 months and memory at age 3 years (Thompson, Fagan, & Fulker, 1991), visual recognition memory between 4 and 7 months and scores on the Peabody Picture Vocabulary Test between 4 and 7.5 years (Fagan & McGrath, 1981), and shorter duration of looking at 25 to 37 weeks and accuracy on a continuous performance test at age 12 years (Sigman, Cohen, Bechwith, Asarnow, & Parmelee, 1991).

Meta-analyses have substantiated the claim of an association between measures of infant attention and later cognitive abilities and IQ. In an early paper, McCall and Carriger (1993) found that infant habituation and recognition memory performance predicted child IQ between ages 2 and 8 years old, with effect sizes ranging from 0.36 to 0.45. A later meta-analysis by Kavšek (2004) also found an overall correlation in the moderate range, $r = .37$, between habituation and dishabituation measures in infancy and cognitive performance in childhood. Furthermore, both meta-analyses indicated that effects were larger for at-risk populations. McCall and Carriger found that correlations between infant measures of attention and childhood IQ were stronger for infants at risk due to preterm status, low socioeconomic status, or health or neurological problem, than nonrisk populations, with the at-risk population scoring lower on both infant and childhood measures. Similarly, Kavšek found that dishabituation measures in infancy, reflecting recognition memory, were stronger predictors of later IQ for samples at risk for a cognitive delay but habituation measures, reflecting encoding speed, were stronger predictors of later IQ for nonrisk samples. High-quality early care and education programs for at-risk children beginning in infancy may influence infant attention, later IQ, and the correlation between the two by counteracting some of the biological and environmental risk factors that children face.

In addition to infant attention, patterns of body movement may also be related to later cognitive and behavioral outcome reflecting self-regulation. Infants show distinct patterns of movement–attention coupling during visual attention as well as around gaze offset that mature between 1 and 3 months of age (Robertson, Bacher, & Huntingon, 2001). For example, infants tend to show a burst of motor activity just prior to gaze offset and a quieting of motor activity beginning just prior to gaze onset. Although the previously discussed research focuses only on how infant attention may be a precursor to later self-regulation, this research suggests that an infant's ability to regulate his or her body movement surrounding episodes of attention, in order to minimize the interruption of attention, may also foreshadow later self-regulation skills. Such close coupling of cognitive and motor abilities early in development is expected, given neurobiological evidence of interrelations between areas of prefrontal cortex associated with executive functions and areas of the cerebellum associated with the coordination of movement (Diamond, 2000). Individual differences in patterns of attention and movement, particularly when infants' body movement is not suppressed during visual attention, are associated with later parent-reported measures of attention in childhood (Friedman, Watamura, & Robertson, 2005). Robertson and Johnson (2009) also speculated that an infant's ability to suppress body movement may facilitate sustained attention and could therefore be associated with a later ability to volitionally control attention. Again, these findings help to substantiate the expectation that measures of infant attention and movement will predict later self-regulation abilities (Diamond, 2000).

Early Care and Education in Infancy and Toddlerhood and the Development of Attention and Self-Regulation

As introduced above, there is accumulating evidence that attention in infancy may be a meaningful precursor to the "full-fledged" cognitive and emotion regulation skills that become increasingly evident in early childhood. We have proposed that many of the long-term positive effects of "gold-standard" early childhood interventions accrue partially as a function of their effects on children's self-regulation skills. As such, intervention research aimed at building these skills in infancy and toddlerhood may find program effects on attention (i.e., orienting, habituation–dishabituation, visual recognition memory, attention–movement coupling) as meaningful early indicators of self-regulation, and, perhaps, cognitive performance in the long term. With the exception of the positive impacts of the Abecedarian and Project Care programs on infant task orientation mentioned above, evidence testing the impacts of high-quality center- or home-based infant/toddler care on attention- or self-regulation-related outcomes is limited. However, there is converging evidence that parenting-based interventions may impact attention-related outcomes in infancy and toddlerhood. A full review of the correlational literature concerning relations between parenting and attention and self-regulation development is beyond the scope of this chapter. Instead, we conclude by briefly examining studies employing randomized trials, to highlight causal effects.

Parenting intervention programs aimed at infants and toddlers have been strongly informed by the concept of caregiver *sensitivity,* discussed commonly in the context of attachment theory (Ainsworth, Blehar, Waters, & Wall, 1978; Bowlby, 1969). Sensitive parenting is typically considered the ability to consistently perceive, accurately interpret, and show contingent and appropriate responses to infant behaviors (Ainsworth et al., 1978; Isabella, 1993). From an attachment perspective, histories of sensitive care are proposed to allow the child to balance exploration and proximity seeking with the caregiver in a way that maintains an equilibrium feeling of emotional security. As such, attachment can also be seen as the "dyadic regulation of emotion" (Schore, 2001, p. 14; Sroufe, 1996).

From a neurocognitive perspective, caregiver sensitivity over the course of the first years of life has been proposed to underlie the development of the neurobiological substrates of self-regulation, namely, as described above, the structure and function of neural circuitry linking subcortical limbic regions with prefrontal cortical regions that underlie executive functions. Specifically, Schore (2001) has proposed that the coordination of these neural systems through secure relationships with caregivers promotes the ability to efficiently evaluate and encode social stimuli, monitor the internal visceral emotional response of the lower limbic regions, and make affective or behavioral adjustments to maintain goal-driven behavior (Schore, 2001). For example, infants who experience consistent, sensitive care in infancy would be expected to monitor the social environment more effectively, interpret social information and their own affective states more accurately, and effectively regulate their affect and behavior more consistently and efficiently than children not receiving such care. Indeed, correlational work suggests that such "secure children" show advantages in each of these domains, compared to their insecure peers (Belsky, Spritz, & Crnic, 1996; Laible & Thompson, 1998; Urban, Carlson, Egeland, & Sroufe, 1991).

Although neural mechanisms through which early intervention effects might be mediated remain to be demonstrated, findings from several randomized clinical control trials indicate that sensitive caregiving has important impacts on attention and self-regulation development in infancy and toddlerhood, particularly for children characterized by high levels of negative emotionality. van den Boom's (1994) seminal intervention work with parents of highly irritable infants was explicitly designed to reflect an attachment perspective. Specifically, intervention parents received three 2-hour one-on-one sensitivity coaching sessions concentrating on effective ways to perceive and interpret infant signaling, and select and implement appropriate responses. This relatively "low-dose" intervention impacted both sensitivity in mothers and multiple attention-related outcomes in infants. Compared to control mothers, mothers who received the intervention showed more sensitive maternal behavior after the intervention, as well as more positive gains in their sensitivity levels over the course of the intervention. Intervention infants fared better on several behavioral outcomes, including two aspects of attention. At the end of the intervention (age 9 months), infants showed decreases in inattentive behavior during free-play tasks (called "non-specific manipulation" by van den Boom [1994, p. 1466]), whereas children in the control group showed increases in inattentive behavior. Similar to the attention-orienting strategies introduced above, infants who received the intervention also showed higher overall levels of self-soothing behavior, as well as more positive gains in these behaviors across the course of the intervention, compared to the average self-soothing *declines* seen for control children.

Landry and colleagues (Landry, Smith, & Swank, 2006; Landry, Smith, Swank, & Guttentag, 2008) tested the effects of a similar sensitivity-based parenting intervention—Play and Learning Strategies (PALS)—with low-income families and also found positive program impacts on maternal behavior and attention-related child outcomes. Across ten 1.5-hour sessions, home visitors worked with intervention-group mothers to develop their abilities to respond contingently and warmly to their infants' needs, maintain and redirect infant attention, and verbally scaffold and encourage positive behaviors. The control group received home visits, with more general support (e.g., developmental screening, pamphlets on development). Across multiple measures of maternal sensitivity and responsivity, mothers receiving the PALS intervention showed greater gains in positive caregiving behaviors across the intervention period compared to mothers in the control group. Infants in the PALS intervention showed similar improvements across several outcomes tapping positive social behaviors. Most importantly for our purposes, infants in the PALS intervention group showed more effective goal-directed behavior during free-play tasks, as well as more positive behavior during interactions with a novel adult—both markers of attention control and self-regulation. A follow-up study of these children, testing intervention "dosing" effects showed additional effects on attention-related outcomes in early childhood (Landry et al., 2008). Specifically, participants in the prior study were randomized to participate in 11 "booster" PALS sessions between the ages of approximately 2.5 and 3 years. Among several other positive impacts, those receiving the extra dose of the PALS intervention in toddlerhood were better at aligning their joint attention and language with their mothers.

Other parenting interventions have shown notable impacts on attention- and self-regulation-related outcomes, such as early developing externalizing problems. In their intervention with mothers of 1- to 3-year-old children at high risk for externalizing problems (i.e., highly overactive, aggressive), van Zeijl and colleagues (2006) similarly adopted a coaching-based approach to improve maternal sensitivity and build child-discipline strategies particular to highly externalizing children. Intervention families received six 1.5-hour sessions in which coaches used videos of the mother–child interactions as a tool to scaffold more effective parenting strategies. Control families received six phone calls, in which they discussed general child-development issues. Compared to control mothers, those who received the intervention showed more positive discipline strategies, and had children who showed larger decreases in their parent-rated overactive behaviors over time.

Taken together, there is a clear indication that changing children's experiences in infancy and toddlerhood can have positive impacts on children's attention, with implications for emerging self-regulations skills. In particular, adult–child interactions marked by consistent and accurate perceptions and contingent and appropriate responses to infant behaviors may lead to dyadic regulatory processes between adult and infant that set the stage for increasingly volitional control of attention. Further, this may be especially important for children growing up in low-income contexts, given the psychosocial and physiological stressors that these children are more apt to face.

Conclusion and Future Directions

A converging body of evidence indicates that high-quality early care and education experiences can have positive long-term impacts on the lives of children growing up in poverty. In particular, these experiences appear to affect a wide array of meaningful life outcomes, ranging from higher levels of academic achievement to lower levels of crime. Such impacts benefit the lives of the children and families receiving intervention, as well as society as a whole. We propose that many of the long-term benefits of early care and education accrue as a function of the way high-quality environments positively impact children's self-regulation development. Although these skills are sometimes referred to as *noncognitive* skills, our growing understanding of the developmental neurobiology of self-regulation makes it clear that self-regulation is a product of transactional processes between bottom-up emotion-based processes, as well as more top-down higher-order cognitive processes (e.g., executive function).

Notably, the importance of self-regulation skills as a mechanism underlying early childhood intervention effects is often inferred rather than measured explicitly. We suggest that direct measures of children's emotion and cognitive regulation skills may be important markers of program success, given the accumulating evidence that self-regulation abilities play a role in a wide array of important developmental outcomes—from academic achievement and social competence to psychopathology. The emerging positive effects of recent early childhood education interventions aimed directly at children's self-regulation skills seem to support this assertion. In the future, follow-up studies will hopefully reveal the degree to which early gains in children's self-regulation abilities translate to long-term impacts on more positive life outcomes.

One limitation to traditional thinking about self-regulation is that researchers have tended to consider it as not being measurable (using executive function and emotion regulation tasks) until children transition into the preschool years. This raises the important question: How might one study program impact self-regulation, when child care and education intervention begins in infancy and toddlerhood? Based on theory and increasing evidence (Posner & Rothbart, 1998, 2007), including the impacts of multiple parenting interventions, we suggest that aspects of children's developing attention skills may serve as important indicators of program effects on children's development of self-regulation in the first few years of life.

The field of developmental cognitive and affective neuroscience is providing valuable insights into the potential mechanisms through which children's environments "get under the skin" to affect self-regulation development. Biological markers, such as those reflecting young children's developing physiological stress systems, as well as measures of brain structure and function, are important potential intermediary mechanisms underlying the way development is impacted by experience. As such, including neurobiological measures in the evaluation of early care and education programs will inform our understanding of program impacts, as well as help to elucidate some of the mechanisms through which these effects manifest over time. Taking this next step will require interdisciplinary partnerships. Yet, we suggest that such partnerships will yield important, novel findings that will inform basic and applied developmental science, and ultimately lead to more effective interventions for children.

REFERENCES

Ainsworth, M. D. S., Blehar, M. C., Waters, E., & Wall, S. (1978). *Patterns of attachment: A psychological study of the strange situation*. Hillsdale, NJ: Erlbaum.

Arnsten, A. F. T. (2000). Through the looking glass: Differential noradrenergic modulation of prefrontal cortical function. *Neural Plasticity, 7*, 133–146.

Bahrick, L. E., Walker, A. S., & Neisser, U. (1981). Selective looking by infants. *Cognitive Psychology, 13*, 377–390.

Barbas, H., & Zikopoulos, B. (2007). The prefrontal cortex and flexible behavior. *Neuroscientist, 13*(5), 532–545.

Barkley, R. A. (1997). *ADHD and the nature of self-control*. New York: Guilford Press.

Barnett, W. S., Jung, K., Yarosz, D. J., Thomas, J., Hornbeck, A., Stechuk, R., et al. (2008). Educational effects of the Tools of the Mind curriculum: A randomized trial. *Early Childhood Research Quarterly, 23*, 299–313.

Belsky, J., Spritz, B., & Crnic, K. (1996). Infant attachment security and affective–cognitive information processing at age 3. *Psychological Science, 7*, 111–115.

Bierman, K. L., Domitrovich, C. E., Nix, R. L., Gest, S. D., Welsh, J. A., Greenberg, M. T., et al. (2008). Promoting academic and social–emotional school readiness: The Head Start REDI program. *Child Development, 79*(6), 1802–1817.

Bierman, K. L., Nix, R. L., Greenberg, M. T., Blair, C., & Domitrovich, C. E. (2008). Executive functions and school readiness intervention: Impact, moderation, and mediation in the Head Start REDI program. *Development and Psychopathology, 20*(3), 821–843.

Blair, C., & Dennis, T. (2010). An optimal balance: Emotion–cognition integration in context. In S. Calkins & M. Bell (Eds.), *Child development at the intersection of cognition and emotion* (pp. 17–36). Washington DC: American Psychological Association.

Blair, C., Granger, D., & Razza, R. P. (2005). Cortisol reactivity is positively related to executive function in preschool children attending Head Start. *Child Development, 76*(3), 554–567.

Blair, C., Granger, D. A., Kivlighan, K. T., Mills-Koonce, R., Willoughby, M., Greenberg, M. T., et al. (2008). Maternal and child contributions to cortisol response to emotional arousal in young children from low-income, rural communities. *Developmental Psychology, 44,* 1095–1109.

Blair, C., Granger, D., Willoughby, M., Mills-Koonce, R., Cox, M., Greenberg, M. T., et al. (2011). Salivary cortisol mediates effects of poverty and parenting on executive functions in early childhood. *Child Development, 82*(6), 1970–1984.

Blair, C., Raver, C. C., Granger, D., Mills-Koonce, R., Hibel, L., & the Family Life Project Investigators. (2011). Allostasis and allostatic load in the context of poverty in early childhood. *Development and Psychopathology, 23*(3), 845–857.

Blair, C., & Razza, R. P. (2007). Relating effortful control, executive function, and false belief understanding to emerging math and literacy ability in kindergarten. *Child Development, 78*(2), 647–663.

Blair, C., & Ursache, A. (2011). A bidirectional model of executive functions and self-regulation. In K. D. Vohs & R. F. Baumeister (Eds.), *Handbook of self-regulation: Research, theory, and applications* (2nd ed., pp. 300–320.). New York: Guilford Press.

Bodrova, E., & Leong, D. J. (2007). Play and early literacy: A Vygotskian approach. In K. A. Roskos & J. F. Christie (Eds.), *Play and literacy in early childhood: Research from multiple perspectives* (2nd ed., pp. 185–200). Mahwah, NJ: Erlbaum.

Bowlby, J. (1969). *Attachment and loss: Vol. 1. Attachment.* New York: Basic Books.

Bredy, T. W., Humpartzoomian, R. A., Cain, D. P., & Meaney, M. J. (2003). Partial reversal of the effect of maternal care on cognitive function through environmental enrichment. *Neuroscience, 118*(2), 571–576.

Buhs, E. S., Ladd, G. W., & Herald, S. L. (2006). Peer exclusion and victimization: Processes that mediate the relation between peer group rejection and children's classroom engagement and achievement? *Journal of Education Psychology, 98*(1), 1–13.

Bull, R., & Scerif, G. (2001). Executive functioning as a predictor of children's mathematics ability: Inhibition, switching, and working memory. *Developmental Neuropsychology, 19*(3), 273–293.

Burchinal, M. R., Campbell, F. A., Bryant, D. B., Wasik, B. H., & Ramey, C. T. (1997). Early intervention and mediating processes in cognitive performance of children of low-income African-American families. *Child Development, 68,* 935–954.

Butcher, P. R., Kalverboer, A. F., & Geuze, R. H. (2000). Infants' shifts of gaze from a central to a peripheral stimulus: A longitudinal study of development between 6 and 26 weeks. *Infant Behavior and Development, 23,* 3–21.

Calkins, S. D., & Leerkes, E. M. (2011). Early attachment processes and the development of emotional self-regulation. In K. D. Vohs & R. F. Baumeister (Eds.), *Handbook of self-regulation: Research, theory and applications* (2nd ed., pp. 355–373). New York: Guilford Press.

Campbell, F. A., Pungello, E. P., Miller-Johnson, S., Burchinal, M., & Ramey, C. T. (2001). The development of cognitive and academic abilities: Growth curves from an early childhood educational experiment. *Developmental Psychology, 37*(2), 231–242.

Carlson, S. M., Mandell, D. J., & Williams, L. (2004). Executive function and theory of mind: Stability and prediction from ages 2 to 3. *Developmental Psychology, 40*(6), 1105–1122.

Consortium for Longitudinal Studies. (1983). *As the twig is bent. . . . Lasting effects of preschool programs.* Hillsdale, NJ: Erlbaum.

Crockenberg, S. C., & Leerkes, E. M. (2004). Infant and maternal behaviors regulate infant reactivity to novelty at 6 months. *Developmental Psychology, 40,* 1123–1132.

Crockenberg, S. C., & Leerkes, E. M. (2006). Infant and maternal behavior moderate reactivity to novelty to predict anxious behavior at 2.5 years. *Development and Psychopathology, 18,* 17–34.

Crockenberg, S. C., Leerkes, E. M., & Bárrig Jó, P. S. (2008). Predicting aggressive behavior in the third year from infant reactivity and regulation as moderated by maternal behavior. *Development and Psychopathology, 20,* 37–54.

Denham, S. A. (2006). Social–emotional competence as support for school readiness: What is it and how do we assess it? *Early Education and Development, 17*(1), 57.

Denham, S. A., Blair, K. A., DeMulder, E., Levitas, J., Sawyer, K., Auerbach-Major, S., et al. (2003). Preschool emotional competence: Pathway to social competence? *Child Development, 74*(1), 238–256.

Diamond, A. (2000). Close interrelation of motor development and cognitive development and of the cerebellum and prefrontal cortex. *Child Development, 71,* 44–56.

Diamond, A., Barnett, W. S., Thomas, J., & Munro, S. (2007). Preschool program improves cognitive control. *Science, 318,* 1387–1388.

Domitrovich, C. E., Cortes, R. C., & Greenberg, M. T. (2007). Improving young children's social and emotional competence: A randomized trial of the preschool "PATHS" curriculum. *Journal of Primary Prevention, 28*(2), 67–91.

Eisenberg, N., Valiente, C., & Eggum, N. D. (2010). Self-regulation and school readiness. *Early Education and Development, 21*(5), 681–698.

Elliott, E. S., & Dweck, C. S. (1988). Goals: An approach to motivation and achievement. *Journal of Personality and Social Psychology, 54*(1), 5–12.

Espy, K. A., McDiarmid, M. M., Cwik, M. F., Stalets, M. M., Hamby, A., & Senn, T. E. (2004). The contribution of executive functions to emergent mathematic skills in preschool children. *Developmental Neuropsychology, 26*(1), 465–486.

Evans, G. W. (2003). A multimethodological analysis of cumulative risk and allostatic load among rural children. *Developmental Psychology, 39*(5), 924–933.

Evans, G. W., & English, K. (2002). The environment of poverty: Multiple stressor exposure, psychophysiological stress, and socioemotional adjustment. *Child Development, 73*(4), 1238–1248.

Fagan, J. F., & McGrath, S. K. (1981). Infant recognition memory and later intelligence. *Intelligence, 5,* 121–130.

Francis, D. D., Diorio, J., Plotsky, P. M., & Meaney, M. J. (2002). Environmental enrichment reverses the effects of maternal separation on stress reactivity. *Journal of Neuroscience: Official Journal of the Society for Neuroscience, 22*(18), 7840–7843.

Friedman, A. H., Watamura, S. E., & Robertson, S. S. (2005). Movement–attention coupling in infancy and attention problems in childhood. *Developmental Medicine and Child Neurology, 47,* 660–665.

Friedman, N. P., Haberstick, B. C., Willcutt, E. G., Miyake, A., Young, S. E., Corley, R. P., et al. (2007). Greater attention problems during childhood predict poorer executive functions in late adolescence. *Psychological Science, 18,* 893–900.

Hamre, B. K., & Pianta, R. C. (2001). Early teacher–child relationships and the trajectory of children's school outcomes through eighth grade. *Child Development, 72*(2), 625–638.

Hamre, B. K., & Pianta, R. C. (2005). Can instructional and emotional support in the first-grade classroom make a difference for children at risk of school failure? *Child Development, 76*(5), 949–967.

Hart, B., & Risley, R. T. (1995). *Meaningful differences in the everyday experience of young American children.* Baltimore: Brookes.

Heckman, J. (2006). Skill formation and the economics of investing in disadvantaged children. *Science, 312,* 1900–1902.

Heckman, J. J., Malofeeva, L., Pinto, R., & Savelyev, P. (2008). *The effect of the Perry preschool program on cognitive and noncognitive skills: Beyond treatment effects.* Unpublished manuscript, University of Chicago, Department of Economics.

Holmes, A., & Wellman, C. L. (2009). Stress-induced prefrontal reorganization and executive dysfunction in rodents. *Neuroscience and Biobehavioral Reviews, 33*(6), 773–783.

Howse, R. B., Calkins, S. D., Anastopoulos, A. D., Keane, S. P., & Shelton, T. L. (2003). Regulatory contributors to children's kindergarten achievement. *Early Education and Development, 14*(1), 101–119.

Hughes, C., & Ensor, R. (2007). Executive function and theory of mind: Predictive relations from ages 2 to 4. *Developmental Psychology, 43*(6), 1447–1459.

Isabella, R. (1993). Origins of attachment: Maternal interactive behavior across the first year. *Child Development, 64,* 605–621.

Johnson, M. H., Posner, M. I., & Rothbart, M. K. (1991). Components of visual orienting in early infancy: Contingency learning, anticipatory looking and disengaging. *Journal of Cognitive Neuroscience, 3,* 335–344.

Kavšek, M. (2004). Predicting later IQ from infant visual habituation and dishabituation: A meta-analysis. *Applied Developmental Psychology, 25,* 369–393.

Kochanska, G., Murray, K. T., & Harlan, E. T. (2000). Effortful control in early childhood: Continuity and change, antecedents, and implications for social development. *Developmental Psychology, 36*(2), 220–232.

Ladd, G. W., Birch, S. H., & Buhs, E. S. (1999). Children's social and scholastic lives in kindergarten: Related spheres of influence? *Child Development, 70*(6), 1373–1400.

Ladd, G. W., Herald, S. L., & Kochel, K. P. (2006). School readiness: Are there social prerequisites? *Early Education and Development, 17*(1), 115–150.

Laible, D., & Thompson, R. (1998). Attachment and emotional understanding in preschool children. *Developmental Psychology, 34*, 1038–1045.

Landry, S. H., Smith, K. E., & Swank, P. R. (2006). Responsive parenting: Establishing early foundations for social, communication, and independent problem-solving skills. *Developmental Psychology, 42*, 627–642.

Landry, S. H., Smith, K. E., Swank, P. R., & Guttentag, C. (2008). A responsive parenting intervention: The optimal timing across early childhood for impacting maternal behaviors and child outcomes. *Developmental Psychology, 44*, 1335–1353.

Liston, C., McEwen, B. S., & Casey, B. J. (2009). Psychological stress reversibly disrupts prefrontal processing and attentional control. *Proceedings of the National Academy of Sciences, 106*(3), 912–917.

Liston, C., Watts, R., Tottenham, N., Davidson, M. C., Niogi, S., Ulug, A. M., et al. (2006). Frontostriatal microstructure modulates efficient recruitment of cognitive control. *Cerebral Cortex, 16*(4), 553–560.

McCall, R. B., & Carriger, M. S. (1993). A meta-analysis of infant habituation and recognition memory performance as predictors of later IQ. *Child Development, 64*(1), 57–79.

McClelland, M. M., Cameron, C. E., Connor, C. M., Farris, C. L., Jewkes, A. M., & Morrison, F. J. (2007). Links between behavioral regulation and preschoolers' literacy, vocabulary, and math skills. *Developmental Psychology, 43*(4), 947–959.

Mischel, W., & Ayduk, O. (2011). Willpower in a cognitive affective processing system: The dynamics of delay of gratification. In K. D. Vohs & R. F. Baumeister (Eds.), *Handbook of self-regulation: Research, theory, and applications* (2nd ed., pp. 83–105). New York: Guilford Press.

Morgan, A. B., & Lilienfeld, S. O. (2000). A meta-analytic review of the relation between antisocial behavior and neuropsychological measures of executive function. *Clinical Psychology Review, 20*, 113–136.

Nigg, J. T., Wong, M. M., Martel, M. M., Jester, J. M., Puttler, L. I., Glass, J. M., et al. (2006). Poor response inhibition as a predictor of problem drinking and illicit drug use in adolescents at risk for alcoholism and other substance use disorders. *Journal of American Academy of Child and Adolescent Psychiatry, 45*, 1–8.

Papies, E., & Aarts, H. (2011). Nonconscious self-regulation, or the automatic pilot of human behavior. In K. D. Vohs & R. F. Baumeister (Eds.), *Handbook of self-regulation: Research, theory, and applications* (2nd ed., pp. 125–142). New York: Guilford Press.

Posner, M. I., & Rothbart, M. K. (1998). Attention, self-regulation, and consciousness. *Philosophical Transactions of the Royal Society of London, B, 353*, 1915–1927.

Posner, M. I., & Rothbart, M. K. (2000). Developing mechanisms of self-regulation. *Development and Psychopathology, 12,* 427–441.

Posner M. I., & Rothbart, M. K. (2007). *Educating the human brain.* Washington, DC: American Psychological Association.

Ramey, C. T., & Campbell, F. A. (1984). Preventive education for high-risk children: Cognitive consequences of the Carolina Abecedarian project. *American Journal of Mental Deficiency, 88*(5), 515–523.

Ramos, B. P., & Arnsten, A. F. T. (2007). Adrenergic pharmacology and cognition: Focus on the prefrontal cortex. *Pharmacology and Therapeutics, 113*(3), 523–536.

Raver, C. C. (2002). Emotions matter: Making the case for the role of young children's emotional development for early school readiness. *Social Policy Report of the Society for Research in Child Development, 16*(3), 1–20.

Raver, C. C., Garner, P., & Smith-Donald, R. (2007). The roles of emotion regulation and emotion knowledge for children's academic readiness: Are the links causal? In B. Pianta, K. Snow, & M. Cox (Eds.), *Kindergarten transition and early school success* (pp. 121–148). Baltimore: Brookes.

Raver, C. C., Jones, S. M., Li-Grining, C., Metzger, M., Champion, K. M., & Sardin, L. (2008). Improving preschool classroom processes: Preliminary findings from a randomized trial implemented in Head Start settings. *Early Childhood Research Quarterly, 23,* 10–26.

Raver, C. C., Jones, S. M., Li-Grining, C., Zhai, F., Metzger, M. W., & Solomon, B. (2009). Targeting children's behavior problems in preschool classrooms: A cluster-randomized controlled trial. *Journal of Consulting and Clinical Psychology, 77*(20), 302–316.

Reynolds, A. J. (1992). Grade retention and school adjustment: An explanatory analysis. *Educational Evaluation and Policy Analysis, 14,* 101–121.

Reynolds, A. J., & Temple, J. A. (2008). Cost-effective early childhood development programs from preschool to third grade. *Annual Review of Clinical Psychology, 4,* 109–139.

Reynolds, A. R., Temple, J., Robertson, D., & Mann, E. (2001). Long-term effects of an early childhood intervention on educational achievement and juvenile arrest: A 15-year follow-up of low-income children in public schools. *Journal of the American Medical Association, 285,* 2339–2346.

Robbins, T. W., & Arnsten, A. F. T. (2009). The neuropsychopharmacology of fronto-executive function: Monoaminergic modulation. *Annual Review of Neuroscience, 32,* 267–287.

Robertson, S. S., Bacher, L. F., & Huntington, N. L. (2001). The integration of body movement and attention in young infants. *Psychological Science, 12*(6), 523–526.

Robertson, S. S., & Johnson, S. L. (2009). Embodied infant attention. *Developmental Science, 12*(2), 297–304.

Rose, S. A., & Feldman, J. F. (1997). Memory and speed: Their role in the relation of infant information processing to later IQ. *Child Development, 68*(4), 630–641.

Rose, S. A., Feldman, J. F., & Jankowski, J. J. (2004). Infant visual recognition memory. *Developmental Review, 24,* 74–100.

Rothbart, M. K., Ellis, L. K., Rueda, M. R., & Posner, M. I. (2003). Developing mechanisms of temperamental effortful control. *Journal of Personality, 71*(6), 1113–1143.

Schore, A. N. (2001). Effects on secure attachment relationship on right brain development, affect regulation, and infant mental health. *Infant Mental Health Journal, 22,* 7–66.

Schweinhart, L. J., Barnes, H. V., & Weikart, D. (1993). *Significant benefits: The High-Scope Perry preschool study through age 27.* Ypsilanti, MI: High/Scope Press.

Schweinhart, L., & Weikart, D. (1984). *Changed lives: The effects of the Perry preschool programs on youths through age 19.* Ypslanti, MI: High/Scope Press.

Seguin, J. R., & Zelazo, P. D. (2005). Executive function in early physical aggression. In R. E. Tremblay, W. W. Hartup, & J. Archer (Eds.), *Developmental origins of aggression.* New York: Guilford Press.

Sethi, A., Mischel, W., Aber, J., Shoda, Y., & Rodriguez, M. (2000). The role of strategic attention deployment in development of self-regulation: Predicting preschoolers' delay of gratification from mother–toddler interactions. *Developmental Psychology, 36,* 767–777.

Sigman, M., Cohen, S. E., Bechwith, L., Asarnow, R., & Parmelee, A. H. (1991). Continuity in cognitive abilities from infancy to 12 years of age. *Cognitive Development, 6,* 47–57.

Sroufe, L. A. (1996). *Emotional development: The organization of emotional life in the early years.* New York: Cambridge University Press.

Stifter, C. A., & Braungart, J. M. (1995). The regulation of negative reactivity: Function and development. *Developmental Psychology, 38,* 448–455.

Tarter, R. E., Kirisci, L., Mezzich, A., Cornelius, J. R., Pajer, K., Vanyukov, M., et al. (2003). Neurobehavioral disinhibition in childhood predicts early age at onset of substance use disorder. *American Journal of Psychiatry, 160*(6), 1078–1085.

Thompson, L. A., Fagan, J. F., & Fulker, D. W. (1991). Longitudinal prediction of specific cognitive abilities from infant novelty preference. *Child Development, 67,* 530–538.

Trentacosta, C. J., & Izard, C. E. (2007). Kindergarten children's emotion competence as a predictor of their academic competence in first grade. *Emotion, 7*(1), 77–88.

Tronick, E. Z. (1982). Affectivity and sharing. In E. Z. Tronick (Ed.), *Social interchange in infancy: Affect, cognition, and communication* (pp. 1–6). Baltimore: University Park Press.

Urban, J., Carlson, E., Egeland, B., & Sroufe, L. A. (1991). Patterns of individual adaptation across childhood. *Development and Psychopathology, 3,* 445–460.

Ursache, A., Blair, C., & Raver, C. C. (2012). The promotion of self-regulation as a means of enhancing school readiness and early achievement in children at risk for school failure. *Child Development Perspectives, 6,* 122–128.

van den Boom, D. C. (1994). The influence of temperament and mothering on attachment and exploration: An experimental manipulation of sensitive responsiveness among lower-class mothers with irritable infants. *Child Development, 65,* 1457–1477.

van Zeijl, J., Mesman, J., Van IJzendoorn, M. H., Bakermans-Kranenburg, M.

J., Juffer, F., Stolk, M. N., et al. (2006). Attachment-based intervention for enhancing sensitive discipline in mothers of 1- to 3-year-old children at risk for externalizing behavior problems: A randomized controlled trial. *Journal of Consulting and Clinical Psychology, 74*(6), 994–1005.

Welsh, J. A., Nix, R. L., Blair, C., Bierman, K. L., & Nelson, K. E. (2010). The development of cognitive skills and gains in academic school readiness for children from low-income families. *Journal of Educational Psychology, 102*(1), 43–53.

Willcutt, E. G., Doyle, A. E., Nigg, J. T., Faraone, S. V., & Pennington, B. F. (2005). Validity of the executive function theory of attention-deficit/hyperactivity disorder: A meta-analytic review. *Biological Psychiatry, 57,* 1336–1346.

Zelazo, P. D., Muller, U., Frye, D., & Marcovitch, S. (2003). The development of executive function in early childhood. *Monographs of the Society for Research in Child Development, 68*(3, Serial No. 274).

Zhai, F., Raver, C. C., & Li-Grining, C. (2011). *Can classroom-based interventions reduce teachers' job stressors? Evidence from a cluster-randomized controlled trial in Head Start settings.* Manuscript submitted for publication.

CHAPTER 7

Temperament as a Tool in Promoting Early Childhood Development

John E. Bates

This chapter describes possible applications of temperament concepts in promoting child development. Temperament concepts, prominent in theories about the origins of children's social and academic behavior characteristics, pertain to individual differences in emotional reactivity and effortful self-regulation (Rothbart & Bates, 2006). Temperament characteristics are linked to biological substrates and are present early in life. They are relatively stable across development, but also may show some development (Bates, Schermerhorn, & Goodnight, 2010) and predict child adjustment (Rothbart & Bates, 2006). To illustrate how temperament concepts can be practically useful, this chapter considers what temperament does in development and how it is defined and measured.

Temperament plays a complex role in children's social development. Temperament may influence caregiving patterns; caregiving patterns may influence change in temperament, or at least its expression; it may directly influence child adjustment; and temperament and caregiving may interact in some ways to influence adjustment (Bates, Schermerhorn, & Petersen, 2012). Temperament could affect the child's experience by influencing the caregiving environment in an active way, such as by shaping the parents' behavior, and could also influence it by shaping the child's cognitive and emotional processing of experiences. As Ellis and Boyce (2008) have argued, particular temperament traits could predispose a child to develop problems in a poor environment but develop better than other children in a good environment. Previous authors have offered insightful educational and clinical applications (e.g., McClowry, Rodriguez, & Koslowitz, 2008; Cameron, Hansen, & Rosen, 1989; Keogh, 2003; Martin, 1989). The current chapter offers more precisely targeted applications, based on the emerging research on how temperament and the environment interact to predict children's adjustment.

Before considering temperament in detail, it may be helpful to consider why we should do so: Is temperament worth it? Temperament concepts do help explain individual differences in child development, but this does not automatically mean that we should invest in them. Temperament-based interventions are plausible, I argue, but they are not necessarily easy to implement. I have learned this with my graduate-student clinicians in a parent behavioral training program for families with oppositional children. Perhaps we could just try harder to find more socially gifted caregivers instead of adding to the training demands of already busy caregivers. Very effective caregivers already, without special training, take advantage of implicit concepts of temperament, effectively adapting their practice to children with diverse personalities and abilities.

Although we certainly should try to recruit caregivers who are naturally effective, this is only a partial answer to providing effective caregiving for challenging children. Such natural talents (whether born or bred) are relatively rare and in demand throughout society, so it is unlikely we would be able to recruit significantly higher numbers of such caregivers. As Rusby, Smolkowski, and Jones (2009) argue in proposing a study of home child care, caregivers can be offered a number of effective strategies, and temperament's implications for adjustment outcomes might be moderated by what the caregivers do. Fortunately, more typical caregivers are often effective, too, especially with the many children with relatively easy temperaments, and sometimes even with those with difficult temperaments. This chapter, using the emerging literature on temperament's interactions with developmental environments, argues that caregivers might be able to adapt caregiving by using temperament tools, or strategies based on a child's temperament, to promote child development.

Temperament tools need further development—the science of applying temperament tools is not far enough advanced to offer detailed, proven strategies. However, temperament tools do show promise. Considerable research has been done, especially in recent years, on the meanings of temperament differences in children.

Assuming, then, that temperament is worth the effort, the first task is to determine the goal of a practical use of temperament. The key goal envisioned here is applied research on growth-promoting and risk-buffering caregiving of young children from low-income families, toward the aims of improved academic and social adjustment outcomes. Since caregiving is the focus, we should first consider strategies used by caregivers that might be amenable to adaptations involving temperament.

Caregiving and Temperament

Caregiving addresses the child's immediate physical, social, and cognitive needs in the context of the child's overarching need to develop. Development can be seen as an integrated, dynamic process (Smith & Breazeal, 2007). For example, a child learning to follow adults' directives such as "Bring me teddy bear" could represent development with motor, socioemotional, and cognitive–language components. Each of these components could pertain critically to the other components. Child temperament might shape and affect the efficacy of caregiving efforts in all domains, including physical, social, and cognitive-developmental. This is the case whether the caregiver's actions in response to temperament are intuitive or deliberate. Sometimes the effects may be positive, as in mothers giving more warmth and attention to a fussy baby than to an average baby (Bates, Olson, Pettit, & Bayles, 1982). Sometimes, they may be negative, as in mothers engaging in more conflict sequences with difficult than with average toddlers (Lee & Bates, 1985).

If temperament is related to caregiving characteristics, as at least some studies indicate (Bates et al., 2012), and if these caregiving characteristics are related to child adjustment outcomes, as many studies show (Rothbaum & Weisz, 1994), then it is reasonable to hypothesize that temperament can have some important influences on children's lives. Influences would be partly through the qualities of caregiving that children elicit, and partly through how different children respond differently to a given kind of caregiving. The outcome would be the trajectory of child adjustment that consists of the child's typical daily transactions with family and other caregivers, teachers, and peers. Findings suggest that child temperament effects upon caregiver behavior are generally small, but this does not mean that temperament has trivial effects. Small differences in child and caregiver dispositions can have cumulative and trajectory-shaping powers (Dodge et al., 2009). Children's temperament characteristics might, through developmental cascades of small influences upon caregiver actions and responses to caregiving, add a substantial force to the development of behavior problems versus positive adjustment.

In effective caregiving, interactions meet the immediate biological and psychosocial needs of the child but also in the longer term, build language, cognitive, and social skills. Most children experience effective caregivers. Nevertheless, even caring adults sometimes find themselves working harder and experiencing less success with particular children. Temperament concepts may help in such instances.

The best understood caregiving context for temperament's influence is parenting. At the broadest level, there are findings of adverse temperament qualities being associated with less ideal parenting, and positive temperament qualities being associated with more ideal parenting (Bates et al., 2012). Mothers do not consistently appear to be influenced by difficult child temperament in their observed warmth and control behaviors at the infancy stage, but by toddlerhood they do appear to be influenced to a moderate degree. Teachers make a lot of decisions about children every day, and some of these decisions would have to be influenced by the teachers' perceptions of children's temperament (Keogh, 2003). Some evidence supports this supposition. Teachers of school-age children are influenced from modest to moderate degrees by child temperament in their warmth and control behaviors (Martin, 1989; Keogh, 2003; Rudasill & Rimm-Kaufman, 2009), in mostly positive ways but sometimes negative ways. A positive effect, such as the teacher giving a temperamentally impulsive child more praise than more well-regulated children, may in the long run be positive or negative, depending on whether it is part of a strategy that effectively builds the child's capacity for skills such as sustained attention.

Successful handling of temperament–environment conflicts, as with successful handling of other conflicts, promotes children's growth. The majority of children develop well despite having some conflicts with the environment and some deficits in environmental resources, but still, substantial numbers have difficulties at multiple steps. As an early step in envisioning temperament applications to caregiving, I suggest particular applications of temperament concepts, offered as research ideas. The ideas are promising, but they would need testing in good prevention science research. If early conflicts involving temperament are resolved more effectively, then temperament does not have to forecast behavior problems. In some cases, it may be crucial to offer extra support to the children whose temperaments might make them less likely to naturally elicit that support, especially in challenging environments. In other cases, it may be more crucial to offer less support, or a different kind of support, to children who are too good at eliciting protective support.

Further Defining Temperament

Temperament is a rubric for describing biologically based, early appearing, stable individual differences in reactivity and self-regulation. As detailed in the chapter by Rothbart and Bates (2006) and a monograph by Rothbart (2011), it has been appreciated for millennia that children have genetic, neural-developmental, psychophysiological, and behavioral variations, and these variations may be summarized in a cross-level way by temperament concepts. Biological factors are involved in differences in emotional reactions, and differences in emotional reactions are closely involved in children's psychosocial adjustment. Biological factors are also involved in differences in self-regulatory cognition and skills that may have even greater connections to adjustment. Emotional expressions are partly a function of self-regulatory traits, too. Part of what makes temperament so useful in developmental models is that it appears relatively early in life and is relatively stable across time (Rothbart & Bates, 2006). However, not all relevant differences are apparent from the beginning of life. The most important example involves differences in self-regulation traits that appear most clearly in late infancy and in toddlerhood. Nevertheless, despite the complexities, temperament concepts provide relatively simple ways of talking about how children differ in their responses.

Standard lists of temperament boil down to three to five dimensions, with some variations depending on developmental stage. This condensation reflects substantial assessment and factor-analytic research (Rothbart & Bates, 2006; Mervielde & De Pauw, 2012). During infancy the key dimensions are (1) negative emotionality, which includes fear, sadness, and frustration/irritability; (2) surgency/extraversion, which includes approach, expressions of joy, activity level, and pleasure in high-intensity events; and (3) orienting/regulation, which includes duration of orienting, cuddliness, soothability, and pleasure in low-intensity events (Rothbart & Bates, 2006). In the first half year, negative emotionality is not well differentiated into its components, but in the second half year, there are clear differences between fearful and angry negative emotionality traits. This is important because the biological systems underlying these two aspects of negative emotionality are at least partially distinct (Rothbart, 2011; Rothbart & Bates, 2006). Fearfulness—as when a child hides behind a caregiver when meeting someone new—is related to Gray's (1991) behavioral inhibition system, a set of neural circuits processing information about possible punishers or dangers, with the behavioral output being inhibition or withdrawal. Anger—as when a child strikes someone who has taken a toy—is often related to frustration, which is related to Gray's behavioral approach system, a set of neural circuits processing information about possible rewards, with the behavioral output being approach, or positive goal pursuit. Frustration responds to blockage of goal pursuit, and may activate not only aggressive approach responses but also rage (related to a third neural system: the fight/flight system). Across the second year, the most notable development is that the infancy-era orienting/regulation dimension becomes effortful control/self-regulation. Frontal circuits that allow the young child to direct attention in an effortful way develop, and the child becomes able to inhibit a dominant response tendency in favor of a subdominant response (Rothbart & Bates, 2006). To the extent that children can direct attention away from attractive or frightening stimuli, they are better able to self-manage their emotional responses to cues for approach and inhibition, and thus independently avoid problematic behaviors. The various genetic processes underlying the neural systems and the neural systems themselves operate in a complex, dynamic equilibrium, just as psychological processes do. Children differ in the relative activity of these emerging biological systems, and thus the behavior differences that we call temperament emerge.

The ancient notion of temperament is of a mixing of biological factors (Rothbart, 2011). We used to think of the biological factors as the four humors: black bile, yellow bile, blood, and phlegm. Now we think of numbers of neurons in particular regions, synaptic connections, and the activity of hormones and neurotransmitters, all supported by the activity of genes in interaction with the many layers of the environment. Many of us like to have a biological image of what underlies the behavior differences we call temperament. But ultimately, for practitioners, the most important guide for practice is the assessment of children's behavior patterns.

Assessing Temperament

Temperament dimensions can be assessed through parent or caregiver reports on standard questionnaires. The specific questionnaire to be used depends on the particular constructs of interest. In my own research with toddlers, I regularly use two questionnaires. I use the toddler form of the Infant Characteristics Questionnaire (Bates, Freeland, & Lounsbury, 1979; Bates & Bayles, 1984; Bates, Pettit, Dodge, & Ridge, 1998), which assesses constructs that are of particular interest in my work on development of behavior problems, including difficultness (i.e., general negative emotionality and negative demands for caregiver attention), unadaptability (i.e., discomfort in novel situations, such as a new person), and resistance to control (i.e., unmanageability, unresponsive to social cues to stop approach behavior). Also, I use a much longer questionnaire, a form of Rothbart's Infant Behavior Questionnaire (the Children's Behavior Questionnaire; Rothbart, Ahadi, Hershey, & Fisher, 2001) that models the big domain of temperament with many facets, but which also can be reduced to the broad factors of surgency/extraversion (i.e., approach, high-intensity pleasure, activity level, and nonshyness), negative affectivity (i.e., discomfort, fear, anger/frustration, sadness, and nonsoothability), and effortful control (i.e., inhibitory control, attentional focusing, low-intensity pleasure, and perceptual sensitivity).

The measures used in an early childhood prevention science research project would depend on the constructs considered important for children's adaptations to the caregiving situations and for caregivers' adaptations to the children. Evidence supports using parents and other caregivers and teachers as sources of information about their children's temperament. On average, caregivers' reports converge with one another to moderate degrees—correlations between mother and teacher are typically in the .20 to .40 range, although sometimes lower, with mother–father correlations sometimes in the .50+ range. There are even some small but plausibly nonzero correlations between the ratings of parents and those of observers (Bates, 1989; Rothbart & Bates, 1998; Rothbart & Bates, 2006). Altogether, findings add up to substantial support for the validity of the measures, especially allowing for (1) differences between situations that would affect child behavior (e.g., mother vs. father at home vs. teacher at school), (2) differences in a rater's amount of experience with this child and other children in the relevant situations, and (3) differences in raters' interpretations of items in the questionnaires. Nevertheless, there is no clear biological reason why children should be expected to be perfectly consistent across these measurement conditions, even if one could produce a perfectly reliable measurement. There appear to be probabilistic elements at every level of a biological system, even though the whole system shows coherence. Another way of putting this is that all temperament measures include a component of error (Bates & Bayles, 1984). The error is not just in the measure but probably also in the child (e.g., acting in a frustrated way on one occasion and in the next, very similar one, not acting upset). As measures add together, however, the errors cancel each other out, yielding a more "true" picture of the child. In this spirit, it is widely recommended (Kagan & Fox, 2006; Rothbart & Bates, 2006) that both parents and teachers complete questionnaires, and whenever possible, that questionnaires be supplemented by direct observations in multiple situations.

An important guide to a measure's meaning is the research evidence on its convergent and divergent validity. Using multiple measures allows for clarification by comparison. When modern temperament measures were first being developed, a number of studies used naturalistic observation to assess temperament, such as during home observations (e.g., Bates & Bayles, 1984). Most observational measurements of temperament in recent years have employed structured situations, usually done in a laboratory, such as when a child is exposed to an unfamiliar, moving robot (e.g., Kochanska, Aksan, & Joy, 2007). One can triangulate on meaningful individual differences in children by considering multiple measures in both naturalistic and structured settings (Bates & Bayles, 1984). For example, one might measure children's initial responses to the laboratory (or clinical) situation or the arrival of an observer at the home, both in the dimension of inhibition and attraction to the novel stimuli. Because some qualities are difficult for observers to see, such as characteristic response to family stress or mother unresponsiveness, one would also ask multiple caregivers for ratings of the child's temperament.

In our work we tend to use two different kinds of observational measures of temperament. The first is structured lab episodes that might elicit interest, joy, fear, and frustration. A widely employed set of such episodes is that of the Laboratory Temperament Assessment Battery (LabTAB) (Goldsmith & Rothbart, 1992). Typically, such episodes are video recorded and then carefully coded. The second is a questionnaire that asks observers, after each visit (usually to the home), to rate the temperament-relevant behaviors seen in the visit. This is not a highly refined method, but it is a relatively economical way to get an observational measure. Such ratings converged with temperament as seen by the primary caregiver (Bates & Bayles, 1984). Much more work is needed on the specific dimensions assessed in this type of measure and on the kinds of observer training that would be best.

Choosing Assessment Methods

Measures should be selected to assess specific temperament constructs of interest, but a handful of temperament scales broadly cover the major domains that are actively considered in current research. A number of different measures have achieved a substantial enough degree of validation to be readily interpretable. Measures of temperament do have validity but they do not necessarily all mean the same thing, even when the names of the scales are similar. The Big Three and Big Five factor-analytic work has provided a handy, well-researched organizing framework for comparisons among temperament constructs (Caspi & Shiner, 2006; Lemery, Goldsmith, Klinnert, & Mrazek, 1999; Mervielde & De Pauw, 2012; Rothbart & Bates, 2006). In selecting a measure, it is good to consider the extent to which it is likely that the specific scales represent more than just a narrow point in time or psychological space. This is partly a function of amount of observation and breadth of situations sampled, but even some short assessments can provide diagnostic value. Studies showing convergence between temperament ratings by caregivers and observers and even physiological measures support the argument that caregiver ratings and observational measures have some validity (Rothbart & Bates, 2006). In the current state of the art, it makes sense to use caregiver questionnaires in many studies, and whenever feasible, both questionnaire measures and observational or structured tests.

Implications of Temperament for Caregiving and Child Adjustment

Effects of temperament on caregiving are important because they might ultimately affect children's adjustment. In recent reviews we have considered how children's temperament differences might affect the qualities of caregiving they receive, especially in the family (Bates & Pettit, 2007; Bates et al., 2010, 2012; Rothbart & Bates, 2006). Here I give a brief overview of some key relationships between temperament and adjustment. Sometimes one would like to think of temperament and adjustment as fundamentally separate things. However, temperament could be conceptualized as a value-neutral set of personality characteristics that create a bias toward a certain kind of behavior, as in a fearless child becoming dangerously or annoyingly heedless of limits and, at the same time, not becoming annoyingly overdependent. It is not customary to think of very young children's behaviors in terms of adjustment or psychopathology. However, we could also think about adjustment or pathology as a set of continuous characteristics that emerge as organized patterns of adaptation in the same ways that other individual difference characteristics of children emerge (Sroufe, 1979). The components may not mean the same thing at an early stage, but many of them are present in some form, such as an early bias to attend to information about possible threats. They organize into more advanced forms as the child's repertoire and opportunities grow, but an essential core of the child remains visible (Patterson, Reid, & Dishion, 1992). Temperament differences are not the same as behavior problems, but they do appear to provide developmental core traits that can be transformed, via experience, into behavior problems.

Particular temperament traits may be viewed as dispositions for adaptive behavior in a *differential linkage pattern*. Findings of longitudinal and cross-sectional studies support a pattern in which the several main temperament traits are most relevant to conceptually analogous traits in the domain of adjustment (Bates, 1989; Bates & Bayles, 1984; Rothbart & Bates, 1998, 2006; Saudino, 2005). *Fearful temperament* is a disposition to respond with inhibition and distress to possible threats. Children who are high on this trait tend to notice and evade risks more than other children. The differential linkage is that early fearfulness is associated with later internalizing problems in adjustment, such as social withdrawal from peers and symptoms of anxiety. As a clinical and theoretical speculation, such development would be especially likely when the fearful temperament is also accompanied by a reasonably high desire to control action, which might command protection from caregivers.

The desire to control is actually a facet of *extraversion or surgency* (Rothbart & Bates, 2006). Children, even at an early age, like to make things happen, as can be seen by the delight shown by a young infant who discovers control of a crib mobile (Watson, 1972). Some children appear to have a stronger disposition to control social attention than others (Spivack, Marcus, & Swift, 1986). This appears to be a component of how mothers explain difficult infants who characteristically fuss and cry a lot—they are seeking attention (Bates, 1989). At an early age, caregivers seem to tolerate this with some forbearance. There is, after all, little else young babies can do to meet their attachment and other regulatory needs (Ainsworth, Blehar, Waters, & Wall, 1978). However, as children get older, their caregivers expect more positive bids and more independence. When children make a lot of negative bids, by age 2 years they may have more conflict with their caregivers (Lee & Bates, 1985; Bates et al., 2010, 2012).

Difficultness is a third, major temperament concept with relevance to adjustment. It is defined in various ways, but according to the mothers we asked (Bates et al., 1979) the core facet is *negative emotionality,* which could contain both fearful and frustrated forms of distress, and which has been found to be equally associated with both externalizing and internalizing problems (Bates, 1989; Rothbart & Bates, 2006; Saudino, 2005). Sometimes negative emotionality is measured as general negative emotionality that involves irritability, expression of distress from fear, social demand, and expression of frustration. Temperament scales and tests, like other psychological tests, rarely tap just one specific theoretically separate element of temperament.

Finally, *effortful control* is another major temperament concept. Early effortful control measures have predicted later adjustment, especially externalizing problems. Effortful control is often evident in the self-regulation of tendencies to approach stimulating objects. In theory (Rothbart & Bates, 2006), effortful control can also be involved in self-regulation of avoidance behavior, too, but there is less empirical evidence of such processes in predicting adjustment.

In brief, the differential linkage pattern suggests that adjustment outcomes of temperament reflect continuity of temperament types—with temperamental tendencies to be fearful in novel situations predicting later internalizing problems, tendencies to be dysregulated in approach predicting later externalizing problems, and tendencies to be high in negative emotionality predictive of both internalizing and externalizing problems.

Caregivers' Responses to Temperament

The adaptive implications of temperament also involve how caregivers respond. We reviewed the evidence on temperament and parenting in a recent chapter (Bates et al., 2012); studies show correlations between child temperament measures and parenting measures. The most compelling evidence of temperament effects is longitudinal and involves controls for initial levels of parenting behavior. This is more feasible in studies of older children than infants, because the parenting repertoire changes rapidly as the child's behavioral repertoire changes from infancy into early childhood. Only a few of the studies have been longitudinal studies, and they are mixed on whether the child's traits lead to parent behavior. Correlational and a few experimental studies do show, nevertheless, a possibility that caregivers' warmth may be elicited by child positive emotionality traits, and that caregivers' negative reactions may be elicited by child negative emotionality/difficultness. Caregivers and teachers typically have less extensive relations with children than do parents, and they strive to maintain a warmly but effectively controlled environment, with room for creativity and growth in child autonomy (Bierman, Nix, Greenberg, Blair, & Domitrovich, 2008; Pianta, Barnett, Burchinal, & Thornburg, 2009). Therefore, one might expect that professional and other secondary caregivers would typically be less susceptible to the effects of child temperament than the average parent. Caregivers are not blank slates for the child to write upon, just as children are not blank slates for the caregivers. Caregivers have many ideas about how to meet children's needs. Nevertheless, based on findings with parents, we could predict that the more tractable and positively emotional children will easily elicit cooperative relations with most caregivers; the more highly fearful children will elicit protective responses, perhaps along with warmth, support, effective exposure, demands, and irritation; and children higher on negative emotionality, especially anger (related to surgency), would sometimes elicit defensive affect, along with effective and ineffective efforts to control the child (Bates et al., 2012). Further research is needed to evaluate the possible effects of temperament listed here, including systematic comparisons of different developmental eras, and some of those studies will need to consider child temperament in child care situations. The prediction is that the findings with parents will generalize, perhaps to an attenuated degree, to findings with other caregivers and teachers. Moreover, if such effects are found, they may prove to act as a mediator in the model of how temperament becomes behavior problem versus positive adjustment. Based on the research we have described, we would expect to find that some elements of children's social experience with caregivers in day care are responses to the child's previous traits, and that the same would apply to peers in the day care.

Now, considering the other direction of influence in the transactional process of children and caregivers, caregivers could also influence the expression and development of child temperament. Studies, including ones with longitudinal designs with controls for initial levels of child temperament, support the possibility that parental warmth and effective control (vs. irritability) promote child positive emotion and self-regulated behavior and reduce expressions of negative emotion and dysregulated behaviors (Bates et al., 2012). I would expect similar effects for nonparental caregivers upon children's expressions of emotionality and self-regulation. More research is needed on how transactional influences of child and caregiver unfold in the development of adjustment. This will not be the whole story, however. More research is also needed on how child temperament and caregiving moderate one another's associations with child adjustment outcomes. What we have already learned about temperament–caregiving interactions and what we might learn through practical experiments is the focus of the rest of the chapter.

Implications of the Interaction of Temperament and Caregiving Environment

The temperament-related effects described previously, between temperament and caregiving, between temperament and behavioral adjustment, and between caregiving and changes in temperament expression, are main effects in the statistical models of the role of temperament. That is, the temperament variables are associated with the other variables in direct, linear ways, such as for every standard deviation unit a baby's negative emotionality is above average there is a certain increase in extra caregiving attention. The main, direct effects involving child temperament, however, are of limited value in and of themselves. Although they are interesting and logically consistent, the relationships are not so strong or consistently found that one would assume that they were present in every child–caregiver relationship. Nor do they directly imply a particular course of action to counter the effects, other than "Don't be adversely influenced by the child's adverse characteristics" or "Do explicitly counter the child's adverse characteristics and encourage positive characteristics." This allows the possibility that the implications of temperament for child development could depend on how the caregiver deals with the child's temperament or how the child's temperament affects developmental implications of caregivers' actions. That is, child temperament and caregiving variables may interact. If we can observe caregiving conditions in which the child's temperamental disposition to behavior problems is and is not associated with behavior problems, we can develop hypotheses about specific caregiving approaches that might be effective social development-promoting responses to the child's temperamental presses.

The recent literature has been suggesting patterns of Child Temperament × Caregiving Interaction in the development of child adjustment (see Bates & Pettit, 2007; Bates et al., 2010, 2012; Rothbart & Bates, 2006; Saudino, 2005; Wachs, 2000, for reviews). For the present purposes, this chapter points to five specific interaction patterns in the literature that could have promise as tools for caregivers—effective ways to work with the child's temperament.

As a foundation for conceptual tools based on the five moderator patterns, we consider some basic principles about the use of temperament concepts: First, how we understand a problem affects what we try to do about it. When parents and teachers have been given temperament explanations for conflicts with their children they have, anecdotally at least, altered their emotions and actions in dealing with challenging behaviors. According to family therapy models, when one puts a familiar sequence in a new frame, it becomes more likely that one will act differently. Many of our standard professional frames are pathology oriented, as when a child is described as having attention-deficit/hyperactivity disorder. Such frames are often insufficient for inspiring effective change. Temperament frames are associated with the pathology frames, but they have independent status, in that they might or might not signify or lead to a behavior problem (Chess & Thomas, 1984). The frame of temperament helps one see the child's tendencies as basic personality that could forecast psychopathology rather than pathology in itself. A second principle is that temperament consists of multiple different concepts operating at multiple levels of child functioning; it is complex. But luckily, if one can keep in mind three or four dimensions of temperament and know what we have learned about them so far, one can have a pretty rich but not overwhelmingly complex model of temperament. The third principle is that temperament concepts are models, not reality. Temperament concepts can help us notice things in reality that we might otherwise miss. The challenge is to avoid letting a model bias us against seeing other important things or letting the model be confused with reality. Temperament interventions can be done in multiple ways, and it will take experimentation to learn the most effective ways for different kinds of caregivers to use them. Given that the most important caregiving approaches would involve authoritative relationships (warmth + effective control), temperament-based interventions could help caregivers interact more positively with a given child, manage more effectively, and be more educationally stimulating. But what specifically might temperament have to do with achieving this caregiving profile? Five interactions between temperament and environment in predicting child adjustment are listed next, along with thoughts toward developing specific caregiver tools. Theoretical and empirical bases are described in more detail in recent chapters (Bates & Pettit, 2007; Bates et al., 2010, 2012; Rothbart & Bates, 2006).

1. *Fearful × Gentle (vs. Harsh) Control → learning the rules and internal self-regulation of behavior.* Kochanska and her colleagues have replicated findings that suggest that children who are high in fearfulness in novel situations are more sensitive to the gentleness of mothers' control techniques during toddlerhood than children who are less fearful in developing self-control (Kochanska, 1997; Kochanska et al., 2007). Even a novelty-anxious child is likely to misbehave sometimes, and these events can be the opportunity for learning about the values and rules of the social group. When mothers' control is harsh, fearful children are slower to develop their internalized self-control than when their mothers' control is gentle. The harshness of mother's control does not matter much for the relatively fearless children. Kochanska's interpretation of this, based on Hoffman's (2000) socialization model, is that harshness produces too much arousal for the fearful child to be able to cognitively process the lessons of the discipline event. Gentle control, on the other hand, leads to more optimal arousal, which provides opportunities to learn from the discipline encounter. Repeated over many such encounters, over many months

of development, such learning or failure to learn could amount to notice-able differences in self-regulation. Thus, it can be hypothesized that it is particularly important to emphasize gentle forms of control when dealing with a temperamentally anxious child. Anecdotally, I have found that this emphasis helps parents deal with oppositional children who are also high in anxiety.

The potential tool: By understanding the model of temperamental fear-fulness and by watching levels of child arousal in management situations, caregivers can distinguish the needs of an annoying or uncooperative child from the child's whims or neurotic needs. When children are high in fear, this is a cue to the caregiver to be firm, but gentle, keeping their arousal at a level where they will most effectively follow the expectations and will be most likely to learn from a conflict and its resolution.

2. *Fearful* × *Not-Too-Nice, Firm Parenting → getting on with it, not being too inhibited.* Another replicated contribution involving early nov-elty fear is the finding that children who are high in novelty distress in infancy, who would otherwise be at elevated risk for internalizing problems via developing a pattern of behavioral inhibition, end up with less behav-ioral inhibition if they are treated in what I characterize as a "not-too-nice way," with relatively strong control (Arcus, 2001; Park, Belsky, Putnam, & Crnic, 1997). The not-too-nice parent is not harsh. Harsh and denigrating parenting may work in the opposite direction (Rubin, Hastings, Stewart, Henderson, & Chen, 1997). One could hypothesize that effective caregiv-ing would desensitize the child to challenges and not reinforce the child's coercively avoidant expressions of novelty distress, and that this would reduce the child's fearful reactions over time. It could be hypothesized that the caregiver who firmly insists on the child adhering to the same rules as others (although in a nonharsh way) and who firmly encourages the child to get past inhibitions due to novel elements of otherwise instructive situations (Chess & Thomas, 1984), would help the child to develop more adaptive ways to deal with novelty than would occur through avoidance and using caregivers as shields.

The potential tool: If a child is intensely reactive to novel people and objects, it may be best not to let the child's reactions and avoidance maneuvers become coercive influences on the caregivers. One would avoid harshness in any event, but one might focus on maintaining a campaign of exposing such a child to mild challenges with pressure and supports to master such challenges. Children sometimes need protection, but children with temperamentally intense and steady reactions to new people, places, and things might actually need less than they demand. A reminder: Here, even if one is managing the child with a matter-of-fact or brusque style, it is important to be well attuned to the child. The caregiver would then be able to expose the child to levels of novelty and social demand that might evoke some distress and resistance but that are tolerable. On occasions when a child gets too upset, it may be time to nurture, reset, and plan the next exposure trial. Over many events, caregiver support and pressure are gradually reduced as the child is more successfully self-managing.

3. *Fearful × Impulsive × Family Stress → risk for externalizing*. This potential tool is more complex and more speculative, based only on two not-yet-published studies of our group. It is based on a model of inhibitory and approach behaviors as products of processing of cues for punishment and cues for reward. This model uses Gray's (1991) model of the behavioral inhibition system (BIS), the behavioral approach system (BAS), and the nonspecific arousal system (NAS), influenced by the activation of the BIS and BAS. It also uses the Newman and Wallace (1993) model of response modulation through attention to peripheral cues during pursuit of goals in mixed-incentive situations. In mixed-incentive situations both punishments and rewards are available, as in most social situations. Some individuals become insensitive to a "stop" cue when they are hot on the pursuit of some goal, such as a young girl playing with an interesting statuette even after her father has told her to put it down. The theoretical model here is of a profile of temperament in which a child is high in both fearful and impulsive temperament traits. Where would this combination of traits be especially risky? We reasoned that it would be in stressful, anxiety-evoking environments, frequently activating the child's fear system, and perhaps also reducing parents' capacity for coregulation efforts with their children. We predicted that in families that experienced high levels of stress, such as from economic problems, illnesses, and relationship interruptions, and in which children had both high-unadaptable (novelty distress) and high resistance to control (impulsive approach) tendencies in early childhood, the children were especially likely to have later externalizing behavior problems. We expected that such children would have chronically high levels of nonspecific arousal as the result of the consequences of family stress in activating the child's BIS, but they would also have relatively high approach and dominance tendencies and/or low self-regulation, so the high levels of nonspecific activation would serve to increase the likelihood of dominant, approach behaviors, or aggressive and uncooperative behaviors. It is also possible that the child's chronically aroused anxiety might interfere with the learning of discipline lessons. In fact, we found especially elevated levels of externalizing behavior when children were high in both unadaptability and resistance to control and were living in stressful families. We found this in two different longitudinal data sets, when modeled in relatively simple models using moderated multiple regression (Bates, Sandy, Dodge, & Pettit, 2000), and when modeled in relatively complex models using structural equations and with teacher reports of externalizing outcomes (Schermerhorn, Bates, Goodnight, Lansford, Dodge, & Pettit, 2011).

How might a caregiver most effectively respond to such a child? One possibility is to focus on helping the child deal with anxiety and nonspecific arousal. A supportive relationship would be the caregiver's goal—responsive to the child's developmental and basic needs, but not to coercive whims, such as angry and fearful demands to stop exposure to social demands, as with the previously mentioned tools. Caregivers know that children can gain much stress reduction from successful interactions with peers and supportive adults. Another focus would be on helping the child to develop better self-regulation. Toward this, in our clinic for families of oppositional children, we sometimes encourage parents to give children tasks that require them to make something or to wait for manageable lengths of time, such as "Please play by yourself for 5 minutes, and then I'll play with you again." Also toward better self-regulation, we often encourage parents to rearrange sleep schedules for their children. This is partly based on research that suggests that children's sleep deficits can relate to their adjustment at preschool, even independent of the effects of family stress and poor child management strategies (Bates, Viken, Alexander, Beyers, & Stockton, 2002). This effect is particularly strong for children high in temperamental resistance to control (Bates, Viken, Staples, & Williams, 2011; also see Goodnight, Bates, Staples, Pettit, & Dodge, 2007). Sleep loss may be viewed as a form of stress, based on Weissbluth's (1989) arguments, and improved sleep as a form of stress reduction. We have even been able to sometimes achieve such improved sleep in otherwise high-stress families, along with correspondingly better child self-regulation in child care or preschool. Much more research is needed (Staples & Bates, 2011), but perhaps some of that research can be in the form of thoughtful experiments in practical settings.

The possible tool: If dealing with a child from a family with high stress who is impulsive and also anxious, one can, of course, work directly on the child's ability to manage impulsive behavior (e.g., by reminding the child of rules, the usual gentle but firm control, executive function training exercises). But this may go faster if the child's overall burden of stress and anxiety is reduced first. This can be done by parents' solving some of their problems, and even if these issues are not solved, by helping the parent to create a zone of warmth and security around the child, especially around child sleep times. Better sleep schedules might allow the child to cope in more cognitively mature ways and elicit more warm, supportive, and fun interactions from others.

4. *Fearless × Positive, Securely Attached Parenting → less externalizing, better "conscience."* The important, complementary piece to Kochanska et al.'s (2007) finding of the Gentle Discipline × Fearful Temperament interaction in prediction of conscience development is the finding that toddlers who are relatively fearless in novel situations, who are highly

approaching, appear to internalize social norms through a different channel than fearful children do. The fearless children do not develop self-control or conscience better with mothers who provide more gentle discipline than with those who are harsher. They do, however, develop self-control better with mothers who maintain a more warmly supportive, enjoyable, securely attached relationship with them. As Hoffman (2000) pointed out, one pathway to socialization is fear of negative consequences of rule violation, and another is desire to maintain a positive relationship. For the fearless child, it appears that the second pathway to socialization is the more important one. We fairly often see children in our clinic whose oppositional, aggressive behavior is accompanied by lack of inhibition in novel situations. An element of the standard parent behavioral training model that seems especially important for such children is Sheila Eyberg's practice of a regular, child-directed, one-on-one playtime (Bagner, Fernandez, & Eyberg, 2004). We ask the parent to provide choices of low-intensity activities that encourage the child's imagination and interactivity, with the parent following and joining in, for example, a game played with toy animals, dolls, small cars, building blocks, or low-mess art supplies. The parent is positively responsive and nondirective, and if the child becomes aggressive, the parent merely withholds attention and reengages when the child's behavior is back within bounds. Oppositional children in general are highly interested in getting responses from other people (Spivack et al., 1986), and this provides a low-conflict opportunity for that. It also provides a platform from which, on other occasions, parents can exercise powerful discipline techniques, such as time out from positive reinforcement, with the child trusting that the parent and child will also share enjoyment, and the current discipline issue being resolved with less effort at dominance by the child. This technique would not be implemented as such in a child care situation, but the teacher of such a fearless, high-approach child might be able to design a regular play session like the one described, involving well-chosen sets of other children to provide a teacher-led, conflict-preventive, fun experience of interactive and imaginative play. The regularity of these play sessions will be key to their value.

We have also seen cases where augmenting the child's own ability to engage in effortful self-control was important to improvement in child behavior. As in cases where the child is both slow to adapt to novelty and hard to manage, we have found that improvements in the child's sleep routine can be helpful in improving self-regulation in cases where the child is fearless, and this is supported by longitudinal research (Bernier, Carlson, Bordeleau, & Carrier, 2010). Aside from the direct effects of sleep on cognitive functioning, which theoretically allow the child to process social information more effectively, the improved sleep routine explicitly involves parents providing a secure relationship to facilitate the child letting go of vigilance (Staples & Bates, 2011; Dahl, 1996). The bedtime routine (which we organize into a "sleep train" and teach via a special video) includes a regular predictable routine that the child likes, such as bathing, pajamas, stories, and then snuggles before lights out. Fearless young children seem to respond well to this.

The possible tools: If dealing with a fearless, all-go, no-stop child, don't expect the usual expressions of disapproval or irritation to be sufficient, so stronger discipline (such as time out) will be necessary. However, as a fulcrum for the lever or stronger discipline, improving the positive aspect of the caregiver–child relationship is important. Take advantage of the child's capacity for enjoyment of social control by having predictable regular occasions where the child gets to lead in positive, mutually enjoyable ways. An oppositional child often plays poorly with other children, and we have usually emphasized one child with one parent, but in an analogous situation with a skilled caregiver and well-chosen peers, the child might find enough enjoyment and grow in capacity for true mutuality. Through such interactions, the fearless child gains interest in others' reactions and learns how to maintain the positive relationship by complying with others' wishes, too. The low-fear, high-approach child in a positive, mutually enjoyable relationship with a caregiver or peer may respond better to low-level discipline lessons in order to maintain the positive relationship. A secure attachment comes from the child's trusting that his or her needs will be met, and this not only involves needs for distress removing but also social and activity needs. Sometimes fearless children do not regularly elicit protective caregiving, but in a secure relationship their social and activity needs will be reliably met, even so. At the same time, this may not be sufficient if the fearless child is highly dysregulated. Such a child may need the help of explicit training in self-regulation skills (e.g., as in "executive function training" programs; e.g., Diamond, Barnett, Thomas, & Munro, 2007), or they may need longer and more regular sleep.

5. Impulsive × Firm Parenting → less externalizing. Children who are high in resistance to control are relatively unresponsive to social cues to inhibit approach behaviors such as "No, no, put that down!" They have elevated risk of showing high levels of externalizing behavior problems. The core challenge in resistant or unmanageable temperament is the lack of effortful control or presence of impulsivity. There is a lack of attention to cues for inhibition. However, we have found, in two separate longitudinal studies, that temperamentally resistant children with mothers active in controlling them are less likely to develop later externalizing problems than those with mothers who are not active in controlling them (Bates et al., 1998). Other studies (reviewed by Bates & Pettit, 2007; Bates et al., 2012) show related kinds of effects involving child self-regulation traits and relevant parenting qualities. We also found that when parents recognize that they have a problem with their child's behavior and they institute a campaign of greater involvement and control to solve the problem, these campaigns yield the biggest results with children who are high in temperamental resistance to control (Goodnight, Bates, Pettit, & Dodge, 2008). Further, we found that parental management practices matter more for the preschool adjustment of temperamentally resistant children (Bates et al., 2011). Prior to encountering these findings, we had been inclined to think of high levels of parental control as restrictiveness, which had been found to be associated with high levels of child behavior problems (Rothbaum & Weisz, 1994). However, by considering maternal control in the context of child temperament and over the course of development, we began to see controlling behavior as sometimes preventing child psychopathology. To apply this temperament–environment interaction pattern, we assess the caregivers' tendencies. If caregivers are already active in their control, we merely try to make that control more efficient—urging them to make their commands clear and heard by the child, picking their battles carefully, and using discipline techniques like withholding attention and time out in more precise ways. If they are inconsistent in their control, however, especially if they avoid control in many situations because they are afraid of setting off child tantrums or other coercive countercontrol efforts (Patterson et al., 1992), we put extra focus on helping them build chains of thought that support their discipline efforts. For example, a caregiver could think, "It's my job to give her active guidance on how to behave in this situation. If she gets mad, I can handle that. I will do one of the things I've practiced, like withhold attention." Also, as with children with other temperament profiles, we often find it useful to emphasize improvements in sleep routines. The child who is getting enough sleep may still have some impulsive and coercive behavior patterns, but it will be easier for them to learn the new expectations if they are well rested and more able to self-regulate their attention and actions. As mentioned, a regular sleep schedule matters more for the adjustment of preschoolers who are high on resistance to control than for those who are more manageable (Bates et al., 2011).

The possible tools: Impulsive children blocked from their goal pursuits often become frustrated and employ coercive countercontrol (e.g., tantrums, disruptive behavior), and in response, caregivers occasionally abandon demands. When caregivers act toward the child in subtly or obviously rejecting ways, or respond to child misbehavior in harsh ways, they may teach more advanced forms of coercion than socially motivated self-regulation and they lose many opportunities for socialization. A caregiver who knows that effective control is especially important for the later adjustment of an impulsive child has a strong rationale for consistent discipline, for persisting in the face of child resistance. Of course, the other elements of effective caregiving, such as warmth and fun, are also important with this kind of child, just as for the others mentioned previously. And finally, we have seen instances where improved sleep routines also appear to promote the child's ability to learn rules and self-regulate.

Conclusion: Implications for Early Development Programs

Child care research has shown that quantities and qualities of early child care have both beneficial and not-so-beneficial influences on young children's development (Pluess & Belsky, 2009). However, such main effects are only part of the story. Consistent with the Temperament × Parenting interaction research I have described, studies are starting to show that child temperament may affect how child care qualities help shape child development. Studies show that for children with high negative emotionality and unadaptability child care qualities matter more (Pluess & Belsky, 2009) and also less (De Schipper, Tavecchio, van IJzendoorn, & van Zeijl, 2004) than for easier children. Such findings have led to some good general suggestions about how to adapt caregiving according to child temperament. Crockenberg (2003) suggested that child care teachers use, essentially, a tag-team approach to maintain sensitive care and foster development of self-regulation with difficult children. Greenspan (2003) advised caregivers to make allowances for child reactivity in order to promote long chains of coregulated behavior. Further research, such as in experimental child care programs, is needed to evaluate these suggestions, as well as the possible tools suggested by the present chapter.

In conclusion, this chapter argues that temperament concepts can be useful in promoting good outcomes and preventing poor outcomes for children. This has been argued elsewhere (Crockenberg, 2003; McClowry et al., 2008; Carey & McDevitt, 1989), but the chapter goes further in suggesting five possible tools, based on Temperament × Environment interaction effects as well as the main effects of child temperament and caregiving environment. One value of a focus on the interactions between temperament and environment is that it allows a more targeted adaptation to challenging temperament than more universal interventions. The basic framework for these potential tools is from research on temperament in development, including a few experiments on how teaching temperament ideas may help in avoiding child problems (e.g., Cameron et al., 1989; McClowry, Snow, Tamis-LeMonda, & Rodriguez, 2010), and from the author's experience with families and teachers. The potential tools involve identification of developmental needs of children in connection with their temperament, plus suggestions for effective approaches to more challenging temperament characteristics. The five include (1) disciplining fearful children in gentle ways, which is fairly standard in high-quality caregiving, but still worth mention; (2) managing fearful children in firm, not-too-nice ways, which is a little more difficult than gentle control; (3) specially attending to children with the temperament profile of fearful plus resistant to control and living in stressed families, giving them, in addition to the standard gentle control, help in reducing their stress–anxiety burden and increasing self-regulation capacity, for example, with better sleep schedule or with executive function training; (4) managing fearless children within warm, involved, fun relationships, and taking advantage of such children's interest in learning discipline as part of learning how to maintain the positive relationships; and finally (5) actively managing and promoting self-regulation capacity with impulsive, high-approach children. Research on these tools could result in advances in effectiveness of caregiving in early childhood.

REFERENCES

Ainsworth, M. D. S., Blehar, M. C., Waters, E., & Wall, S. (1978). *Patterns of attachment: A psychological study of the Strange Situation*. Hillsdale, NJ: Erlbaum.

Arcus, D. (2001). Inhibited and uninhibited children: Biology in the social context. In T. D. Wachs & G. A. Kohnstamm (Eds.), *Temperament in context* (pp. 43–60). Mahwah, NJ: Erlbaum.

Bagner, D. M., Fernandez, M. A., & Eyberg, S. M. (2004). Parent–child interaction therapy and chronic illness: A case study. *Journal of Clinical Psychology in Medical Settings, 11*(1), 1–6.

Bates, J. E. (1989). Applications of temperament concepts. In G. A. Kohnstamm, J. E. Bates, & M. K. Rothbart (Eds.), *Temperament in childhood* (pp. 322–355). Chichester, UK: Wiley.

Bates, J. E., & Bayles, K. (1984). Objective and subjective components in mothers' perceptions of their children from age 6 months to 3 years. *Merrill-Palmer Quarterly, 30,* 111–130.

Bates, J. E., Freeland, C. B., & Lounsbury, M. L. (1979). Measurement of infant difficultness. *Child Development, 50,* 794–803.

Bates, J. E., Olson, S. L., Pettit, G. S., & Bayles, K. (1982). Dimensions of individuality in the mother–infant relationship at six months of age. *Child Development, 53,* 446–461.

Bates, J. E., & Pettit, G. S. (2007). Temperament, parenting, and socialization. In J. E. Grusec & P. D. Hastings (Eds.), *Handbook of socialization: Theory and research* (pp. 153–177). New York: Guilford Press.

Bates, J. E., Pettit, G. S., Dodge, K. A., & Ridge, B. (1998). Interaction of temperamental resistance to control and restrictive parenting in the development of externalizing behavior. *Developmental Psychology, 34*(5), 982–995.

Bates, J. E., Sandy, J. M., Dodge, K. A., & Pettit, G. S. (2000, October–November). *Child and adolescent adjustment as a function of child temperament and family stress*. Paper presented at the First Expert Workshop on Personality Psychology, Ghent University, Belgium.

Bates, J. E., Schermerhorn, A. C., & Goodnight, J. A. (2010). Temperament and personality through the lifespan. In M. E. Lamb & A. Freund (Eds.), *Handbook of lifespan development* (pp. 208–253). Hoboken, NJ: Wiley.

Bates, J. E., Schermerhorn, A. C., & Petersen, I. T. (2012). Temperament and parenting in developmental perspective. In M. Zentner & R. L. Shiner (Eds.), *Handbook of temperament*. New York: Guilford Press.

Bates, J. E., Viken, R. J., Alexander, D. B., Beyers, J., & Stockton, L. (2002). Sleep and adjustment in preschool children: Sleep diary reports by mothers relate to behavior reports by teachers. *Child Development, 73*(1), 62–74.

Bates, J. E., Viken, R. J., Staples, A. D., & Williams, N. (2011). *Children's temperament moderates the relationship between sleep and preschool adjustment*. Unpublished manuscript, Indiana University.

Bernier, A., Carlson, S. M., Bordeleau, S., & Carrier, J. (2010). Relations between physiological and cognitive regulatory systems: Infant sleep regulation and subsequent executive functioning. *Child Development, 81*(6), 1739–1752.

Bierman, K. L., Nix, R. L., Greenberg, M. T., Blair, C., & Domitrovich, C. E. (2008). Executive functions and school readiness intervention: Impact, moderation, and mediation in the Head Start REDI program. *Development and Psychopathology, 20*, 821–843.

Cameron, J. R., Hansen, R., & Rosen, D. (1989). Preventing behavioral problems in infancy through temperament assessment and parental support programs. In W. B. Carey & S. C. McDevitt (Eds.), *Clinical and educational applications of temperament research* (pp. 155–165). Berwyn, PA: Swets North America.

Carey, W. B., & McDevitt, S. C. (Eds.). (1989). *Clinical and educational applications of temperament research*. Berwyn, PA: Swets North America.

Caspi, A., & Shiner, R. L. (2006). Personality development. In W. Damon & R. Lerner (Series Eds.) & N. Eisenberg (Vol. Ed.), *Handbook of child psychology: Vol. 3. Social, emotional, and personality development* (6th ed., pp. 300–365). New York: Wiley.

Chess, S., & Thomas, A. (1984). *Origins and evolution of behavior disorders*. New York: Brunner/Mazel.

Crockenberg, S. C. (2003). Rescuing the baby from the bathwater: How gender and temperament (may) influence how child care affects child development. *Child Development, 74*(4), 1034–1038.

Dahl, R. (1996). The regulation of sleep and arousal: Development and psychopathology. *Development and Psychopathology, 8*(1), 3–27.

De Schipper, J. C., Tavecchio, L. W. C., van IJzendoorn, M. H., & van Zeijl, J. (2004). Goodness-of-fit in center day care: Relations of temperament, stability, and quality of care with the child's adjustment. *Early Childhood Research Quarterly, 19*, 257–272.

Diamond, A., Barnett, W. S., Thomas, J., & Munro, S. (2007, November). Preschool program improves cognitive control. *Science, 318*(30), 1387–1388.

Dodge, K. A., Malone, P. S., Lansford, J. E., Miller, S., Pettit, G. S., & Bates, J. E. (2009). A dynamic cascade model of the development of substance-use onset. *Monographs of the Society for Research in Child Development, 74*(3, Serial No. 294).

Ellis, B. J., & Boyce, W. T. (2008). Biological sensitivity to context. *Current Directions in Psychological Science, 17*, 183–187.

Goldsmith, H. H., & Rothbart, M. K. (1992). *Laboratory Temperament Assessment Battery (LAB-TAB—Pre- and Locomotor Versions*. University of Oregon, Eugene.

Goodnight, J. A., Bates, J. E., Pettit, G. S., & Dodge, K. A. (2008). Parents' campaigns to reduce their children's conduct problems: Interactions with temperamental resistance to control. *European Journal of Developmental Science,* 2(1/2), 100–119.

Goodnight, J. A., Bates, J. E., Staples, A. D., Pettit, G. S., & Dodge, K. A. (2007). Temperamental resistance to control increases the association between sleep problems and externalizing behavior development. *Journal of Family Psychology,* 21(1), 39–48.

Gray, J. A. (1991). The neuropsychology of temperament. In J. Strelau & A. Angleitner (Eds.), *Explorations in temperament: International perspectives on theory and measurement* (pp. 105–128) New York: Plenum Press.

Greenspan, S. I. (2003). Child care research: A clinical perspective. *Child Development,* 74(4), 1064–1068.

Hoffman, M. L. (2000). *Empathy and moral development: Implications for caring and justice.* New York: Cambridge University Press.

Kagan, J., & Fox, N. A. (2006). Biology, culture, and temperamental biases. In N. Eisenberg, W. Damon, & R. M. Lerner (Eds.), *Handbook of child psychology: Vol. 3. Social, emotional, and personality development* (6th ed., pp. 167–225). Hoboken, NJ: Wiley.

Keogh, B. (2003). *Temperament in the classroom.* Baltimore: Brookes.

Kochanska, G. (1995). Children's temperament, mothers' discipline, and security of attachment: Multiple pathways to emerging internalization. *Child Development,* 66, 597–615.

Kochanska, G. (1997). Multiple pathways to conscience for children with different temperaments: From toddlerhood to age 5. *Developmental Psychology,* 33(2), 228–240.

Kochanska, G., Aksan, N., & Joy, M. E. (2007). Children's fearfulness as a moderator of parenting in early socialization: Two longitudinal studies. *Developmental Psychology,* 43, 222–237.

Lee, C. L., & Bates, J. E. (1985). Mother–child interaction at age two years and perceived difficult temperament. *Child Development,* 56, 1314–1325.

Lemery, K. S., Goldsmith, H. H., Klinnert, M. D., & Mrazek, D. A. (1999). Developmental models of infant and childhood temperament. *Developmental Psychology,* 35, 189–204.

Martin, R. P. (1989). Temperament and education: Implications for underachievement and learning disabilities. In W. B. Carey & S. C. McDevitt (Eds.), *Clinical and educational applications of temperament research* (pp. 37–51). Berwyn, PA: Swets North America.

McClowry, S. G., Rodriguez, E. T., & Koslowitz, R. (2008). Temperament-based intervention: Re-examining goodness of fit. *European Journal of Developmental Science,* 2(1/2), 120–135.

McClowry, S. G., Snow, D. L., Tamis-LeMonda, C. S., & Rodriguez, E. T. (2010). Testing the efficacy of INSIGHTS on student disruptive behavior, classroom management, and student competence in inner city primary grades. *School Mental Health,* 2, 23–35.

Mervielde, I., & De Pauw, S. W. (2012). Models of child temperament. In M. Zentner & R. L. Shiner (Eds.), *Handbook of temperament.* New York: Guilford Press.

Newman, J. P., & Wallace, J. F. (1993). Diverse pathways to deficient self-regulation: Implications for disinhibitory psychopathology in children. *Clinical Psychology Review, 13*, 699–720.

Park, S.-Y., Belsky, J., Putnam, S., & Crnic, K. (1997). Infant emotionality, parenting, and 3-year inhibition: Exploring stability and lawful discontinuity in a male sample. *Developmental Psychology, 33*, 218–227.

Patterson, G. R., Reid, J. B., & Dishion, T. J. (1992). *Antisocial boys.* Eugene, OR: Castalia.

Pianta, R. C., Barnett, W. S., Burchinal, M., & Thornburg, K. R. (2009). The effects of preschool education: What we know, how public policy is or is not aligned with the evidence base, and what we need to know. *Psychological Science in the Public Interest, 10*(2), 49–88.

Pluess, M., & Belsky, J. (2009). Differential susceptibility to rearing experience: The case of childcare. *Journal of Child Psychology and Psychiatry, 50*(4), 396–404.

Rothbart, M. K. (2011). *Becoming who we are.* New York: Guilford Press.

Rothbart, M. K., Ahadi, S. A., Hershey, K. L., & Fisher, P. (2001). Investigations of temperament at three to seven years: The Children's Behavior Questionnaire. *Child Development, 72*(5), 1394–1408.

Rothbart, M. K., & Bates, J. E. (1998). Temperament. In W. Damon (Ed.) & N. Eisenberg (Vol. Ed.), *Handbook of child psychology: Vol 3. Social, emotional, and personality development* (5th ed., pp. 105–176). Hoboken, NJ: Wiley.

Rothbart, M. K., & Bates, J. E. (2006). Temperament. In N. Eisenberg, W. Damon, & R. M. Lerner (Eds.), *Handbook of child psychology: Vol 3. Social, emotional, and personality development* (6th ed., pp. 99–166). Hoboken, NJ: Wiley.

Rothbaum, F., & Weisz, J. (1994). Parental caregiving and child externalizing behavior in nonclinical samples: A meta-analysis. *Psychological Bulletin, 116*(1), 55–74.

Rubin, K. H., Hastings, P. D., Stewart, S. L., Henderson, H. A., & Chen, X. (1997). The consistency and concomitants of inhibition: Some of the children, all of the time. *Child Development, 68*, 467–483.

Rudasill, K. M., & Rimm-Kaufman, S. E. (2009). Teacher–child relationship quality: The roles of child temperament and early teacher–child interactions. *Early Childhood Quarterly, 24*, 107–120.

Rusby, J. C., Smolkowski, K., & Jones, L. B. (2009). *Efficacy trial of carescapes: Promoting social development in home-based child care.* Eugene: Oregon Research Institute grant, funded by National Center for Special Education.

Saudino, K. J. (2005). Behavioral genetics and child temperament. *Developmental and Behavioral Pediatrics, 26*, 214–223.

Schermerhorn, A. C., Bates, J. E., Goodnight, J. A., Lansford, J. E., Dodge, K. A., & Pettit, G. S. (2011). *Temperament moderates associations between exposure to stress and children's externalizing problems.* Manuscript submitted for publication.

Smith, L. B., & Breazal, C. (2007). The dynamic lift of developmental process. *Developmental Science, 10*(1), 61–68.

Spivack, G., Marcus, J., & Swift, M. (1986). Early classroom behaviors and later misconduct. *Developmental Psychology, 22*, 124–131.

Sroufe, L. A. (1979). The coherence of individual development: Early care, attachment, and subsequent developmental issues. *American Psychologist, 34,* 834–841.

Staples, A. D., & Bates, J. E. (2011). Children's sleep deficits and cognitive and behavioral adjustment. In M. El-Sheikh (Ed.), *Sleep and development: Familial and socio-cultural considerations* (pp. 133–164). New York: Oxford University Press.

Wachs, T. D. (2000). *Necessary but not sufficient: The respective roles of single and multiple influences on individual development.* Washington, DC: American Psychological Association.

Watson, J. S. (1972). Smiling, cooing and "the game." *Merrill–Palmer Quarterly, 18*(4), 323–339.

Weissbluth, M. (1989). Sleep-loss stress and temperamental difficultness: Psychobiological processes and practical considerations. In G. A. Kohnstamm, J. E. Bates, & M. K. Rothbart (Eds.), *Temperament in childhood* (pp. 357–375). Chichester, UK: Wiley.

CHAPTER 8

Leveraging Attachment Research to Re-vision Infant/Toddler Care for Poor Families

Lisa J. Berlin

Questions about the role of nonparental care in children's well-being informed the development of Bowlby's attachment theory (1969/1982) and remain pertinent today. In the United States in 2005, 51% of all infants and toddlers (between birth and age 3) received at least some nonparental care and 20% received center-based care (Child Trends, 2010). These rates are generally higher for poor families. In the more than 40 years since Bowlby's first writings, attachment research has made enormous contributions to understanding early parenting and the role of infant–parent relationships in human development. In the interest of "re-visioning" high-quality, center-based care for poor infants and toddlers, this chapter examines three main issues. First, I discuss infant–parent attachment and its role in child development. Second, I review several areas of research on attachment and early child care. Third, drawing on this research, I make a series of recommendations for the development of state-of-the art, center-based care for infants and toddlers. Included in these recommendations is a discussion of the role of attachment-based intervention. Throughout, I emphasize research and implications for low-income children.

Infant–Parent Attachment and Its Role in Child Development

According to attachment theory, the infant–parent attachment is an evolutionarily adaptive relationship, a key function of which is to protect

178

the child (Bowlby, 1969/1982). Rather than describing a child as being attached or not, attachment theory and research focus on the *security* of the relationship between the child and parent, developed during the first year of life through repeated daily caregiving interactions. Bowlby (1973) asserted that daily interactions between infants and parents lead the infant to develop expectations about the parent's caregiving that are gradually organized into secure or insecure internal working models of the caregiver, of the self in relation to this caregiver, and of the attachment relationship as a whole. In this section, I discuss research addressing (1) the origins of infant–parent attachment security, (2) infant–parent attachment security in poor families, (3) the concordance of infant–caregiver attachments, and (4) the outcomes of infant–parent attachment security.

Origins of Infant–Parent Attachment Security

The hypothesized driving role of parenting in the development of the child's attachment has been widely examined and integrated into a "transmission model" (van IJzendoorn, 1995). According to the transmission model, parenting behaviors both contribute directly to the quality of the child–parent attachment and are informed largely by the parent's own attachment security. In particular, parents' own internal working models are believed to guide their parenting behaviors by directing the parent's sensitivity and responsiveness to their child's needs (Ainsworth, Blehar, Waters, & Wall, 1978; Main, 1990).

A sensitive parent is open to the full range of his or her child's needs and responds contingently to these needs, potentiating a secure child attachment (Ainsworth et al., 1978). A secure child–parent attachment is in turn characterized by the child's use of the parent as a haven of safety when distressed and secure base from which to explore (Ainsworth, 1963). Conversely, an insensitive parent misunderstands his or her child's needs, and responds only selectively to them, potentiating an insecure child attachment. An insecure child–parent attachment is characterized by the child's limited capacity to use the parent as a haven of safety or base from which to explore.

The most widely used and well-validated assessment of infant–parent security is the laboratory Strange Situation procedure (Ainsworth et al., 1978). A meta-analysis of 2,000 Strange Situations found that 62% of infants in middle-class, nonclinical, North American samples were classified secure (van IJzendoorn, Schuengel, & Bakermans-Kranenburg, 1999). Infant attachment security is also assessed with the Attachment Q-Set (Waters, Vaughn, Posada, & Kondo-Ikemura, 1995). Adult attachment security is assessed through the semistructured Adult Attachment Interview (George, Kaplan, & Main, 1996) and through self-report (see Mikulincer & Shaver, 2007).

Through two meta-analyses, van IJzendoorn (1995; De Wolff & van IJzendoorn, 1997) has provided strong support for direct links between (1) parents' attachment security and their sensitive parenting behaviors, (2) parents' attachment security and their child's attachment to them, and (3) parents' sensitive behaviors and their child's attachment to them. Moreover, a growing body of randomized trials testing attachment-based interventions is demonstrating that experimentally induced increases in mothers' sensitive parenting behaviors can increase the likelihood of infant attachment security (Berlin, Zeanah, & Lieberman, 2008).

At the same time, it is important to note that sensitive parenting behaviors have been found to account for a relatively small proportion of the association between parental and child attachment security (van IJzendoorn, 1995). Thus, sensitive parenting, at least as typically measured, does not appear to be the principal mediator of the effects of parental working models on child security. Recent research is expanding conceptualizations of adult attachment to include the construct of "reflective functioning" (Slade, Grienenberger, Bernbach, Levy, & Locker, 2005) and is examining specific types of insensitive parenting behaviors rather than the absence of parental sensitivity (Lyons-Ruth, Bronfman, & Parsons, 1999). Recent research is also examining infants' genetic predispositions in interaction with parenting behaviors (Belsky & Pleuss, 2009). In these "Gene × Parenting" studies, genetic predispositions are often linked—though not limited to—some aspects of infant temperament. These developing areas of research, in concert with a growing understanding of attachment security as determined by multiple, co-occurring factors, are deepening the understanding of the origins of attachment security (Belsky & Fearon, 2008).

It is also important to note that associations between infant temperament and infant–parent attachment have been thoroughly researched (Vaughn, Bost, & van IJzendoorn, 2008). The widely shared conclusion is that infant temperament does not directly affect the security of infant–parent attachment. Infant temperament can affect the way attachment security or insecurity is expressed, however (i.e., temperament is associated with attachment subclassifications; Belsky & Rovine, 1987).

Infant–Parent Attachment Security in Poor Families

In attachment studies with high-risk families, family income is typically one of several risk factors. Family income in and of itself has received scant attention as a predictor of infant–parent attachment security. Two sets of relevant findings, however, have come from the large-scale National Institute of Child Health and Human Development Study of Early Child Care (NICHD SECC; NICHD Early Child Care Research Network, 2005). First, this study found that infants from lower-income families were more likely to be insecurely attached than infants from higher-income families. Second, African American 2-year-olds were found to have significantly lower security scores (according to the Attachment Q-Set) than white 2-year-olds (Bakermans-Kranenburg, van IJzendoorn, & Kroonenberg, 2004). African American mothers, who had significantly lower incomes than white mothers, were observed to be less sensitive than white mothers during the first 2 years of their child's life. Finally, in a mediated model, low income decreased maternal sensitivity, which in turn decreased toddler attachment security. Poverty, thus, may reduce the prevalence of attachment security through its negative effects on maternal sensitivity, likely due in turn to the increased stress and mental health challenges experienced by poor mothers (e.g., Linver, Brooks-Gunn, & Kohen, 2002). It is also notable that De Wolff and van IJzendoorn's (1997) meta-analysis found that socioeconomic status (SES) moderated the association between maternal sensitivity and infant attachment security such that this association was stronger in middle-class than lower-class samples. In the context of the multiple stressors associated with family poverty, maternal sensitivity may play a lesser role in the development of attachments in low-income than higher-income families.

Concordance of Infant–Caregiver Attachments

Bowlby (1969/1982) and other theorists have been clear in stating that an infant can form an attachment to more than one caregiver at a time. Observational studies support this claim (e.g., Ainsworth, 1967). Associations among infants' multiple attachments are less clear, however. If the quality of an infant's attachment to the parent reflects the quality of interaction with that parent, then the infant's attachments across parents would be similar only to the extent that the two sets of interactions were similar, and neither attachment relationship would influence the formation of the other. At the same time, according to Bowlby's concept of "monotropy" (1969/1982), infants tend to have a principal attachment figure who is sought preferentially as a secure base in times of trouble. It may be that the infant's attachment to the principal attachment figure influences the formation of the infant's attachments to other caregivers.

Numerous studies have examined the associations among infants' attachments to different caregivers, including mothers, fathers, and child care providers (e.g., Ahnert, Pinquart, & Lamb, 2006; Fox, Kimmerly, & Schafer, 1991). Although some studies have indicated that an infant can form different types of attachments to different caregivers, there is stronger evidence of concordance, especially between parents, as demonstrated by two meta-analyses (Fox et al., 1991; van IJzendoorn & De Wolff, 1997).

Fox and colleagues highlighted the possibilities of (1) caregivers' shared child-rearing values and practices, and (2) infants' characteristics as contributors to concordant attachment classifications. Further study of the associations among early attachments is required.

One question regarding infants' relationships with their child care providers, discussed more in the next section, is the extent to which the typical approaches to understanding infant–parent relationships should extend to the study of infant–provider relationships. Certainly (secure and insecure) attachments between infants and their providers can and do form, but, in many cases, especially in the context of center-based care, the lenses through which infant–caregiver relationships are viewed may need adjusting.

Outcomes of Infant–Parent Attachment Security

During the past 40 years, studies of attachment have repeatedly demonstrated associations between an infant's attachment security and multiple aspects of early and later development, especially early development, and especially in the domains of social and psychological functioning. For example, numerous inquiries have indicated positive associations between infant–parent attachment and the qualities of friendships in children as young as 2 and as old as 12 (e.g., Pierrehumbert, Iannotti, Cummings, & Zahn-Waxler, 1989; Youngblade & Belsky, 1992). Numerous studies have also illustrated associations between a secure child–mother attachment and more harmonious interactions with peers, higher regard from peers, fewer behavior problems in preschool and elementary school, and peer competence during adolescence (Berlin, Cassidy, & Appleyard, 2008; Thompson, 2008). For longer-term outcomes, associations with early attachment appear increasingly less likely to be direct and more likely to operate through other relationships and social cognitions (Carlson, Sroufe, & Egeland, 2004).

It is relevant to the purposes of the current chapter to note that the associations between infant–parent attachment and subsequent child development can vary depending on family risk. In the NICHD SECC, for example, at age 3, the associations between attachment and social competence were moderated by a composite measure of family risk, which included family income, maternal education, maternal depression, and parenting stress (Belsky & Fearon, 2002). Specifically, for all attachment groups, as family risk increased, social competence declined linearly, and at the highest level of risk, there were no attachment group differences in social competence. Thus, to the extent that family risk includes low income, attachment security may play a different role in the development of social competence for low-income versus higher-income children.

Summary

Infant–parent attachment security plays a major role in human development. Attachment security appears less prevalent in lower-income than higher-income families. Maternal sensitivity is a key driver of infant attachment security, but plays a lesser role among lower- versus higher-income families. Likewise, infant–parent attachment security is a key predictor of child outcomes, but appears to play a lesser role among higher-risk (including poor) families. Infants can form attachments to multiple caregivers, including child care providers. Indeed, the importance of the quality of child care providers' caregiving is a recurring theme in the research addressing attachment and early child care, discussed next.

Research on Attachment and Early Child Care

In this section I consider three areas of research addressing attachment and early child care. First, I discuss research on the associations among early child care, maternal sensitivity, and infant–parent attachment security. Second, I discuss infants' and toddlers' attachments to their child care providers. Third, I discuss the factors that promote child care providers' sensitive and supportive caregiving behaviors.

Associations among Early Child Care, Maternal Sensitivity, and Infant–Parent Attachment Security

Echoing some of Bowlby's (1969/1982) original concerns, initial studies of the associations between early child care and infant–parent attachment security hypothesized and found a greater prevalence of insecure attachments among infants who had experienced more than 20 hours per week of child care during their first year of life (e.g., Belsky & Rovine, 1988). These early studies typically did not factor in child care quality or family characteristics associated with child care quality or attachment security, however. Since then, larger and more carefully controlled studies have offered a more nuanced view. The largest U.S. study of early child care is the well-known NICHD SECC that has followed 1,153 children from infancy through adolescence and includes rigorous longitudinal assessments of child care quality, amount, timing, and type, and equally comprehensive measurement of child and family development (NICHD Early Child Care Research Network, 2005).

Among the first questions addressed by the NICHD study was the extent to which the Strange Situation procedure, which includes two brief infant–parent separations to help activate the infant's attachment system, is as valid (i.e., equally activating) for infants who typically experience more routine separations as it is for those who do not (NICHD Early Child Care Research Network, 1997). First, analyses compared infants who had experienced "low-intensity" child care (fewer than 10 hours per week; n = 251) to those who had experienced "high-intensity" child care (more than 30 hours per week; n = 263). There were no differences between the low-intensity and high-intensity groups in infant distress during the Strange Situation. Likewise, there were no group differences in the confidence ratings of the coders who quantified the Strange Situation videos. Thus, there was no evidence that the Strange Situation is less valid for infants who typically experience more separations due to more time spent in child care. Moreover, consistent with the existing literature on the origins of infant–parent attachment security, the NICHD SECC found that the main predictors of infant–mother attachment quality at age 15 months were maternal sensitivity observed at ages 6 and 15 months and mothers' self-reported psychological adjustment (mental health and personality), collected when infants were 1, 6, and 15 months old (NICHD Early Child Care Research Network, 1997). It is also notable that mothers who reported stronger beliefs in the benefits of maternal employment for children's development were also observed to interact less sensitively with their infants, to have infants who started child care earlier in life, spent more time in care, and received lower-quality care, and to have infants who were more likely to be insecurely attached to them.

The NICHD SECC did *not* find evidence that early child care affects infant–parent attachment (NICHD Early Child Care Research Network, 1997). Of all infants assessed in the Strange Situation at age 15 months, 62% were classified secure. Of five key indicators of infant's child care experiences assessed when infants were 5 and 14 months old—child care type, quantity, quality, the infant's age of entry, or the stability of child care arrangements—none was related to the rate of infant–mother attachment security. Thus, in and of itself, infants' participation in early child care did not appear to affect infant–mother attachment security.

Similarly, a study of 70 German 15-month-olds during the transition to center-based care found no evidence that initiating care, though clearly stressful, increased the likelihood that infants would be insecurely attached to their mothers 2 months later (Ahnert, Gunnar, Lamb, & Barthel, 2004). Interestingly, infants were more likely to stay secure or to change from insecure to secure depending on the number of days, during the first month, that their mothers spent in the child care centers with them. Attachment security was maintained or increased when mothers spent more days with their infants during this transition period. Although these findings are based on a relatively small sample and require replication, they begin to suggest that a center's transition practices may affect the developing infant–mother attachment.

Child care practices and quality are also highlighted by findings of interactions among child care quantity, quality, maternal sensitivity, and attachment security that have emerged from the NICHD study. These findings qualify some of the initial lack of main effects of child care on attachment. For example, when infants spent more than 10 hours per week in care *and* were observed to have mothers who interacted less sensitively with them, the infants were more likely to be insecurely attached (NICHD Early Child Care Research Network, 1997). Similar findings were obtained in this sample at age 3 (NICHD Early Child Care Research Network, 2001). Interaction effects were small, however, and require replication, especially with a more diverse sample (Howes & Spieker, 2008).

Child care quality in the NICHD study was defined according to observations of child care providers' positive behaviors toward the infants in their care. Positive caregiving in turn reflected caregivers' greater sharing of positive affect, positive physical contact, responsivity, and stimulation of cognitive development, and lesser detachment and flatness of affect (NICHD Early Child Care Research Network, 1997). Findings indicated that when maternal sensitivity was lower, if child care quality was relatively high, children were more likely to be securely attached than when maternal sensitivity and child care quality were both relatively low (NICHD Early Child Care Research Network, 1997). By the time children were 3, although higher quantity (more hours) of care continued to be related to lower maternal sensitivity, there was also some evidence that higher child care quality predicted increases in maternal sensitivity (NICHD Early Child Care Research Network, 1999). Thus, higher child care quality, defined in terms of positive caregiving, may serve a compensatory role in the development of attachment, especially when maternal sensitivity is initially relatively low.

Likewise, an analysis of 64 poor children from the longitudinal Minnesota Study of Risk and Adaptation found that participation in infant child care had positive effects on later socioemotional development for those infants who had been insecurely attached to their mothers at age 1 (Egeland & Hiester, 1995). These results must be interpreted with caution because of the small sample and the fact that child care quality was not measured. Nonetheless, the findings again suggest a compensatory effect of child care for more vulnerable children.

Complementary findings have come from a large Israeli study of early child care that sampled 758 participants of varying SES (Sagi, Koren-Karie, Gini, Ziv, & Joels, 2002). Unlike the NICHD study, the Haifa (Israeli) study did find an effect of early child care on infant attachment security. Infants who received center-based care, in particular, were less likely to be securely attached at age 1 (54%) than infants who received either parental care or another type of nonparental care (75%). This effect was directly attributable to widely implemented center-based care with average infant–caregiver ratios of eight infants per caregiver. These high ratios severely compromised caregivers' physical and psychological availability. Among infants placed with professional child care providers in centers or other settings, those who experienced infant–caregiver ratios of three or fewer infants per caregiver were more likely to be securely attached than infants who experienced higher ratios (i.e., 72% and 57%, respectively). Also noted in the Haifa study for those infants in center-based care was that the usual association between maternal sensitivity and infant attachment security was not obtained (Aviezer, Sagi-Schwartz, & Koren-Karie, 2003). This finding suggests that these infants' attachment systems were overwhelmed and distorted by regularly occurring experiences of insufficient positive interactions with their child care providers.

In a subsequent analysis that combined data from the NICHD SECC and the Haifa study, higher infant–caregiver ratios predicted a lower likelihood of attachment security (Love et al., 2003). Thus, although in the NICHD study alone, child care experiences did not appear to affect infant–mother attachment security, when the Haifa data were included, thus broadening (downward) the range of child care quality, child care quality related directly to attachment security. These findings again highlight the importance of child care quality—defined in terms of caregivers' physical and psychological availability—for the key developmental indicator of infant–mother attachment security. Longer-term findings from the NICHD SECC as well as numerous studies of the quality of child care for preschoolers also repeatedly link child care providers' physical availability and positive interactions with the children in their care to better child outcomes including fewer behavior problems and more advanced academic, language, and social skills (e.g., Burchinal, Vandergrift, Pianta, & Mashburn, 2010; Mashburn et al., 2008; NICHD Early Child Care Research Network, 2002).

The compelling body of research pointing to the importance of child care providers' behaviors is made even more striking by considering the NICHD Early Child Care Research Network (2000) report estimating that positive caregiving across child care settings was very uncharacteristic or somewhat uncharacteristic for 61% of U.S. children between the ages of 1 and 3, and highly characteristic or somewhat characteristic for only 39% (NICHD Early Child Care Research Network, 2000; see also Pianta, Barnett, Burchinal, & Thornburg, 2009). Thus, a critical feature of good child care may be missing or incompletely implemented in the majority of U.S. child care settings.

In sum, the associations among early child care, maternal sensitivity, and infant–parent attachment security appear to hinge largely on the quality of care. Perhaps especially relevant to low-income infants and toddlers are the findings suggesting that higher-quality child care may help to compensate for initial low maternal sensitivity and/or attachment insecurity (NICHD Early Child Care Research Network, 1997, 1999; Egeland &

Hiester, 1995). To the extent that poverty and its co-occurring stressors can impede parental sensitivity and attachment security, high-quality child care may serve an especially important function for poor infants and toddlers. Child care quality, in turn, appears to hinge largely on low infant–caregiver ratios and on caregivers' sensitive and supportive behaviors. Increasing concern about child care providers' behaviors has motivated two interrelated areas of research, considered next: first, the study of infants' and toddlers' attachments to their child care providers; and second, factors that promote providers' positive caregiving behaviors.

Infants' and Toddlers' Attachments to Child Care Providers

Numerous studies have examined infants' and toddlers' relationships with their child care providers through the lenses of attachment theory and research, which seems appropriate given the intimacy and daily caregiving interactions that define early child care. At the same time, some caution may be required, given typically less continuity in caregiver providers than parents, and because group child care (including family care) is often quite different than parental care in its temporal rhythms, child–adult ratios, and actual sensitivity of the care provided. For example, a German study that included extensive observational data confirmed that the quality of care provided to 12- to 24-month-old toddlers by mothers was higher than that provided by child care providers (Ahnert, Rickert, & Lamb, 2000). Thus, the unique role(s) of early child care providers must be considered (Howes, 1999). As discussed next, as a whole, the research into infant/toddler attachments to child care providers again points to the importance of child care providers' sensitive and positive caregiving behaviors. This research also illustrates the importance of considering child care type when examining infant–provider relationships.

Earlier, small-scale studies suggested the relevance of attachment constructs for understanding infant–provider relationships. For example, one study found that 9-year-old children's perceptions of their friendships were predicted by the security of their attachments to their child care providers, measured with the Attachment Q-Set, during toddlerhood (when the mean age of the children was 21 months) and/or preschool (when the mean age of the children was 30 months; Howes, Hamilton, & Philipsen, 1998). Another study also used the Attachment Q-Set to examine 12- to 19-month-old infants' relationships with their child care providers in family child care settings and found that attachment security was predicted by the degree of the caregiver's involvement with the infant (Elicker, Fortner-Wood, & Noppe, 1999).

A more recent meta-analysis examined the attachments of 2,867 infants and toddlers, whose mean age was 30 months, to their child care providers across multiple types of care (Ahnert et al., 2006). First, the meta-analysis revealed a higher proportion of secure attachments to parents (60 and 66% to mothers and fathers, respectively) than to providers (42%). Interestingly, children of lower-SES parents were more likely to be classified as insecurely attached to their child care provider than were children of higher-SES parents. A history of child care instability also predicted attachment insecurity.

Second, there was a higher proportion of secure attachments to providers among children who received home-based care as opposed to center-based care. An important qualifier of these results is that attachment security for all of the children in home-based care was assessed with the Attachment Q-Set, whereas attachment security for the children in center-based care was assessed with the Attachment Q-Set or the Strange Situation. It is quite possible that the structure of home-based care is more conducive to the development of a secure attachment than is center-based care, and that more secure attachments did develop within the home- versus center-based programs. It is also possible that there was measurement bias, if the Attachment Q-Set was a more sensitive measure of a secure child–provider relationship in home- versus center-based care. Likewise, it is possible that the Strange Situation was a less appropriate measure of the infant–provider relationship in the context of center-based care, as might be inferred from a second set of findings regarding "group-focused sensitivity."

Ahnert and her colleagues (2006) reliably classified observations of caregiving into two types: individual-focused sensitivity and group-focused sensitivity. Individual-focused sensitivity referred to one-on-one responsiveness to individual needs, whereas group-focused sensitivity referred to caregivers' child-oriented attitudes and positive involvement while supervising a group of children. The meta-analysis revealed that care providers' group-focused sensitivity was associated with infant/toddler attachment security, whereas individual-focused sensitivity was not. Moreover, group-focused sensitivity was not affected by group size and child–adult ratios, whereas individual-focused sensitivity declined as group size and child–adult ratios increased. Thus, perhaps infant–provider relationships, which may or may not be attachments per se, are driven more by caregivers' general attitudes and collective behaviors toward all of the children in their care than by caregivers' behaviors toward particular children. Individual-focused sensitivity in turn may be most appropriate to consider when conceptualizing infant–parent and/or infant–provider relationships that are characterized by individual caregiving (e.g., an infant's relationship with her nanny).

In sum, given the importance of child care providers' positive caregiving behaviors, the nature of the *relationship* between infants and their child care providers is equally critical to understand. Paralleling the research on infant–parent attachment, infant–provider attachment security appears less prevalent among infants from lower-income than higher-income families. At the same time, the extent to which an infant forms an attachment to a particular provider, and the extent to which that relationship (attachment or otherwise) is affected by group size, child–caregiver ratio, and caregivers' individual- or group-focused sensitivity appear to vary importantly according to child care type. For center-based care, care providers' group-focused sensitivity may be especially important. Although generally not distinguishing individual- versus group-focused sensitivity, the research into the factors that promote child care providers' sensitive and supportive caregiving behaviors is discussed next.

Factors That Promote Child Care Providers' Sensitive and Supportive Caregiving Behaviors

Research findings to date concerning the factors that promote child care providers' positive caregiving behaviors identify sensitivity-promoting conditions, as well as raise questions about some caregiver characteristics that deserve greater attention. Findings to date are highly consistent in pointing to low child–adult ratios as the single most important factor predicting providers' sensitivity and supportiveness toward the children in their care, regardless of child age (e.g., Pianta et al., 2009; NICHD Early Child Care Research Network, 2000). Results from two NICHD studies are especially informative about caregiving for infants and toddlers, per se. The first study, focusing on 6-month-olds, identified smaller group sizes, lower child–adult ratios, and caregivers' more child-centered (less authoritarian) child-rearing beliefs as predictors of observed positive caregiving behaviors, regardless of child care type (*N* = 576; NICHD Early Child Care Research Network, 1996). The highest ratings and frequencies of positive caregiving behaviors were made for individual care settings (e.g., care provided by a grandfather or nanny), whereas the lowest ratings and frequencies were made for center-based settings. There was also some indication that, in child care centers, there was more positive caregiving when infants were grouped in classrooms with infants only, or with infants and toddlers, as opposed to when the groups also included preschoolers. The safety, cleanliness, and level of stimulation within child care settings were also positively associated with positive caregiving behaviors.

These findings were replicated and extended by another set of analyses of the NICHD sample, at ages 15, 24, and 36 months (NICHD Early Child Care Research Network, 2000). In this study, regardless of child age *or* child care type, smaller group sizes, lower child–adult ratios, and caregivers' less authoritarian child-rearing beliefs again predicted observed positive caregiving behaviors. Again, the lowest ratings and frequencies were made for center-based settings, with typically higher child–adult ratios. Interestingly, however, and reminiscent of the Ahnert et al. (2006) findings concerning group-focused sensitivity discussed earlier, child–adult ratios were less predictive of positive caregiving in child care centers and in family care settings than they were in individual care arrangements. Also, the strength of most predictors waned as children aged, so that factors such as group size and child care type contributed less to the positive caregiving of 36-month-olds compared to 15- and 24-month olds. Arguably, as children became more self-sufficient and involved with their peers, positive caregiving was easier to provide and less dependent on the characteristics of the setting or the provider.

From the perspective of attachment theory and research, however, the characteristics of the provider deserve further consideration. As noted, when children were 6, 15, 24, and 36 months old, more child-centered beliefs predicted more positive caregiving. Of all types of child care providers, center-based caregivers had the highest levels of education and the most child-centered beliefs about child rearing. These beliefs, however, did not elevate the quality of center-based caregiving to the levels observed in other settings. Moreover, caregivers' specialized training in child care and child development was not consistently related to positive caregiving behaviors. Taken together, these findings suggest that there may be some deficits in typical caregiver hiring or training protocol, a point echoed by recent studies of preschool quality (e.g., Early et al., 2007). Another (not mutually exclusive) possibility is that positive caregiving derives most from sources other than training.

A consideration of attachment research's "transmission model" leads to an argument for the closer scrutiny of caregivers' own attachment security as drivers of child-rearing behaviors (i.e., operating as parents' attachment security does). For example, might not a child care provider with secure working models be more likely to provide sensitive care to infants than a provider with an unresolved history of trauma and/or insecure working models of attachment? Such questions have not, to my knowledge, been addressed in the child care literature. Several studies in related areas, however, have begun to suggest that caregivers' own attachment orientations may factor into the care they provide.

Two studies have examined the adult attachment styles of providers of early home visiting services for high-risk families with infants (Burrell et al., 2009; McFarlane et al., 2010). In one study, home visitors' self-reported attachment anxiety was related to indicators of burnout, whereas attachment avoidance was associated with a shorter tenure as a home visitor (Burrell et al., 2009). In the second study, home visitors who reported more attachment avoidance were also more likely to respond to mothers' mental health problems and to domestic violence, whereas home visitors who reported more attachment anxiety were less likely to respond to these issues (McFarlane et al., 2010). Home visitors' attachment styles also interacted with mothers' attachment styles in ways that appeared to affect program implementation. For example, when either home visitors or mothers reported higher levels of attachment anxiety, more home visits were provided. Moreover, mothers who reported higher levels of attachment anxiety were less trusting of home visitors who were also higher on attachment anxiety, and more trusting of home visitors who were higher on attachment avoidance (McFarlane et al., 2010).

Interactions between providers' and clients' attachment states of mind have also emerged from two studies of case managers and their severely mentally ill clients (Dozier, Cue, & Barnett, 1994; Tyrell, Dozier, Teague, & Fallot, 1999). In one study, case managers who were more preoccupied (i.e., anxious) were found to intervene with their clients in greater depth than did case managers who were more dismissing (i.e., avoidant). More secure case managers were less likely to attend to dependency needs for their more preoccupied clients versus their more dismissing clients (Dozier et al., 1994). In the second study, stronger therapeutic alliances were formed when case managers and their clients had opposing attachment inclinations: case managers who were less avoidant worked better with clients who were more avoidant, whereas case managers who were more avoidant worked better with clients who were less avoidant (Tyrrell et al., 1999).

Last, it is also relevant to note that in a study of foster infants and their foster mothers, foster infants were more likely to be securely attached to foster mothers with secure versus insecure states of mind with respect to attachment (Dozier, Stovall, Albus, & Bates, 2001). Thus, even for infants who experienced disrupted and often traumatic early attachments, foster caregivers' own attachment security appeared to play a decisive role in the care provided to their foster infants. A related study of foster mothers' child-rearing attitudes highlighted the importance of their commitment to their foster child, defined in terms of caring for their foster child unconditionally, as opposed to viewing foster care as temporary and best implemented at arms' length (Dozier & Lindhiem, 2006). Higher levels of commitment were predictive of greater relationship stability, including fewer placement disruptions and a greater likelihood of adoption. Similar findings have emerged from a study of Romanian foster infants (Smyke, Zeanah, Fox, Nelson, & Guthrie, 2010).

Thus, there appear to be two main avenues toward promoting child care providers' sensitive and supportive caregiving behaviors. The first pertains to the structural features of the setting, with low ratios being the most consistently implicated feature. Small group sizes, homogeneous groupings (with respect to child age), cleanliness, and level of stimulation are also associated with more positive caregiving behaviors. The second, less explored, avenue pertains to caregivers' own attachment security. The studies to date of attachment security in early home visitors, case managers, and foster parents all suggest a contribution of caregivers' attachment security to the quality of the helping relationships in which they are engaged. Taken together, they argue for a closer consideration of child care providers' own attachment security, and of how this security may factor into their individual- and/or group-focused sensitivity.

Summary

Taken as a whole, the research on infant–parent attachment and early child care is expansive, yet also converging. The literature repeatedly points to the importance of child care quality, defined in terms of low child–caregiver ratios and caregivers' sensitive and supportive behaviors. For center-based child care providers, group-focused sensitivity may be especially important for engendering trust and security among the infants and toddlers in their care. In addition, a gradual transition into child care has been associated, albeit preliminarily, to infants' attachment security. Finally, child care providers' own attachment security merits further consideration as a contributing factor in their caregiving behaviors. Along with the other bodies of research being culled for the present volume, the research on attachment and child care can and should be brought to bear on the development of state-of-the-art, center-based care for poor infants and toddlers.

Lessons from Attachment Research for Infant/Toddler Care for Poor Families

The principal implication from the research on attachment and child care for "re-visioning" infant/toddler care for poor families centers on promoting and maintaining child care providers' sensitive and supportive caregiving behaviors. In this section I provide practical suggestions for how this might be accomplished, through targeted hiring, attachment-based training, support and supervision, coordinating child care and family perspectives, and integrating attachment-based intervention.

Targeted Hiring

After establishing strong structural features (i.e., low ratios, small groups), developing hiring criteria for child care providers provides the first opportunity for a child care program to establish positive caregiving practices. From the perspective of attachment research, hiring childcare providers should include a careful consideration of the extent to which caregivers can be open and contingently responsive to the full range of infants' needs. Given the frequency with which infants cry, and the importance of comforting behaviors to the development of attachment security, caregivers' capacities to be consistently responsive to infants' distress should be considered especially closely. A caregiver's level of education, degree of specialized training, and prior work experience may be less important to these capacities than their own attachment orientations. In the course of implementing and disseminating the Attachment and Biobehavioral Catch-Up (ABC) intervention program for mothers and infants, Dozier and her colleagues (Dozier, Lindhiem, & Ackerman, 2005) have developed hiring procedures that include questions about prospective interventionists' own values and states of mind with respect to attachment (M. Dozier, personal communication, April, 2009). Similar practices could be considered when hiring infant and toddler child care providers.

Hiring procedures to assess prospective providers' capacities might also include questions about their commitment to the infants in their care. For example, to what extent do providers believe they should care for children as if they were their own? Conversely, to what extent do providers refrain from becoming invested, on the basis of the short-term nature of the relationship with the children in their care? Hiring procedures might also include prospective providers viewing and responding to videotaped Strange Situation procedures. For example, to what extent do providers believe that an infant classified as insecure–avoidant is strategically avoidant versus happily independent? Finally, a secondary level of screening could include actual observations of infant–caregiver interaction in a typical center setting. These observations could be coded with the same types of measures used to quantify caregiver behaviors in the NICHD SECC and similar studies.

Attachment-Based Training

A second opportunity to promote child care providers' positive caregiving behaviors can come from attachment-based training. Such training would teach the basics of attachment theory and research, such as the concept that responding to crying infants does not "spoil" them but rather builds security and actually reduces crying during toddlerhood. Such training could also cover the attachment "transmission model," and the role of caregivers' own attachment security in the care they provide. As discussed more below, protocol from interventions designed to support infant–parent attachment security may be usefully adapted for such training purposes.

Support and Supervision (Nurturing the Nurturers)

Strong support of child care providers serves the interrelated functions of maintaining quality and minimizing staff turnover. Attachment perspectives emphasize the emotionally demanding nature of providing early child care and related early intervention services. Approaches to staff support highlight parallel process and reflective supervision. Parallel process refers to the supervisor–supervisee (provider) relationship serving as a model for the provider's relationship with the child. In this vein, Pawl has offered the "platinum rule" of supervision: "Do unto others as you would have them do unto others" (Pawl & St. John, 1998). Reflective supervision focuses on the emotional content of working with young children and their families, including the thoughts and feelings evoked in providers by this intimate and emotionally challenging work (Heller & Gilkerson, 2009). In a similar vein, Lantieri's Inner Resilience programs emphasize the need to support teachers' emotional development and self-care, with obvious applications to child care providers and early intervention staff (Lantieri, 2008).

Coordinating Child Care and Family Perspectives

Given that parental and nonparental caregivers are the critical players in infants' and toddlers' daily lives, communication and coordination between child care providers and the families they serve is crucial (Ahnert & Lamb, 2003). Although a high degree of agreement with respect to child-rearing values and practices is ideal, often providers and parents have different perspectives. Communicating and coordinating these perspectives facilitates a more coherent experience for the child. High agreement between caregivers, in fact, predicts fewer behavior problems in child care (Elicker, Noppe, Noppe, & Fortner-Wood, 1997). Conversely, disjointed approaches (e.g., to sleeping, crying, and/or discipline) can create confusion for children as well as build resentment between caregivers.

One perspective that may be particularly useful to consider concerns the mother's (or primary caregiver's) state of mind with respect to attachment. Several studies have shown that mothers' attachment security can moderate the effectiveness of early intervention (e.g., Duggan, Berlin, Cassidy, Burrell, & Tandon, 2009). For example, in a recent study of 947 participants from the national randomized trial of Early Head Start (EHS), my colleagues and I found more negative parenting outcomes for mothers who entered the program with more self-reported attachment avoidance or attachment anxiety (Berlin et al., 2011). One interpretation of these findings was that the less secure mothers in this study may also have been less receptive to—and/or too anxious to "take in"—EHS providers' input on early parenting, which typically emphasized the importance of parents' responsiveness to infants' cues and needs. Thus, one practical implication of these findings is that it may be valuable for programs to screen incoming parents' attachment avoidance and anxiety and to use this information to inform plans for child care–family coordination.

One area in which child care–family coordination may be especially valuable concerns infants' transitions into care. As noted earlier, a gradual transition into child care has been associated with infants' attachment security (Ahnert et al., 2004). This finding, while preliminary, suggests the importance of a carefully orchestrated and gradual transition into care. For example, initially, centers might slowly increase the duration of time per day that an infant spends in care. In addition, mothers or other primary caregivers could spend time with the infant in the child care setting until the infant becomes well acclimated. This would have the added advantage of acclimating the child's mother/caregiver to the child care setting as well. Finally, consistent procedures for soothing infants' separation distress could be implemented such as a caregiver holding the infant and telling the infant that his or her mother will be back soon. Parents may need help with separation distress as well, and could be asked to say one warm "good-bye" and then depart quickly. If possible, a one-way mirror or viewing area where parents can observe their children without being seen by them may be helpful.

Integrating Attachment-Based Intervention

As noted earlier, there is a growing number of attachment-based interventions that are not only derived from attachment theory but also supported by randomized trials (Berlin, Zeanah, et al., 2008). Some of these interventions are relatively brief and could be implemented in conjunction with center-based care. For example, Dozier's ABC program consists of 10 sessions (Dozier et al., 2005). While brief, the ABC program is also intensive, addressing four themes: (1) the importance of parental nurturance; (2) following the child's lead; (3) the importance of nonthreatening, nonfrightening caregiving behavior; and (4) "overriding" one's own history and/ or non-nurturing instincts. In a randomized trial with foster infants and their foster parents, the ABC program showed positive effects on infant–parent attachment security and infant biobehavioral regulation (Dozier et al., 2006, 2009). Findings from a second randomized trial, with neglected infants and their biological mothers, have indicated positive impacts on maternal sensitivity and infant attachment (Dozier & Peloso, 2009). The ABC program could be adapted for training child care providers, to promote and maintain their supportive caregiving behaviors. Moreover, in the spirit of offering comprehensive early intervention and coordinating child care and family perspectives, many child care programs include a parenting component. Thus, the ABC program could also be implemented as a short-term supplement to ongoing center-based care. Moreover, using the same protocol for providing attachment-based training for child care providers and for parents could synergistically support an overarching attachment-based culture of caregiving.

In sum, the research on attachment and child care can be taken to offer several suggestions for "re-visioning" infant/toddler care for poor families. In the short term, translating research to practice can be challenging and labor-intensive. In the long term, however, more scientifically informed services for some of America's most vulnerable citizens also promise some of the greatest returns.

ACKNOWLEDGMENTS

The writing of this chapter was supported by National Institute of Mental Health Grant No. K01MH70378 awarded to Lisa J. Berlin, and National Institute on Drug Abuse Grant No. P30DA023026 awarded to the Duke University Transdisciplinary Prevention Research Center. The content is solely the responsibility of the author and does not necessarily represent the official views of the National Institutes of Health.

REFERENCES

Ahnert, L., Gunnar, M. R., Lamb, M. E., & Barthel, M. (2004). Transition to child-care: Associations with infant–mother attachment, infant negative emotion, and cortisol elevation. *Child Development, 75,* 639–650.

Ahnert, L., & Lamb, M. E. (2003). Shared care: Establishing a balance between home and child care settings. *Child Development, 74,* 1044–1049.

Ahnert, L., Pinquart, M., & Lamb, M. E. (2006). Security of children's relationships with nonparental care providers: A meta-analysis, *Child Development, 77,* 664–679.

Ahnert, L., Rickert, H., & Lamb, M. E. (2000). Shared caregiving: Comparisons between home and child care settings. *Developmental Psychology, 36,* 339–351.

Ainsworth, M. D. S. (1963). The development of infant–mother interaction among the Ganda. In B. M. Foss (Ed.), *Determinants of infant behavior* (pp. 67–104). New York: Wiley.

Ainsworth, M. D. S. (1967). *Infancy in Uganda: Infant care and the growth of love.* Baltimore: Johns Hopkins Press.

Ainsworth, M. D. S., Blehar, M. C., Waters, E., & Wall, S. (1978). *Patterns of attachment.* Hillsdale, NJ: Erlbaum.

Aviezer, O., Sagi-Schwartz, A., & Koren-Karie, N. (2003). Ecological constraints on the formation of infant–mother attachment relations: When maternal sensitivity becomes ineffective. *Infant Behavior and Development, 26,* 285–299.

Bakermans-Kranenburg, M. J., van IJzendoorn, M. H., & Kroonenberg, P. M. (2004). Differences in attachment security between African-American and white children: Ethnicity or socio-economic status? *Infant Behavior and Development, 27,* 417–433.

Belsky, J., & Fearon, R. M. (2002). Infant–mother attachment security, contextual risk, and early development: A moderational analysis. *Development and Psychopathology, 14,* 293–310.

Belsky, J., & Fearon, R. M. P. (2008). Precursors of attachment security. In J.

Cassidy & P. R. Shaver (Eds.), *Handbook of attachment: Theory, research, and clinical applications* (2nd ed., pp. 295–316). New York: Guilford Press.

Belsky, J., & Pluess, M. (2009). Beyond diathesis stress: Differential susceptibility to environmental influences. *Psychological Bulletin, 135,* 885–908.

Belsky, J., & Rovine, M. (1987). Temperament and attachment security in the Strange Situation: An empirical rapprochement. *Child Development, 58,* 787–795.

Belsky, J., & Rovine, M. (1988). Nonmaternal care in the first year of life and security of infant–parent attachment. *Child Development, 59,* 157–167.

Berlin, L. J., Cassidy, J., & Appleyard, K. (2008). The influence of early attachments on other relationships. In J. Cassidy & P. R. Shaver (Eds.), *Handbook of attachment: Theory, research, and clinical applications* (2nd ed., pp. 333–347). New York: Guilford Press.

Berlin, L. J., Whiteside-Mansell, L., Roggman, L. A., Green, B. L., Robinson, J., & Spieker, S. (2011). Testing maternal depression and attachment style as moderators of Early Head Start's effects on parenting. *Attachment and Human Development, 13,* 49–67.

Berlin, L. J., Zeanah, C. H., & Lieberman, A. F. (2008). Prevention and intervention programs for supporting early attachment security. In J. Cassidy & P. R. Shaver (Eds.), *Handbook of attachment: Theory, research, and clinical applications* (2nd ed., pp. 745–761). New York: Guilford Press.

Bowlby, J. (1969/1982). *Attachment and loss: Vol. 1. Attachment.* New York: Basic Books.

Bowlby, J. (1973). *Attachment and loss: Vol. 2. Separation.* New York: Basic Books.

Burchinal, M., Vandergrift, N., Pianta, R. C., & Mashburn, A. J. (2010). Threshold analysis of association between child care quality and child outcomes for low-income children in pre-kindergarten programs. *Early Childhood Research Quarterly, 25,* 166–176.

Burrell, L., McFarlane, E., Tandon, D., Fuddy, L., Leaf, P., & Duggan, A. (2009). Home visitor relationship security: Association with perceptions of work, satisfaction, and turnover. *Journal of Human Behavior in the Social Environment, 19,* 592–610.

Carlson, E. A., Sroufe, L. A., & Egeland, B. (2004). The construction of experience: A longitudinal study of representation and behavior. *Child Development, 75,* 66–83.

Child Trends. (2010). *Child care.* Retrieved from *www.childtrendsdatabank.org/pdf/21_PDF.*

De Wolff, M. S., & van IJzendoorn, M. H. (1997). Sensitivity and attachment: A meta-analysis on parental antecedents of infant attachment. *Child Development, 68,* 571–591.

Dozier, M., Cue, K. L., & Barnett, L. (1994). Clinicians as caregivers: Role of attachment organization in treatment. *Journal of Consulting and Clinical Psychology, 62,* 793–800.

Dozier, M., & Lindhiem, O. (2006). This is my child: Differences among foster parents in commitment to their young children. *Child Maltreatment, 11,* 338–345.

Dozier, M., Lindhiem, O., & Ackerman, J. P. (2005). Attachment and biobehavioral catch-up. In L. J. Berlin, Y. Ziv, L. Amaya-Jackson, & M. T. Greenberg (Eds.), *Enhancing early attachments: Theory, research, intervention and policy* (pp. 178–194). New York: Guilford Press.

Dozier, M., Lindhiem, O., Lewis, E., Bick, J., Bernard, K., & Peloso, E. (2009). Effects of a foster parent training program on young children's attachment behaviors: Preliminary evidence from a randomized clinical trial. *Child and Adolescent Social Work Journal, 26,* 321–332.

Dozier, M., & Peloso, E. (2009, April). Effects of a randomized attachment-based intervention for parents in the child welfare system on parenting and child attachment. In L. J. Berlin (Chair), *Attachment-based assessment and treatment in child maltreatment prevention.* Symposium conducted at the biennial meeting of the Society for Research in Child Development, Denver, CO.

Dozier, M., Peloso, E., Lindhiem, O., Gordon, M. K., Manni, M., Sepulveda, S., et al. (2006). Developing evidence-based interventions for foster children: An example of a randomized clinical trial with infants and toddlers. *Journal of Social Issues, 62,* 767–785.

Dozier, M., Stovall, K., Albus, K., & Bates, B. (2001). Attachment for infants in foster care: The role of caregiver state of mind. *Child Development, 72,* 1467–1477.

Duggan, A., Berlin, L. J., Cassidy, J., Burrell, L., & Tandon, D. (2009). Testing maternal depression and attachment insecurity as moderators of home visiting impacts for at-risk mothers and infants. *Journal of Consulting and Clinical Psychology, 77,* 788–799.

Early, D. M., Maxwell, K., Burchinal, M., Alva, S., Bender, R. H., Bryant, D., et al. (2007). Teachers' education, classroom quality, and young children's academic skills: Results from seven studies of preschool programs. *Child Development, 78,* 558–580.

Egeland, B., & Hiester, M. (1995). The long-term consequences of infant day-care and mother–infant attachment. *Child Development, 66,* 474–485.

Elicker, J., Fortner-Wood, C., & Noppe, I. C. (1999). The context of infant attachment in family child care. *Journal of Applied Developmental Psychology, 20,* 319–336.

Elicker, J., Noppe, I. C., Noppe, L. D., & Fortner-Wood, C. (1997). The parent–caregiver relationship scale: Rounding out the relationship system in infant child care. *Early Education and Development, 8,* 83–100.

Fox, N. A., Kimmerly, N. L., & Schafer, W. D. (1991). Attachment to mother/attachment to father: A meta-analysis. *Child Development, 62,* 210–225.

George, C., Kaplan, N., & Main, M. (1996). *Adult Attachment Interview protocol* (3rd ed.). Unpublished manuscript, University of California at Berkeley.

Heller, S. S., & Gilkerson, L. (Eds.). (2009). *A practical guide to reflective supervision.* Washington, DC: Zero to Three.

Howes, C. (1999). Attachment relationships in the context of multiple caregivers. In J. Cassidy & P. R. Shaver (Eds.). *Handbook of attachment: Theory, research, and clinical applications* (pp. 671–687). New York: Guilford Press.

Howes, C., Hamilton, C. E., & Philipsen, L. C. (1998). Stability and continuity of child-caregiver and child-peer relationships. *Child Development, 69,* 418–426.

Howes, C., & Spieker, S. (2008). Attachment relationships in the context of multiple caregivers. In J. Cassidy & P. R. Shaver (Eds.), *Handbook of attachment: Theory, research, and clinical applications* (2nd ed., pp. 317–332). New York: Guilford Press.

Lantieri, L. (2008). *Building emotional intelligence.* Boulder, CO: Sounds True.

Linver, M., Brooks-Gunn, J., & Kohen, D. (2002). Family processes as pathways from income to young children's development. *Developmental Psychology, 38,* 719–734.

Love, J., Harrison, L., Sagi-Schwartz, A., van IJzendoorn, M., Ross, C., Ungerer, J. A., et al. (2003). Child care quality matters: How conclusions may vary with context. *Child Development, 74,* 1021–1033.

Lyons-Ruth, K., Bronfman, E., & Parsons, E. (1999). Frightened, frightening, and atypical maternal behavior and disorganized infant attachment strategies. In J. Vondra & D. Barnett (Eds.), Atypical patterns of infant attachment: Theory, research, and current directions. *Monographs of the Society for Research in Child Development, 64*(3, Serial No. 258).

Main, M. (1990). Cross-cultural studies of attachment organization: Recent studies, changing methodologies, and the concept of conditional strategies. *Human Development, 33,* 48–61.

Mashburn, A. J., Pianta, R. C., Hamre, B. K., Downer, J. T., Barbarin, O. A., Bryant, D., et al. (2008). Measures of classroom quality in prekindergarten and children's development of academic, language, and social skills. *Child Development, 79,* 732–749.

McFarlane, E., Burrell, L., Fuddy, L., Tandon, D., Derauf, D. C., Leaf, P., et al. (2010). Associations of home visitors' and mothers' attachment style with family engagement. *Journal of Community Psychology, 38,* 541–556.

Mikulincer, M., & Shaver, P. R. (2007). *Attachment in adulthood: Structure, dynamics, and change.* New York: Guilford Press.

NICHD Early Child Care Research Network. (1996). Characteristics of infant child care: Factors contributing to positive caregiving. *Early Childhood Research Quarterly, 11,* 269–306.

NICHD Early Child Care Research Network. (1997). The effects of infant child care on infant–mother attachment security: Results of the NICHD Study of Early Child Care. *Child Development, 68,* 860–879.

NICHD Early Child Care Research Network. (1999). Child care and mother–child interaction in the first 3 years of life. *Developmental Psychology, 35,* 1399–1413.

NICHD Early Child Care Research Network. (2000). Characteristics and quality of child care for toddlers and preschoolers. *Applied Developmental Science, 4,* 116–135.

NICHD Early Child Care Research Network. (2001). Child-care and family predictors of preschool attachment and stability from infancy. *Developmental Psychology, 37,* 847–862.

NICHD Early Child Care Research Network. (2002). Structure → process →

outcome: Direct and indirect effects of caregiving quality on young children's development. *Psychological Science, 13*, 199–206.

NICHD Early Child Care Research Network. (Eds.). (2005). *Child care and child development: Results from the NICHD Study of Early Child Care and Youth Development.* New York: Guilford Press.

Pawl, J., & St. John, M. (1998). *How you are is as important as what you do.* Washington, DC: Zero to Three.

Pianta, R. C., Barnett, W. S., Burchinal, M., & Thornburg, K. R. (2009). The effects of preschool education: What we know, how public policy is or is not aligned with the evidence base, and what we need to know. *Psychological Science in the Public Interest, 10*(2), 49–88.

Pierrehumbert, B., Iannotti, R., Cummings, E. M., & Zahn-Waxler, C. (1989). Social functioning with the mother and peer at 2 and 5 years of age: The influence of attachment. *International Journal of Behavioral Development, 12*, 85–100.

Sagi, A., Koren-Karie, N., Gini, M., Ziv, Y., & Joels, T. (2002). Shedding further light on the effects of various types and quality of early child care on infant–mother attachment relationship: The Haifa study of early child care. *Child Development, 73*, 1166–1186.

Slade, A., Grienenberger, J., Bernbach, E., Levy, D., & Locker, A. (2005). Maternal reflective functioning, attachment, and the transmission gap: A preliminary study. *Attachment and Human Development, 7*, 283–298.

Smyke, A. T., Zeanah, C. H., Fox, N. A., Nelson, C. A., & Guthrie, D. (2010). Placement in foster care enhances quality of attachment among young institutionalized children. *Child Development, 81*, 212–223.

Thompson, R. A. (2008). Early attachment and later development: Familiar questions, new answers. In J. Cassidy & P. R. Shaver (Eds.), *Handbook of attachment: Theory, research, and clinical applications* (2nd ed., pp. 348–365). New York: Guilford Press.

Tyrrell, C. L., Dozier, M., Teague, G. B., & Fallot, R. D. (1999). Effective treatment relationships for persons with serious psychiatric disorders: The importance of attachment states of mind. *Journal of Consulting and Clinical Psychology, 67*, 725–733.

van IJzendoorn, M. H. (1995). Adult attachment representations, parental responsiveness, and infant attachment: A meta-analysis on the predictive validity of the Adult Attachment Interview. *Psychological Bulletin, 117*, 387–403.

van IJzendoorn, M. H., & De Wolff, M. S. (1997). In search of the absent father—Meta-analysis of infant–father attachment: A rejoinder to our discussants. *Child Development, 68*, 604–609.

van IJzendoorn, M. H., Schuengel, C., & Bakermans-Kranenburg, M. J. (1999). Disorganized attachment in early childhood: Meta-analysis of precursors, concomitants, and sequelae. *Development and Psychopathology, 11*, 225–250.

Vaughn, B. E., Bost, K. K., & van IJzendoorn, M. H. (2008). Attachment and temperament: Additive and interactive influences on behavior, affect, and cognition during infancy and childhood. In J. Cassidy & P. R. Shaver (Eds.),

Handbook of attachment: Theory, research and clinical applications (2nd ed., pp. 192–216). New York: Guilford Press.

Waters, E., Vaughn, B. E., Posada, G., & Kondo-Ikemura, K. (Eds.). (1995). Caregiving, cultural, and cognitive perspectives on secure-base behavior and working models: New growing points on attachment theory and research. *Monographs of the Society for Research in Child Development, 60*(2–3, Serial No. 244).

Youngblade, L. M., & Belsky, J. (1992). Parent–child antecedents of 5-year-olds' close friendships: A longitudinal analysis. *Developmental Psychology, 28,* 700–713.

PART IV

HEALTH AND PHYSICAL DEVELOPMENT

CHAPTER 9

Nutrition and Physical Activity

Robert C. Whitaker and Rachel A. Gooze

Health and developmental scientists have long recognized that proper nutrition is a requirement for children's healthy development and that infants and toddlers living in poverty are at higher risk for poor nutrition (Karp, Cheng, & Meyers, 2005). Presently, obesity is the most common health consequence of poor nutrition in this population of children. Because obesity is thought to result primarily from an imbalance of energy intake and expenditure, this chapter discusses obesity prevention strategies for child care in two areas—nutrition and physical activity.

This chapter has three major sections. In the background section, we review the definition and prevalence of obesity in U.S. infants and toddlers, with a focus on children living in poverty. We also provide a rationale for a focus on obesity prevention when developing model child care programs for infants and toddlers living in poverty. In the middle section, we summarize the most relevant scientific findings in childhood obesity prevention *and* their implications for model child care programs. We begin the section by presenting a framework for evaluating the scientific evidence. We then present a set of evidence-based principles that can be used to develop obesity prevention practices in child care, separately discussing the areas of nutrition and physical activity. The chapter concludes with our summary of key opportunities, challenges, and future scientific directions in obesity prevention for those designing child care programs for infants and toddlers in poverty.

The Definition of Obesity in Infants and Toddlers

Obesity is an excess amount of body fat that is associated with physical or psychological morbidity. Clinically, the diagnosis of obesity requires both a direct measure of fatness and an assessment of morbidity. However, the definition of obesity in infants and toddlers for epidemiologic purposes involves an indirect measure of body fat, based on the measurement of weight and length, and no assessment of fatness-related morbidity.

Body fatness in infants and toddlers is usually assessed indirectly by using an index of weight relative to length—either the body mass index (BMI), which is the weight in kilograms divided by the length in meters squared (kg/m^2), or the weight-for-length percentile, in which the child's weight is compared to the weight of all children that length in a reference population. These two indices are expressed relative to a reference population, such as that established by the Centers for Disease Control and Prevention (CDC) (Kuczmarski et al., 2002) or the World Health Organization (WHO) (World Health Organization, 2006). The tracking of the U.S. childhood obesity epidemic has been based on the CDC growth reference. This reference was established by aggregating data from nationally representative, cross-sectional surveys of weight and length in U.S. children between 1971 and 1994. Using this historical reference makes it possible for more than 5% of U.S. children to now have a BMI ≥95th percentile.

Recently, the CDC suggested revisions to both the terminology (Ogden & Flegal, 2010) and reference population to be used (Grummer-Strawn, Reinold, & Krebs, 2010) in defining children as having elevated body weight relative to their length. For all children under 24 months of age, BMI should be compared to the WHO growth reference. This reference is based on a longitudinal study of exclusively or predominantly breastfed infants in six countries, conducted between 1997 and 2003.[1] In addition, the CDC now suggests that the term "obese" be used to describe children ≥24 months of age whose BMI exceeds the age and sex-specific 95th percentile. Although there is no agreed-upon term to describe children younger than 24 months of age with a BMI or weight-for-length ≥95th percentile, we will use the term "obese" to refer to these children.

The Prevalence of Obesity among U.S. Infants and Toddlers Living in Poverty

The most recent estimates from the CDC indicate that the prevalence of obesity is 10.4% among children 2 to 5 years of age (BMI ≥95th percentile of the 2000 CDC growth reference; Ogden, Carroll, Curtin, Lamb, & Flegal, 2010) and 10.1% among children 6 to 23 months of age (weight-for-length ≥95th percentile of the CDC growth reference; Centers for Disease

Control and Prevention, 2010). Since 1980, the prevalence of obesity has approximately doubled among U.S. infants and toddlers.

Although the increased prevalence of obesity has affected both boys and girls and all racial/ethnic groups, those children living in low-income households appear to be at a higher risk for obesity. For example, in 2008 the prevalence of obesity among children enrolled in the Special Supplemental Nutrition Program for Women, Infants, and Children (WIC) was 14.6% among children 2 to 4 years of age (Sharma et al., 2009). In young children, the relationship between obesity and household income is complex. Children living in households between 50 and 185% of the federal poverty threshold (all WIC-eligible income levels) have a higher prevalence of obesity than children living in households above and below these income levels (Anderson & Whitaker, 2010; Whitaker & Orzol, 2006). Among preschool-age children, obesity is more common among Native American, Hispanic, and non-Hispanic black children than among non-Hispanic white and Asian children (Anderson & Whitaker, 2009). However, the differences in obesity prevalence by race and ethnicity at preschool age are not accounted for either by household income or the level of maternal education, and the relationship between obesity and these two socioeconomic indicators is different across racial/ethnic groups (Whitaker & Orzol, 2006).

Rationale for a Focus on Obesity Prevention

Clinical and public health experts now agree that obesity prevention efforts should begin at or before birth (Barlow, 2007; Institute of Medicine, 2005). There are three major reasons to support this recommendation. First, obese children are more likely to become obese adults (Singh, Mulder, Twisk, van Mechelen, & Chinapaw, 2008), and this association is even stronger if the child has an obese parent. For example, a 4-year-old with a BMI ≥85th percentile but without an obese parent has a 24% risk of adult obesity, but this child's risk climbs to 62% if the child has at least one obese parent (Whitaker, Wright, Pepe, Seidel, & Dietz, 1997). The modifying effect of parental obesity on the tracking of obesity from early childhood to adulthood is an even more serious problem for low-income children. One-third of mothers enrolled in WIC are obese at the time of conception and 41% of their offspring already have a BMI ≥85th percentile by 4 years of age (Whitaker, 2004). Second, there are well-established health consequences of obesity across the life course (Daniels, 2009; Must et al., 1999). These include the metabolic consequences of obesity, which can be seen in early childhood (Freedman, Dietz, Srinivasan, & Berenson, 1999) and which lead to an increased risk later in life of diabetes (Colditz, Willett, Rotnitzky, & Manson, 1995), cardiovascular disease (Baker, Olsen, & Sorensen, 2007), and some forms of cancer (Flegal, Graubard, Williamson,

& Gail, 2007). The consequences of obesity are costly at the individual and societal level, reducing the length and quality of life (Fontaine & Barofsky, 2001; Olshansky et al., 2005) and increasing health care costs (Finkelstein, Ruhm, & Kosa, 2005). Finally, obesity is difficult to treat once it is present (Wadden & Butryn, 2003).

In early childhood, parents[2] are responsible for shaping children's home environments and they are the adults with the largest sphere of influence over children's food intake, activity, and weight. Infants and toddlers living in poverty, however, are spending increasing amounts of time in child care (Laughlin, 2010). Therefore, in this population of children, child care programs are a potentially important venue for implementing obesity prevention efforts (Story, Kaphingst, & French, 2006). Model child care programs for this population have the capacity to engage parents as partners and to influence the child's home environment through parent education and support, without which successful obesity prevention is unlikely (Gooze, Hughes, Finkelstein, & Whitaker, 2010). These programs reach children early in life when health behaviors are being shaped. Child care programs serving children in poverty are also eligible to access other federal programs, such as the Child and Adult Care Food Program (CACFP) and WIC, whose resources are now being deployed to prevent childhood obesity.

Relevant Scientific Findings and Implications for Program Design

There are very few randomized trials that have evaluated interventions to prevent obesity in children under 36 months of age (Ciampa et al., 2010; Hesketh & Campbell, 2010). Most of the scientific evidence supporting potential obesity prevention practices that might be used in child care settings for infants and toddlers arises from observational studies in children of this age, experimental studies in older children, or logical inferences about changes in children's environments that would support healthy body weight by balancing energy intake and expenditure. Given this state of the science, we use a framework in which we consider evidence that a given obesity prevention practice, if adopted in the child care setting, (1) might prevent obesity, (2) might benefit some aspect of health or well-being other than obesity prevention, and (3) is unlikely to cause harm (Whitaker, 2010).

The development of this framework for evaluating evidence was motivated by a body of research showing that mothers with overweight preschool-age children do not think that their children are overweight (Baughcum, Chamberlin, Deeks, Powers, & Whitaker, 2000). Among low-income mothers, this paradox arises because they view the definition, causes, and consequences of obesity differently than health professionals (Jain et al.,

2001). These mothers often feel conflicted about their children's weight. They see feeding and rapid weight gain in their infants and toddlers as reflecting their love and nurturance and feel blamed about their children's weight on account of their own weight or parenting skills (Hughes, Sherman, & Whitaker, 2010). Most importantly, these mothers indicate that they are more concerned about their children's cognitive, social, and emotional development than about obesity. Like parents, those designing model child care programs want to address multiple outcomes for children and have limited resources. To work on preventing obesity, like all other goals in children's development, the programs must address the skills and perceptions of staff and parents. This is especially important because child care providers[3] and parents may share cultural beliefs that are not always consistent with obesity prevention (Hughes, Gooze, Finkelstein, & Whitaker, 2010).

There have been a number of recent reviews of obesity prevention practices for child care and early childhood education programs (McWilliams et al., 2009; Trost, Ward, & Senso, 2010). In addition, the Institute of Medicine (IOM, 2011a) has recently published a report with policy recommendations for obesity prevention in children younger than 5 years of age, with recommendations that apply to child care programs. Many of these IOM recommendations align with child care polices already in place in a number of cities (New York City Board of Health, 2006) and states (Benjamin, Cradock, Walker, Slining, & Gillman, 2008). Our purpose is not to restate existing policy and practice recommendations and their rationale. Instead, we discuss *principles* that we feel are the most relevant to guiding the selection of obesity prevention practices in child care programs for infants and toddlers living in poverty. These seven principles are discussed in two major categories—feeding and eating (nutrition) and gross motor development and movement experiences (physical activity). In accordance with our framework, we selected these seven principles because they are consistent with the science supporting practices to prevent obesity and to also enhance cognitive, social, and emotional outcomes.

Feeding and Eating

Enhance Children's Self-Regulation Capacity through Responsive Feeding

The importance of self-regulation capacity for children's learning was emphasized in Chapter 6, but self-regulation capacity also appears to be critical for obesity prevention. The balance between energy intake and expenditure is controlled by the brain (Warne, 2009). For survival, infants are born with some innate ability to maintain energy balance and healthy body weight by responding to their internal hunger and satiety cues. The system that regulates food intake is affected by interrelated physiologic systems that affect learning, such as those regulating sleep (Vgontzas & Bixler, 2008), mood (Calabrese, Molteni, Racagni, & Riva, 2009), and motor activity (Vgontzas, Bixler, & Chrousos, 2006). Although the functioning of these systems at birth varies due to genetics and effects of the intrauterine environment, the postnatal environment plays a major role in shaping children's ability to regulate their food intake and body weight. In this regard, how adults interact with infants and toddlers, especially during feeding, may have lifelong implications for children's obesity risk.

There is epidemiological evidence that interventions to increase self-regulation in children might also have beneficial impacts on children's weight. Using data from the National Institute of Child Health and Human Development's Study of Early Child Care and Youth Development, two reports have shown that 3- to 5-year-olds who perform better on laboratory-based measures of self-regulation gain weight less rapidly (Francis & Susman, 2009) between 3 and 12 years of age and have a lower risk of obesity in preadolescence (Seeyave et al., 2009). The laboratory measures used in these studies were delay of gratification tasks and suggest that the general ability to control impulses may be important for weight regulation, presumably because of the child's ability to control the impulse to eat. With regard to attention, a dimension of self-regulation, children (Waring & Lapane, 2008) and adults (Pagoto et al., 2009) with attention-deficit/hyperactivity disorder (ADHD) are more likely to be obese. It is not known whether the risk for obesity arises from inattention per se, or the related disposition to addiction and low impulse control. If inattention is involved, obesity may arise in part from inattention to internal or external cues to stop eating.

In addition to delay of gratification and attention, emotion regulation (Thompson, 1994) is another dimension of self-regulation that appears to be closely linked to appetite regulation. Besides the well-established link between depressive symptoms and appetite (Markowitz, Friedman, & Arent, 2008), there is emerging evidence that disinhibited eating may result from difficulties regulating negative emotions, such as fear, sadness, anxiety, and anger (Ganley, 1989; Macht, 2008). For children living in poverty, this pathway to obesity could be especially important. These children experience high levels of stress, and eating is one way that both parents and children may address the negative emotions that arise from this stress (Hughes, Sherman, et al., 2010; Dallman et al., 2003). Furthermore, children living in low-income households and neighborhoods may consume palatable, high-calorie, nutrient-poor foods because they are the most accessible and affordable (Drewnowski & Darmon, 2005).

Responsive feeding leads to healthy appetite regulation (Eneli, Crum, & Tylka, 2008) in the same way that responsive caregiving by adults enhances children's self-regulation (Vygotsky, 1978). Responsive feeding is characterized by the ability of adults to recognize and respond to children's behavioral cues of hunger and satiety and to distinguish these cues from those that arise from other emotional or physiologic states. In practice, this means feeding to address a child's hunger rather than to soothe an upset child or reward the child's behavior. Responsive feeding also means never forcing a child to eat or withholding food as a punishment.

A responsive feeding style is important for infants and toddlers for several reasons. First, for infants and toddlers, there is virtually no eating without being fed by an adult, and for adults, feeding cannot be disentangled from the other adult–child interactions that constitute caregiving at this age. Second, eating and feeding are two parts of a dyadic adult–child interaction in which the child's eating behavior affects the adult's feeding behaviors and vice versa. Third, the systems in the brain that regulate both emotion and appetite are developing concurrently at this age. Many of the behavioral cues for internal states of hunger and satiety in infants and toddlers are difficult to distinguish from cues of emotional distress that are not hunger related. Determining whether a crying infant is hungry, tired, or frustrated is challenging, but the decision about whether to feed or hold the distressed baby sends the infant a signal that affects how that infant interprets his or her own physiological and emotional states.

Breast feeding is one responsive feeding practice that may prevent obesity and contribute to the child's general capacity for self-regulation. Most observational studies suggest that breast feeding provides a modest protection against the development of obesity (Owen, Martin, Whincup, Smith, & Cook, 2005). A large randomized trial in Belarus to promote breast feeding resulted in clinically meaningful differences in breast-feeding exposure between treatment and control groups. Although there were positive impacts of the intervention on children's cognition at age 6.5 years (Kramer, Aboud, et al., 2008), there were no impacts on obesity (Kramer et al., 2007) or behavior problems (Kramer, Fombonne, et al., 2008). These findings notwithstanding, compared to bottle feeding, breast feeding may allow infants to have more control over the initiation and termination of feedings and, thereby, enhance the development of their ability to regulate food intake in response to physiological signals of hunger and satiety (Li, Fein, & Grummer-Strawn, 2010).

Because of the many health benefits of breast feeding for mother and child (Kramer, 2010), it is the recommended method of infant feeding (American Academy of Pediatrics, 2005a) and model child care programs for infants and toddlers in poverty must be designed to fully support breast feeding. They should ideally have facilities for mothers (and staff) to pump and store breast milk and to breast-feed their infants. Coordination and even colocation of child care with WIC services and the use of lactation consultants and peer counselors to support breast feeding are useful strategies for increasing the duration of breast feeding (U.S. Department of Agriculture,

Food and Nutrition Service, 2010). To avoid overfeeding when giving formula or breast milk with a bottle, child care providers must be trained to recognize infants' hunger and satiety cues. Use of a bottle beyond infancy, including the practice of putting the child to bed with a bottle, is associated with later obesity (Kimbro, Brooks-Gunn, & McLanahan, 2007) and is also a risk factor for dental caries (Tinanoff & Palmer, 2000).

Decide What, When, and Where Children Eat and Let Children Decide How Much to Eat

The focus of many childhood obesity prevention efforts has been on what and how much children eat. With few exceptions, there is little evidence showing that the consumption of any particular foods either promotes or prevents the development of obesity in children (Davis et al., 2007). There is general agreement, however, that children should consume limited amounts of foods that are high in calories but low in nutrients (e.g., desserts, candy, sugar-sweetened beverages, and salty snacks), consume dairy and meat products that are low in saturated fat, and be encouraged to eat fruits, vegetables, and whole grains. The IOM recently revised the nutrition recommendations for the CACFP (Institute of Medicine, 2011b), and model child care programs for infants and toddlers living in poverty should follow these recommendations. Perhaps the most significant change in these recommendations is to limit the consumption of sugar-sweetened beverages, including 100% fruit juice. The IOM recommendations are based on the accumulating scientific evidence that these beverages may promote obesity and dental caries (Gortmaker, Long, & Wang, 2009).

For young children, there is increasing evidence that a promising obesity prevention strategy is to focus more on how much children eat than on what they eat (Sherry, 2005). Secular trends in portion sizes have been widely noted (Smiciklas-Wright, Mitchell, Mickle, Goldman, & Cook, 2003). Laboratory-based experimental studies with preschool-age children suggest that their energy intakes increase by up to one-third when entrée portion size is doubled (Fisher, Liu, Birch, & Rolls, 2007; Fisher, Rolls, & Birch, 2003; Rolls, Engell, & Birch, 2000). However, there have not yet been any intervention studies outside the laboratory to test the impact of reducing young children's portion sizes on their energy intakes or weight. Promising interventions involve decreasing both the unit size of foods offered (e.g., a smaller-sized sandwich or pancake) and the size of the eating implements (e.g., smaller cups, bowls, plates, and utensils; Wansink, van Ittersum, & Painter, 2006). The utility of these strategies is based on experiments with adults who have been shown to choose larger portions and to eat more when presented with foods in larger unit sizes (Rolls, Roe, Kral, Meengs, & Wall, 2004) and when using larger eating implements (Wansink et al., 2006).

At the present time, the safest way to ensure that children receive appropriate portion sizes is for adults to feed children small portion sizes and then offer the children more food if they want it. An example of such an approach, even in infancy, is to prepare four- to six-ounce bottles of formula rather than eight-ounce bottles and to give the infant more if he or she appears hungry (Whitaker, 2010). There also appears to be no harm in using small eating implements. Beyond their effects on preventing overfeeding and overeating, smaller eating implements may enhance children's fine-motor coordination and their sense of mastery and autonomy. These same obesity and nonobesity outcomes might also arise by allowing toddlers to begin serving their own portions from serving bowls (Fisher, 2007).

Because infants and toddlers must rely on adults to obtain food, the adult–child feeding relationship must be negotiated. In this relationship, a "division of labor" framework has become a widely suggested way to prevent obesity, though it has not undergone rigorous evaluation. This framework holds that adults should decide what, when, and where children eat but that children should decide how much to eat (Satter, 1986). There is controversy over whether obesity can be prevented when adults relinquish control over how much children eat (Kirschenbaum & Kelly, 2009). The success of this strategy appears to depend on two assumptions: (1) children are born with a healthy appetite regulation system that will prevent them from undereating and/or overeating, and (2) adults will provide young children with healthy food choices. When child care programs follow the recent IOM recommendations for CACFP food options, it seems both safe and developmentally optimal to follow the "division of labor" framework. This framework allows adults to use feeding as an opportunity to enhance children's self-regulation. By providing the structure and context for eating, adults let children focus on their internal hunger and satiety cues. Providing meals and snacks at regular intervals, minimizing distractions during eating, not using food as a reward or punishment, and avoiding cues to overeat, such as large eating implements or portion sizes, are all adult responsibilities that can support children in their developmentally critical responsibility—deciding how much to eat.

Model Moderation and Routine

In learning to eat, as in learning within other domains of development, children learn by watching others. Children are particularly influenced by watching adults to whom they have strong emotional bonds and on whom they are highly dependent. Therefore, shaping healthy eating patterns in children is not just about how adults feed children but about how adults model eating. Eating is a skill in which children become competent by watching competent adults (Satter, 2007). Because eating is inherently a social activity with hedonic rewards, it should be a pleasure for children.

Child care providers who are competent eaters are able to convey to children the pleasure of eating while still demonstrating moderation.

Young children will often not accept a new food without multiple exposures to it (Birch, McPhee, Shoba, Pirok, & Steinberg, 1987). For many children, accommodating to a novel sensory experience requires adult encouragement and support, and young children's acceptance of unfamiliar foods, such as fruits and vegetables, is positively influenced by the affect and modeling of adults (Birch & Fisher, 1998). A strong affective context for eating is when food is used for celebration. Given the near universal use of food across cultures and human history to celebrate and to express love and nurturance, trying to separate feeding and eating from the pleasures of social connection is not a sustainable obesity prevention strategy in child care. Competent adult eating involves the ability to not overeat in social situations. It is important for child care providers to model this behavior and to respect the manner in which food is used in different cultures and families. This means showing children ways in which social connection can be celebrated with and without food and being mindful about how food can shape children's behavior.

Incorporating feeding and eating into daily routines is an aspect of modeling that is important for children's development and may also help prevent obesity. Eating meals family style, which is a long-standing program performance criterion in Head Start and Early Head Start (U.S. Department of Health and Human Services, 2008), gives child care providers the opportunity to serve as positive role models by consuming the same foods that the children consume. It also allows child care providers to model and support language development through dialogue with the children during mealtimes. In addition to mealtimes, children can also learn skills by helping grow and prepare food. Gardens in child care settings provide toddlers with the opportunity for outdoor movement, sensory contact with the natural world, and knowledge about where food comes from. Participation in food preparation by toddlers can enhance their fine-motor skills and increase their familiarity with and acceptance of a variety of unfamiliar foods. Whether this "ground to mouth" exposure to food prevents childhood obesity has not been empirically demonstrated. However, this type of holistic exposure to food is a useful consideration for model child care programs because of its potential combination of obesity and nonobesity benefits.

Gross-Motor Development and Movement Experiences

Integrate Movement Experiences into Existing Activities

It is more intuitive to those caring for infants and toddlers to focus on enhancing gross-motor development than on increasing levels of physical activity. As with cognitive development, experience and modeling increases motor skills, and skills beget skills. Therefore, from the perspective of obesity prevention, supporting gross-motor development in infants and toddlers is a logical step in increasing activity-related energy expenditure. There is some evidence that infants with more advanced gross-motor skills move more and have a lower risk of obesity (Slining, Adair, Goldman, Borja, & Bentley, 2010) and that infant movement and fatness are inversely associated (Wells & Ritz, 2001). However, the true causal direction of the relationship between skill, movement, and obesity is unlikely to be disentangled.

Developmental scientists have long emphasized the complementary nature of different streams of development (Thelen, Schoner, Scheier, & Smith, 2001). Infants and toddlers are physically active by nature and learn through movement. It is through movement that infants and toddlers explore their environment to obtain the sensory experiences that stimulate their cognitive development (Bushnell & Boudreau, 1993). Motor development can be viewed as a helpful foundation for the development of language, self-regulation, and executive function. For example, as children's verbal language is developing, they communicate through movement. For children to develop the capacity for cooperative and dramatic play, they must first develop motor skills that allow them to recognize where their body is in space (in relation to self and others) and to plan, inhibit, and execute motor activities, integrating fine- and gross-motor skills, such as object manipulation through reaching and hand movement.

Unfortunately, with the increasing focus on school readiness, there has been more emphasis on children's development in the cognitive, social, and emotional domains than in the motor domain. A major aspect of obesity prevention in infant/toddler care should be renewed attention to children's motor development. The natural propensity of infants and toddlers to move should not be viewed as a marker of inattention and poor impulse control. Rather, this tendency means it is necessary to integrate movement experiences into activities designed to support children's cognitive, social, and emotional development. Doing so may help prevent obesity by increasing children's energy expenditure.

Despite some existing guidelines (American Academy of Pediatrics, 2010; National Association for Sport and Physical Education, 2002), there is not ample empirical evidence upon which to base a recommendation for a minimum amount of time each day in which children younger than 36 months of age should be physically active. Children younger than 36 months do not have the capacity for bouts of intense, sustained movement or for sustained periods of sitting or standing still. For this reason alone, allocating a certain number of minutes of "physical activity" is not a useful approach to enhancing motor development and preventing obesity in infants and toddlers. Instead, model child care settings should be designed to allow children to move freely in the type, frequency, and intensity of movement to which they are naturally inclined. This design does not need to compete with structured or adult-guided activities focused on enhancing cognitive, social, or emotional development. For example, allowing children to dance to music, to stand rather than sit, to move while listening, and to do rather than watch may help prevent obesity and enhance attention or learning.

As with feeding, eating, and appetite regulation, children's motor development is influenced by adult–child interaction. By joining children in their movement experiences and doing so with a positive affect, adults can affect gross motor development and activity levels. Infants and toddlers can learn movement skills and be encouraged to move by watching adults move. Even when working with infants, adults should spend some time on the floor or ground with them to optimize adult–infant interaction and to encourage infants to explore their environments. Child care providers should avoid disciplining toddlers for being too physically active, and should also avoid withholding movement opportunities as a form of discipline. This type of discipline communicates a confusing message to toddlers whose innate tendency is to stimulate their own development by moving.

Avoid Unnecessary Restriction of Children's Movement

Ensuring children's physical safety is a primary responsibility of any child care program and safety is a particular concern from the time infants learn to crawl through the toddler years. An unintentional negative consequence of fulfilling this safety responsibility is the unnecessary restriction of children's movement. Even with favorable staff-to-child ratios, it is often most convenient to ensure the safety of infants and toddlers by keeping them in equipment that restrains their movement. The unnecessary use of car seats, infant seats, cribs, high chairs, and strollers may potentially inhibit movement, energy expenditure, and even cognitive and social development. Equipment should generally be used only for its primary purpose—car seats for car travel, cribs for sleeping, high chairs for eating, and strollers for moving children who cannot feasibly walk. Although there have been no experimental studies that examine whether avoiding the unnecessary use of restraining equipment in child care impacts body weight, motor development, or injury, using this equipment only as needed is a logical way to stimulate gross motor development. Furthermore, ensuring children's safety without these devices might lead to more adult–child interaction, which could have benefits on development in nonmotor domains.

Even from the time of birth, it is important for awake infants to have regular opportunities to be in the prone position and to move freely under adult supervision to explore their environment. There is evidence that gross-motor development is enhanced by placing awake infants in the prone position (Jennings, Sarbaugh, & Payne, 2005; Kuo, Liao, Chen, Hsieh, & Hwang, 2008). In addition, prone positioning can prevent positional skull deformity, which is an unintended negative consequence of the effort to prevent sudden infant death syndrome by placing young infants in the supine position for sleep (American Academy of Pediatrics, 2005b).

Design of Indoor and Outdoor Spaces That Encourage Children's Movement

There are a number of reasons that child care providers should regularly take children outdoors. Several observational studies support the conventional wisdom that children move more when they are outdoors than when they are indoors (Baranowski, Thompson, DuRant, Baranowski, & Puhl, 1993; Boldemann et al., 2006; Klesges, Eck, Hanson, Haddock, & Klesges, 1990). However, there has only been one randomized trial to increase outdoor time in young children, and there was no impact on physical activity levels (Alhassan, Sirard, & Robinson, 2007). Outdoor time can benefit children by increasing their contact with the natural world. Most of the research on the relationship between children's well-being and contact with nature has been conducted in older children, but research is now emerging on this subject in younger children. After older children with ADHD are exposed to green outdoor activities, parents report fewer symptoms (Kuo & Taylor, 2004) and the children perform better on tests of concentration (Taylor & Kuo, 2009). Preschool children's level of attention is also associated with exposure to green outdoor environments (Martensson et al., 2009). With regard to mood, the association between stressful life events and psychological distress is less among older children who have greater exposure to natural environments (Wells & Evans, 2003). These findings about attention and mood are relevant because both areas are related to each other, to learning, and to the stress of living in poverty.

Empirical studies of the relationship between the amount and quality of preschool-age children's movement and the characteristics of their play spaces suggest that model child care programs should consider how their indoor and outdoor spaces are designed. Incorporating natural elements (e.g., mounds and uneven terrain, open grassy areas, large climbing rocks, and shade trees) into outdoor play spaces may enhance children's movement, coordination, and balance (Cosco, Moore, & Islam, 2010; Fjortoft, 2001). In contrast to the design of most existing playgrounds, large fixed play structures, such as swings and slides, may actually decrease rather than increase children's movement. In contrast, more portable play equipment, such as balls, hoops, and wheeled toys (wagons or tricycles) are associated with higher levels of movement in young children (Bower et al., 2008; Dowda et al., 2009). In addition, having "loose parts" outdoors, such as buckets, digging tools, and toys, increases opportunities for creative play.

For reasons of safety and convenience, adults are often reluctant to take infants outdoors. While there is not empirical evidence to suggest that infants move more outdoors, outdoor environments can be designed to allow infants to move safely, even before they crawl. By providing shade from direct sun when needed and a secure perimeter (also requirements for toddlers), child care centers can allow infants to regularly spend time outdoors. Outdoors, infants can experience more varied and natural stimulation to all of their senses than they can indoors.[4]

Like children's movement outdoors, their movement indoors is also associated with elements of design. For example, movement indoors is increased when there is more portable play equipment and more open space. Especially for toddlers who are trying to develop awareness of their own bodies in space, adequate space indoors is important for encouraging vigorous gross-motor movement without injury to self and others. For infants, their movement is also affected by the sensory properties of indoor surfaces and materials that encourage them to explore their surroundings. For example, walking is encouraged by the availability of safe fixed structures on which infants can pull themselves up to stand and cruise.

Children's indoor and outdoor play spaces should ideally be contiguous and located at ground level so that toddlers can safely navigate between these spaces with limited adult supervision. Although this is a rare design feature, it affords benefits for the children and child care providers. Children's access to the outdoors is increased by its proximity to the indoor settings. The time spent in transition between these spaces is minimized and children feel greater autonomy when moving between indoor and outdoor spaces with limited adult assistance. The application of this design feature also reflects the principal of universal design, which allows individuals of varying physical abilities to have autonomy and safety (Preiser & Ostroff, 2001). Finally, the proximity of indoor and outdoor spaces usually means that the outdoor environment and its natural elements can be seen from indoors. These views can increase children's sense of wonder and curiosity about changes of weather, season, and daylight. Seeing the outdoors may also reduce anxiety and improve attention (Taylor, Kuo, & Sullivan, 2002).

Be Intentional about Inactive Time, Especially Screen Time and Sleep

Direct measurement of preschool-age children by accelerometry suggests that children this age are inactive (sitting, standing, or lying still) for half of every hour spent in child care in which they are not sleeping or eating (Institute of Medicine, 2011a). What children do with this half of their time clearly affects their development, but it may also affect their risk of obesity. Whether it is optimal for children to spend this much time inactive is an empirical question that has not been addressed. For infants and toddlers living in poverty, unsafe neighborhood and housing conditions, single parenting, and complex work schedules may all lead to this population of children having limited opportunities for movement and outdoor play. Thus, to prevent obesity, it may be necessary to minimize inactive time in child care.

However, it is not only the duration of inactive time, but also the content and context of that time that is important. From the perspective of preventing obesity as well as optimizing cognitive, social, and emotional development of infants and toddlers living in poverty, there is no compelling reason for child care programs serving this population to include any screen time, such as the use of television, videos, DVDs, or computers. Children learn language, emotional literacy, and self-regulation best from face-to-face interactions with responsive adults and not from watching or interacting with adults on screens. Beginning in infancy, there are substantial disparities in media exposure between children by level of maternal education (Certain & Kahn, 2002), and removing screen time from child care could reduce that disparity. Although there is little evidence among infants and toddlers that screen-viewing time is associated with obesity, there is experimental evidence in older children showing that television viewing causes obesity (Epstein et al., 2008; Robinson, 1999). The primary mechanism of this causal relationship in older children appears to be through the effect of food advertisement on children's food requests and consumption (McGinnis et al., 2006). Evidence for the importance of this mechanism in preschool-age children is now accumulating (Harris et al., 2010).

The most recent development in the understanding of childhood obesity is that short sleep duration is associated with obesity. Several prospective observational studies (Chen, Beydoun, & Wang, 2008), including two involving infants (Bell & Zimmerman, 2010; Taveras, Rifas-Shiman, Oken, Gunderson, & Gillman, 2008), support this finding. It is not clear that the association between short sleep duration and obesity is a causal one; however, the association suggests that all of the daily activities of infants and toddlers, not just their eating and active play, may be relevant for obesity prevention. Aside from its potential impact on obesity, short sleep duration in older children has been associated with functional impairments, such as problems with attention, aggression, and mood (Gregory, Van der Ende, Willis, & Verhulst, 2008). Although children spend over half of their lives asleep between birth and 24 months of age, relatively little research has been done to establish what adults should do to help infants and toddlers develop healthy sleep quality and duration. We do know, however, that developing healthy sleep regulation, like appetite regulation, requires adult support. Awaiting further research, child care programs should consider such practices as establishing consistent nap schedules and reducing sensory stimulation (e.g., light and noise) around nap time (Mindell, Meltzer, Carskadon, & Chervin, 2009).

Opportunities, Challenges, and Future Directions

Success in preventing early childhood obesity is most likely to happen if there are coordinated efforts between the child care and home settings. This requires child care providers and parents to work together on a shared set of goals and practices. Model child care programs can provide opportunities for this collaboration between staff and parents (Gooze et al., 2010). In this collaboration, there is a chance to emphasize those practices in child care and at home that might help prevent obesity while also benefiting other aspects of children's development (Whitaker, 2011). Whether the practice is for adults to limit children's TV viewing or to join children in eating meals and playing outdoors, highlighting nonobesity benefits may help both child care providers and parents initiate and maintain these practices. Obesity prevention should not and need not be seen as a separate set of activities in child rearing. Obesity prevention can be integrated with the three central activities that occupy infants and toddlers—eating, playing, and sleeping. Engaging in these activities in healthy environments and guided by emotionally supportive adults leads not only to optimal development but also healthy weight.

Potential Challenges

Along with the opportunities for obesity prevention afforded by child care settings, there are also challenges, such as engaging and empowering child care providers and parents to work together and to act as positive role models for healthy behavior. A central challenge is finding the time for child care providers and parents to meet with each other so that they can develop a trusting relationship and identify a set of shared goals and practices to support children's development. The subject of obesity is a sensitive one and many parents are defensive and feel blamed by professionals (Chamberlin, Sherman, Jain, Powers, & Whitaker, 2002; Jain et al., 2001). When a child or parent is obese, there may be a tendency for professionals to focus on the child's or family's current or future health problems rather than on positive aspects of the child's current functioning. An emphasis on fitness, fatness, and energy balance should not overshadow discussions about opportunities for developing the child's motor skills, self-regulation, social skills, or autonomy (Burdette & Whitaker, 2005).

As infants and toddlers develop health-related behaviors, they mimic adults. Child care providers must join children in their eating and movement and be positive role models. For child care providers to feel comfortable in this role, model programs should also be prepared to invest in staff- and parent-wellness programs. For example, teachers' lack of comfort with their body weight and physical coordination is a potential barrier to encouraging children's physical activity (Hughes, Gooze, et al., 2010).

Another challenging area is the co-occurrence of food insecurity and obesity. In the United States, approximately 23% of children younger than 6 years of age live in food-insecure households (Nord, Coleman-Jensen, Andrews, & Carlson, 2010), which means that, owing to a lack of money, families have limited or uncertain availability of nutritionally adequate and safe food (Life Sciences Research Office, 1990). In 2009, 46% of U.S. households with incomes below 130% of the poverty threshold and with children younger than 5 years of age were food insecure (Nord et al., 2010), making the co-occurrence of food insecurity and obesity common within the homes of young children living in poverty. Obesity and food insecurity can occur in the same classroom and even in the same child, and child care providers can feel caught between the challenges of helping children learn to consume age-appropriate portion sizes and ensuring that children have enough to eat. Addressing food insecurity is no less important than addressing obesity in early child care settings because food insecurity is associated with behavior problems in young children independent of its association with maternal anxiety and depression (Whitaker, Phillips, & Orzol, 2006).

Lack of training is a major obstacle for early child care providers (Hughes, Gooze, et al., 2010). Degree programs, certification, continuing education, and consultation services for child care providers should include content on obesity prevention in infants and toddlers, and how to counsel parents in this area. Specifically, child care providers need more training on responsive feeding practices, evaluating and encouraging children's gross-motor development (including for children with physical disabilities), and integrating obesity prevention into activities that are primarily designed to enhance children's cognitive, social, and emotional development.

Finally, there are substantial costs to consider (Hughes, Gooze, et al., 2010). It is estimated that the application of the IOM dietary recommendations for CACFP will increase food costs alone by 31–44% (Institute of Medicine, 2011b). Staff time for training, wellness programs, and parent meetings often requires hiring substitute staff, which is costly for programs. It can also be very costly to alter or increase indoor and outdoor spaces to enhance children's opportunities for movement.

Future Scientific Directions

Obesity prevention is increasingly informed by developmental science. Future research in these areas appears most promising for informing the development of model child care programs for children living in poverty.

First, it is likely that more will be understood about the importance of sleep duration and quality in children's development, not just their metabolism and energy balance. Given the differences that already exist in the duration and quality of children's sleep according to household income (Anderson & Whitaker, 2010), sleep may become an important area for addressing poverty-related disparities in child well-being. Thus, child care providers for infant and toddlers in poverty will need to consider how best to address the development of sleep patterns that optimize children's health and development.

Second, much has been learned from research in adults showing how the social and environmental context of eating influences food consumption (Wansink, 2006). It is likely that a great deal will be learned by applying this research to very young children. Obesity prevention strategies in the future, while still emphasizing responsive feeding, are likely to place even more emphasis on removing environmental cues to overeating, such as large portion sizes and eating implements, that can interfere with children's innate ability to regulate their own energy intake.

Finally, there is the role of stress reduction in obesity prevention. Considerable attention is already being paid to the role of poverty-related stress in children's environments and how this may impact cognitive, social, and emotional development (National Scientific Counsel on the Developing Child, 2005). In the future, more is likely to be learned about the potential impact of this stress on obesity and the mechanisms by which this occurs (Bjorntorp & Rosmond, 2000; Tsigos & Chrousos, 2006). In response to the broad array of health and developmental impacts of poverty-related stress, child care programs will need to consider new ways in which they may buffer that stress through staff–child interactions and the design of indoor and outdoor environments. There are promising but underexamined approaches to buffering this stress that could also prevent obesity. These approaches include dance, massage therapy, mindfulness-based practices for toddlers, such as yoga, and the design of facilities that reduce unnecessary noise and increase children's contact with the natural world. Finally, recent work showing the association of poor early maternal–child relationship quality with obesity in preschool-age children (Anderson & Whitaker, 2011) and in adolescents (Anderson, Gooze, Lemeshow, & Whitaker, 2012) raises the possibility that the primary prevention of obesity may also arise from warm and responsive care from adults, which has been a longstanding focus of applied developmental science.

ACKNOWLEDGMENTS

The writing of this chapter was supported by Grant No. R01DK088913 from the National Institutes of Health. The content is solely the responsibility of the authors and does not necessarily represent the official views of the National Institutes of Health.

NOTES

1. Because these children were all exclusively or predominantly breastfed, this is now considered by many to be a growth "standard" rather than a growth reference, and it establishes sex-specific BMI percentiles from birth to 60 months.
2. Throughout, the term "parents" is meant to also include other primary caregivers, such as grandparents, foster parents, and legal guardians.
3. Throughout, the term "child care providers" is meant to also include early childhood educators.
4. In addition, exposure to sunlight is necessary for adequate vitamin D synthesis and bone health, especially for infants who are breast fed, have pigmented skin, or reside in higher latitudes (Wagner, Greer, & Committee on Nutrition, 2008).

REFERENCES

Alhassan, S., Sirard, J. R., & Robinson, T. N. (2007). The effects of increasing outdoor play time on physical activity in Latino preschool children. *International Journal Pediatric Obesity, 2*(3), 153–158.

American Academy of Pediatrics, American Public Health Association, National Resource Center for Health and Safety in Child Care and Early Education. (2010). *Preventing childhood obesity in early care and education programs.* Washington, DC: U.S. Department of Health and Human Services, Health Resources and Services Administration, Maternal and Child Health Bureau.

American Academy of Pediatrics, Section on Breastfeeding. (2005a). Breastfeeding and the use of human milk. *Pediatrics, 115*(2), 496–506.

American Academy of Pediatrics, Task Force on Sudden Infant Death Syndrome. (2005b). The changing concept of sudden infant death syndrome: Diagnostic coding shifts, controversies regarding the sleeping environment, and new variables to consider in reducing risk. *Pediatrics, 116*(5), 1245–1255.

Anderson, S. E., Gooze, R. A., Lemeshow, S., & Whitaker, R. C. (2012). Quality of early maternal–child relationship and risk of adolescent obesity, *Pediatrics, 129*(1), 132–140.

Anderson, S. E., & Whitaker, R. C. (2009). Prevalence of obesity among US preschool children in different racial and ethnic groups. *Archives of Pediatrics and Adolescent Medicine, 163*(4), 344–348.

Anderson, S. E., & Whitaker, R. C. (2010). Household routines and obesity in U.S. preschool-aged children. *Pediatrics, 125*(3), 420–428.

Anderson, S. E., & Whitaker, R. C. (2011). Attachment security and obesity in U.S. preschool-aged children. *Archives of Pediatrics and Adolescent Medicine, 165*(3), 235–242.

Baker, J. L., Olsen, L. W., & Sorensen, T. I. (2007). Childhood body-mass index and the risk of coronary heart disease in adulthood. *New England Journal of Medicine, 357*(23), 2329–2337.

Baranowski, T., Thompson, W. O., DuRant, R. H., Baranowski, J., & Puhl, J. (1993). Observations on physical activity in physical locations: Age, gender, ethnicity, and month effects. *Research Quarterly for Exercise and Sport, 64*(2), 127–133.

Barlow, S. E. (2007). Expert committee recommendations regarding the prevention, assessment, and treatment of child and adolescent overweight and obesity: Summary report. *Pediatrics, 120*(Suppl. 4), S164–S192.

Baughcum, A. E., Chamberlin, L. A., Deeks, C. M., Powers, S. W., & Whitaker, R. C. (2000). Maternal perceptions of overweight preschool children. *Pediatrics, 106*(6), 1380–1386.

Bell, J. F., & Zimmerman, F. J. (2010). Shortened nighttime sleep duration in early life and subsequent childhood obesity. *Archives of Pediatrics and Adolescent Medicine, 164*(9), 840–845.

Benjamin, S. E., Cradock, A., Walker, E. M., Slining, M., & Gillman, M. W. (2008). Obesity prevention in child care: A review of U.S. state regulations. *BMC Public Health, 8,* 188.

Birch, L. L., & Fisher, J. O. (1998). Development of eating behaviors among children and adolescents. *Pediatrics, 101*(3, Pt. 2), 539–549.

Birch, L. L., McPhee, L., Shoba, B. C., Pirok, E., & Steinberg, L. (1987). What kind of exposure reduces children's food neophobia? Looking vs. tasting. *Appetite, 9*(3), 171–178.

Bjorntorp, P., & Rosmond, R. (2000). The metabolic syndrome—A neuroendocrine disorder? *British Journal of Nutrition, 83*(Suppl. 1), S49–S57.

Boldemann, C., Blennow, M., Dal, H., Martensson, F., Raustorp, A., Yuen, K., et al. (2006). Impact of preschool environment upon children's physical activity and sun exposure. *Preventive Medicine, 42*(4), 301–308.

Bower, J. K., Hales, D. P., Tate, D. F., Rubin, D. A., Benjamin, S. E., & Ward, D. S. (2008). The childcare environment and children's physical activity. *American Journal of Preventive Medicine, 34*(1), 23–29.

Burdette, H. L., & Whitaker, R. C. (2005). Resurrecting free play in young children: Looking beyond fitness and fatness to attention, affiliation, and affect. *Archives of Pediatrics and Adolescent Medicine, 159*(1), 46–50.

Bushnell, E. W., & Boudreau, J. P. (1993). Motor development and the mind: The potential role of motor abilities as a determinant of aspects of perceptual development. *Child Development, 64*(4), 1005–1021.

Calabrese, F., Molteni, R., Racagni, G., & Riva, M. A. (2009). Neuronal plasticity: A link between stress and mood disorders. *Psychoneuroendocrinology, 34*(Suppl. 1), S208–S216.

Centers for Disease Control and Prevention. (2010). *Prevalence of overweight infants and children less than 2 years of age: United States, 2003–2004*: NCHS Health E-Stat. Retrieved from *www.cdc.gov/nchs/hestat/overweight/ overweight_child_under02.htm*.

Certain, L. K., & Kahn, R. S. (2002). Prevalence, correlates, and trajectory of television viewing among infants and toddlers. *Pediatrics, 109*(4), 634–642.

Chamberlin, L. A., Sherman, S. N., Jain, A., Powers, S. W., & Whitaker, R. C.

(2002). The challenge of preventing and treating obesity in low-income, pre-school children: Perceptions of WIC health care professionals. *Archives of Pediatrics and Adolescent Medicine, 156*(7), 662–668.

Chen, X., Beydoun, M. A., & Wang, Y. (2008). Is sleep duration associated with childhood obesity? A systematic review and meta-analysis. *Obesity (Silver Spring), 16*(2), 265–274.

Ciampa, P. J., Kumar, D., Barkin, S. L., Sanders, L. M., Yin, H. S., Perrin, E. M., et al. (2010). Interventions aimed at decreasing obesity in children younger than 2 years: A systematic review. *Archives of Pediatrics and Adolescent Medicine, 164*(12), 1098–1104.

Colditz, G. A., Willett, W. C., Rotnitzky, A., & Manson, J. E. (1995). Weight gain as a risk factor for clinical diabetes mellitus in women. *Annals of Internal Medicine, 122*(7), 481–486.

Cosco, N. G., Moore, R. C., & Islam, M. Z. (2010). Behavior mapping: A method for linking preschool physical activity and outdoor design. *Medicine and Science in Sports and Exercise, 42*(3), 513–519.

Dallman, M. F., Pecoraro, N., Akana, S. F., La Fleur, S. E., Gomez, F., Houshyar, H., et al. (2003). Chronic stress and obesity: A new view of "comfort food." *Proceedings of the National Academy of Sciences, 100*(20), 11696–11701.

Daniels, S. R. (2009). Complications of obesity in children and adolescents. *International Journal of Obesity (London), 33*(Suppl. 1), S60–S65.

Davis, M. M., Gance-Cleveland, B., Hassink, S., Johnson, R., Paradis, G., & Resnicow, K. (2007). Recommendations for prevention of childhood obesity. *Pediatrics, 120*(Suppl. 4), S229–S253.

Dowda, M., Brown, W. H., McIver, K. L., Pfeiffer, K. A., O'Neill, J. R., Addy, C. L., et al. (2009). Policies and characteristics of the preschool environment and physical activity of young children. *Pediatrics, 123*(2), e261–e266.

Drewnowski, A., & Darmon, N. (2005). The economics of obesity: Dietary energy density and energy cost. *American Journal of Clinical Nutrition, 82*(Suppl. 1), S265–S273.

Eneli, I. U., Crum, P. A., & Tylka, T. L. (2008). The trust model: A different feeding paradigm for managing childhood obesity. *Obesity (Silver Spring), 16*(10), 2197–2204.

Epstein, L. H., Roemmich, J. N., Robinson, J. L., Paluch, R. A., Winiewicz, D. D., Fuerch, J. H., et al. (2008). A randomized trial of the effects of reducing television viewing and computer use on body mass index in young children. *Archives of Pediatrics and Adolescent Medicine, 162*(3), 239–245.

Finkelstein, E. A., Ruhm, C. J., & Kosa, K. M. (2005). Economic causes and consequences of obesity. *Annual Review of Public Health, 26,* 239–257.

Fisher, J. O. (2007). Effects of age on children's intake of large and self-selected food portions. *Obesity (Silver Spring), 15*(2), 403–412.

Fisher, J. O., Liu, Y., Birch, L. L., & Rolls, B. J. (2007). Effects of portion size and energy density on young children's intake at a meal. *American Journal of Clinical Nutrition, 86*(1), 174–179.

Fisher, J. O., Rolls, B. J., & Birch, L. L. (2003). Children's bite size and intake of an entree are greater with large portions than with age-appropriate or self-selected portions. *American Journal of Clinical Nutrition, 77*(5), 1164–1170.

Fjortoft, I. (2001). The natural environment as a playground for children: The impact of outdoor play activities in pre-primary school children. *Early Childhood Education Journal, 29*(2), 111–117.

Flegal, K. M., Graubard, B. I., Williamson, D. F., & Gail, M. H. (2007). Cause-specific excess deaths associated with underweight, overweight, and obesity. *Journal of the American Medical Association, 298*(17), 2028–2037.

Fontaine, K. R., & Barofsky, I. (2001). Obesity and health-related quality of life. *Obesity Reviews, 2*(3), 173–182.

Francis, L. A., & Susman, E. J. (2009). Self-regulation and rapid weight gain in children from age 3 to 12 years. *Archives of Pediatrics and Adolescent Medicine, 163*(4), 297–302.

Freedman, D. S., Dietz, W. H., Srinivasan, S. R., & Berenson, G. S. (1999). The relation of overweight to cardiovascular risk factors among children and adolescents: The Bogalusa Heart Study. *Pediatrics, 103,* 1175–1182.

Ganley, R. M. (1989). Emotion and eating in obesity: A review of the literature. *International Journal of Eating Disorders, 8*(3), 343–361.

Gooze, R. A., Hughes, C. C., Finkelstein, D. M., & Whitaker, R. C. (2010). Reaching staff, parents, and community partners to prevent childhood obesity in Head Start, 2008. *Preventing Chronic Disease, 7*(3), A54.

Gortmaker, S., Long, M., & Wang, C. (2009). The negative impact of sugar-sweetened beverages on children's health. Retrieved from *www.rwjf.org/files/research/20091203herssb.pdf.*

Gregory, A. M., Van der Ende, J., Willis, T. A., & Verhulst, F. C. (2008). Parent-reported sleep problems during development and self-reported anxiety/depression, attention problems, and aggressive behavior later in life. *Archives of Pediatrics and Adolescent Medicine, 162*(4), 330–335.

Grummer-Strawn, L. M., Reinold, C., & Krebs, N. F. (2010). Use of World Health Organization and CDC growth charts for children aged 0–59 months in the United States. *Morbidity and Mortality Weekly Report, 59*(RR-9), 1–15.

Harris, J. L., Schwartz, M. B., Brownell, K. D., Sarda, V., Ustjanauskas, A., Javadizadeh, J., et al. (2010). *Fast food FACTS: Evaluating fast food nutrition and marketing to youth.* New Haven, CT: Rudd Center for Food Policy and Obesity.

Hesketh, K. D., & Campbell, K. J. (2010). Interventions to prevent obesity in 0–5 year olds: An updated systematic review of the literature. *Obesity (Silver Spring), 18*(Suppl. 1), S27–S35.

Hughes, C. C., Gooze, R. A., Finkelstein, D. M., & Whitaker, R. C. (2010). Barriers to obesity prevention in Head Start. *Health Affairs (Millwood), 29*(3), 454–462.

Hughes, C. C., Sherman, S. N., & Whitaker, R. C. (2010). How low-income mothers with overweight preschool children make sense of obesity. *Qualitative Health Research, 20*(4), 465–478.

Institute of Medicine. (2005). *Preventing childhood obesity: Health in the balance.* Washington, DC: National Academies Press.

Institute of Medicine. (2011a). *Early childhood obesity prevention policies.* Washington, DC: National Academies Press.

Institute of Medicine. (2011b). *Child and Adult Care Food Program: Aligning dietary guidance for all.* Washington, DC: National Academies Press.

Jain, A., Sherman, S. N., Chamberlin, L. A., Carter, Y., Powers, S. W., & Whitaker, R. C. (2001). Why don't low-income mothers worry about their preschoolers being overweight? *Pediatrics, 107*(5), 1138–1146.

Jennings, J. T., Sarbaugh, B. G., & Payne, N. S. (2005). Conveying the message about optimal infant positions. *Physical and Occupational Therapy in Pediatrics, 25*(3), 3–18.

Karp, R. J., Cheng, C., & Meyers, A. F. (2005). The appearance of discretionary income: Influence on the prevalence of under- and over-nutrition. *International Journal for Equity in Health, 4*, 10.

Kimbro, R. T., Brooks-Gunn, J., & McLanahan, S. (2007). Racial and ethnic differentials in overweight and obesity among 3-year-old children. *American Journal of Public Health, 97*(2), 298–305.

Kirschenbaum, D. S., & Kelly, K. P. (2009). Five reasons to distrust the trust model. *Obesity (Silver Spring), 17*(6), 1107–1111.

Klesges, R. C., Eck, L. H., Hanson, C. L., Haddock, C. K., & Klesges, L. M. (1990). Effects of obesity, social interactions, and physical environment on physical activity in preschoolers. *Health Psychology, 9*(4), 435–449.

Kramer, M. S. (2010). "Breast is best": The evidence. *Early Human Development, 86*(11), 729–732.

Kramer, M. S., Aboud, F., Mironova, E., Vanilovich, I., Platt, R. W., Matush, L., et al. (2008). Breastfeeding and child cognitive development: New evidence from a large randomized trial. *Archives of General Psychiatry, 65*(5), 578–584.

Kramer, M. S., Fombonne, E., Igumnov, S., Vanilovich, I., Matush, L., Mironova, E., et al. (2008). Effects of prolonged and exclusive breastfeeding on child behavior and maternal adjustment: Evidence from a large, randomized trial. *Pediatrics, 121*(3), e435–e440.

Kramer, M. S., Matush, L., Vanilovich, I., Platt, R. W., Bogdanovich, N., Sevkovskaya, Z., et al. (2007). Effects of prolonged and exclusive breastfeeding on child height, weight, adiposity, and blood pressure at age 6.5 y: Evidence from a large randomized trial. *American Journal of Clinical Nutrition, 86*(6), 1717–1721.

Kuczmarski, R. J., Ogden, C. L., Guo, S. S., Grummer-Strawn, L. M., Flegal, K. M., Mei, Z., et al. (2002). 2000 CDC growth charts for the United States: Methods and development. *Vital Health Statistics 11,*(246), 1–190.

Kuo, F. E., & Taylor, A. F. (2004). A potential natural treatment for attention-deficit/hyperactivity disorder: Evidence from a national study. *American Journal of Public Health, 94*(9), 1580–1586.

Kuo, Y. L., Liao, H. F., Chen, P. C., Hsieh, W. S., & Hwang, A. W. (2008). The influence of wakeful prone positioning on motor development during the early life. *Journal of Developmental and Behavioral Pediatrics, 29*(5), 367–376.

Laughlin, L. (2010). *Who's minding the kids? Child care arrangements: Spring 2005 and Summer 2006.* Washington, DC: U.S. Census Bureau, Current Population Reports, 70–121. Retrieved from *www.census.gov/prod/2010pubs/p70-121.pdf.*

Li, R., Fein, S. B., & Grummer-Strawn, L. M. (2010). Do infants fed from bottles lack self-regulation of milk intake compared with directly breastfed infants? *Pediatrics, 125*(6), e1386–e1393.

Life Sciences Research Office, Federation of American Societies for Experimental

Biology. (1990). Core indicators of nutritional state for difficult-to-sample populations. *Journal of Nutrition, 120*(Suppl. 11), 1559–1600.

Macht, M. (2008). How emotions affect eating: A five-way model. *Appetite, 50*(1), 1–11.

Markowitz, S., Friedman, M. A., & Arent, S. M. (2008). Understanding the relation between obesity and depression: Causal mechanisms and implications for treatment. *Clinical Psychology: Science and Practice, 15,* 1–20.

Martensson, F., Boldemann, C., Soderstrom, M., Blennow, M., Englund, J. E., & Grahn, P. (2009). Outdoor environmental assessment of attention promoting settings for preschool children. *Health and Place, 15*(4), 1149–1157.

McGinnis, J. M., Gootman, J. A., Kraak, V. I., Institute of Medicine, Food and Nutrition Board, Board on Children, Youth, and Families, et al. (2006). *Food marketing to children and youth: Threat or opportunity?* Washington, DC: National Academies Press.

McWilliams, C., Ball, S. C., Benjamin, S. E., Hales, D., Vaughn, A., & Ward, D. S. (2009). Best-practice guidelines for physical activity at child care. *Pediatrics, 124*(6), 1650–1659.

Mindell, J. A., Meltzer, L. J., Carskadon, M. A., & Chervin, R. D. (2009). Developmental aspects of sleep hygiene: Findings from the 2004 National Sleep Foundation Sleep in America Poll. *Sleep Medicine, 10*(7), 771–779.

Must, A., Spadano, J., Coakley, E. H., Field, A. E., Colditz, G., & Dietz, W. H. (1999). The disease burden associated with overweight and obesity. *Journal of the American Medical Association, 282*(16), 1523–1529.

National Association for Sport and Physical Education. (2002). *Active start: A statement of physical activity guidelines for children from birth to age 5* (2nd ed.). Reston, VA: National Association for Sport and Physical Education.

National Scientific Council on the Developing Child. (2005). *Excessive stress disrupts the architecture of the developing brain: Working paper #3.* Cambridge, MA: Center on the Developing Child.

New York City Board of Health. (2006). *Notice of adoption of amendments to article 47 of the New York City Health Code, daycare services.* New York: Department of Health and Mental Hygiene. *www.nyc.gov/html/doh/downloads/pdf/public/notice-hc-20060615-art47.pdf.*

Nord, M., Coleman-Jensen, A., Andrews, M. S., & Carlson, S. J. (2010). *Household food security in the United States, 2009. Economic research report no. 108.* Alexandria, VA: U.S. Department of Agriculture, Economic Research Service.

Ogden, C. L., Carroll, M. D., Curtin, L. R., Lamb, M. M., & Flegal, K. M. (2010). Prevalence of high body mass index in U.S. children and adolescents, 2007–2008. *Journal of the American Medical Association, 303*(3), 242–249.

Ogden, C. L., & Flegal, K. M. (2010). Changes in terminology for childhood overweight and obesity. *National Health Statistics Reports, 25,* 1–5.

Olshansky, S. J., Passaro, D. J., Hershow, R. C., Layden, J., Carnes, B. A., Brody, J., et al. (2005). A potential decline in life expectancy in the United States in the 21st century. *New England Journal of Medicine, 352*(11), 1138–1145.

Owen, C. G., Martin, R. M., Whincup, P. H., Smith, G. D., & Cook, D. G. (2005). Effect of infant feeding on the risk of obesity across the life course: A quantitative review of published evidence. *Pediatrics, 115*(5), 1367–1377.

Pagoto, S. L., Curtin, C., Lemon, S. C., Bandini, L. G., Schneider, K. L., Bodenlos, J. S., et al. (2009). Association between adult attention deficit/hyperactivity disorder and obesity in the U.S. population. *Obesity (Silver Spring), 17*(3), 539–544.

Preiser, W. F. E., & Ostroff, E. (Eds.). (2001). *Universal design handbook.* New York: McGraw-Hill.

Robinson, T. N. (1999). Reducing children's television viewing to prevent obesity: A randomized controlled trial. *Journal of the American Medical Association, 282*(16), 1561–1567.

Rolls, B. J., Engell, D., & Birch, L. L. (2000). Serving portion size influences 5-year-old but not 3-year-old children's food intakes. *Journal of the American Dietetic Association, 100*(2), 232–234.

Rolls, B. J., Roe, L. S., Kral, T. V., Meengs, J. S., & Wall, D. E. (2004). Increasing the portion size of a packaged snack increases energy intake in men and women. *Appetite, 42*(1), 63–69.

Satter, E. M. (1986). The feeding relationship. *Journal of the American Dietetic Association, 86*(3), 352–356.

Satter, E. M. (2007). Eating competence: Definition and evidence for the Satter Eating Competence model. *Journal of Nutrition Education and Behavior, 39*(Suppl. 5), S142–S153.

Seeyave, D. M., Coleman, S., Appugliese, D., Corwyn, R. F., Bradley, R. H., Davidson, N. S., et al. (2009). Ability to delay gratification at age 4 years and risk of overweight at age 11 years. *Archives of Pediatrics and Adolescent Medicine, 163*(4), 303–308.

Sharma, A. J., Grummer-Strawn, L. M., Dalenius, K., Galuska, D., Anandappa, M., Borland, E., et al. (2009). Obesity prevalence among low-income, preschool-aged children—United States, 1998–2008. *Morbidity and Mortality Weekly Report, 58,* 669–773.

Sherry, B. (2005). Food behaviors and other strategies to prevent and treat pediatric overweight. *International Journal of Obesity (London), 29*(Suppl. 2), S116–S126.

Singh, A. S., Mulder, C., Twisk, J. W., van Mechelen, W., & Chinapaw, M. J. (2008). Tracking of childhood overweight into adulthood: A systematic review of the literature. *Obesity Reviews, 9*(5), 474–488.

Slining, M., Adair, L. S., Goldman, B. D., Borja, J. B., & Bentley, M. (2010). Infant overweight is associated with delayed motor development. *Journal of Pediatrics, 157*(1), 20–25, e21.

Smiciklas-Wright, H., Mitchell, D. C., Mickle, S. J., Goldman, J. D., & Cook, A. (2003). Foods commonly eaten in the United States, 1989–1991 and 1994–1996: Are portion sizes changing? *Journal of the American Dietetic Association, 103*(1), 41–47.

Story, M., Kaphingst, K. M., & French, S. (2006). The role of child care settings in obesity prevention. *Future of Children, 16*(1), 143–168.

Taveras, E. M., Rifas-Shiman, S. L., Oken, E., Gunderson, E. P., & Gillman, M. W. (2008). Short sleep duration in infancy and risk of childhood overweight. *Archives of Pediatrics and Adolescent Medicine, 162*(4), 305–311.

Taylor, A. F., & Kuo, F. E. (2009). Children with attention deficits concentrate better after walk in the park. *Journal of Attention Disorders, 12*(5), 402–409.

Taylor, A. F., Kuo, F. E., & Sullivan, W. C. (2002). Views of nature and self-discipline: Evidence from inner city children. *Journal of Environmental Psychology, 22*(1–2), 49–63.

Thelen, E., Schoner, G., Scheier, C., & Smith, L. B. (2001). The dynamics of embodiment: A field theory of infant perseverative reaching. *Behavioral and Brain Sciences, 24*(1), 1–34, discussion 34–86.

Thompson, R. A. (1994). Emotion regulation: A theme in search of definition. *Monographs of the Society for Research and Child Development, 59*(2–3), 25–52.

Tinanoff, N., & Palmer, C. A. (2000). Dietary determinants of dental caries and dietary recommendations for preschool children. *Journal of Public Health Dentistry, 60*(3), 197–206.

Trost, S. G., Ward, D. S., & Senso, M. (2010). Effects of child care policy and environment on physical activity. *Medicine and Science of Sports and Exercise, 42*(3), 520–525.

Tsigos, C., & Chrousos, G. P. (2006). Stress, obesity, and the metabolic syndrome: Soul and metabolism. *Annals of the New York Academy of Sciences, 1083,* xi–xiii.

U.S. Department of Agriculture, Food and Nutrition Service. (2010). *WIC breastfeeding peer counseling study final implementation report.* Alexandria, VA: Author.

U.S. Department of Health and Human Services, Administration for Children and Families. (2008). *Office of Head Start legislation & regulations. Head Start program performance standards (45 CFR part 1304).* Washington, DC: U.S. Department of Health and Human Services.

Vgontzas, A. N., & Bixler, E. O. (2008). Short sleep and obesity: Are poor sleep, chronic stress, and unhealthy behaviors the link? *Sleep, 31*(9), 1203.

Vgontzas, A. N., Bixler, E. O., & Chrousos, G. P. (2006). Obesity-related sleepiness and fatigue: The role of the stress system and cytokines. *Annals of the New York Academy of Sciences, 1083,* 329–344.

Vygotsky, L. S. (1978). *Mind in society.* Cambridge, MA: Harvard University Press.

Wadden, T. A., & Butryn, M. L. (2003). Behavioral treatment of obesity. *Endocrinology and Metabolism Clinics of North America, 32*(4), 981–1003.

Wagner, C. L., Greer, F. R., & Committee on Nutrition, Section on Breastfeeding. (2008). Prevention of rickets and vitamin D deficiency in infants, children, and adolescents. *Pediatrics, 122*(5), 1142–1152.

Wansink, B. (2006). *Mindless eating: Why we eat more than we think.* New York: Bantam Books.

Wansink, B., van Ittersum, K., & Painter, J. E. (2006). Ice cream illusions: Bowls, spoons, and self-served portion sizes. *American Journal of Preventive Medicine, 31*(3), 240–243.

Waring, M. E., & Lapane, K. L. (2008). Overweight in children and adolescents in relation to attention-deficit/hyperactivity disorder: Results from a national sample. *Pediatrics, 122*(1), e1–e6.

Warne, J. P. (2009). Shaping the stress response: Interplay of palatable food choices, glucocorticoids, insulin and abdominal obesity. *Molecular and Cellular Endocrinology, 300*(1–2), 137–146.

Wells, J. C., & Ritz, P. (2001). Physical activity at 9–12 months and fatness at 2 years of age. *American Journal of Human Biology, 13*(3), 384–389.

Wells, N. M., & Evans, G. W. (2003). Nearby nature: A buffer of life stress among rural children. *Environment and Behavior, 35*(3), 311–330.

Whitaker, R. C. (2004). Predicting preschooler obesity at birth: The role of maternal obesity in early pregnancy. *Pediatrics, 114*(1), e29–e36.

Whitaker, R. C. (2010). The infancy of obesity prevention. *Archives of Pediatrics and Adolescent Medicine, 164*(12), 1167–1169.

Whitaker, R. C. (2011). The childhood obesity epidemic: Lessons for preventing socially determined health conditions. *Archives of Pediatrics and Adolescent Medicine, 165*(11), 973–975.

Whitaker, R. C., & Orzol, S. M. (2006). Obesity among U.S. urban preschool children: Relationships to race, ethnicity, and socioeconomic status. *Archives of Pediatrics and Adolescent Medicine, 160*(6), 578–584.

Whitaker, R. C., Phillips, S. M., & Orzol, S. M. (2006). Food insecurity and the risks of depression and anxiety in mothers and behavior problems in their preschool-aged children. *Pediatrics, 118*(3), e859–e868.

Whitaker, R. C., Wright, J. A., Pepe, M. S., Seidel, K. D., & Dietz, W. H. (1997). Predicting obesity in young adulthood from childhood and parental obesity. *New England Journal of Medicine, 337*(13), 869–873.

World Health Organization. (2006). *WHO child growth standards: Height-for-age, weight-for-age, weight-for-length, weight-for-height and body mass index-for-age: Methods and development.* Geneva, Switzerland: Author.

CHAPTER 10

Impact of Early Childhood on Health throughout the Lifespan

Barry S. Zuckerman

The epidemiology of children's diseases has changed in the past 30 years. The development and widespread dissemination of vaccines have resulted in significant decreases in common infectious diseases such as mumps, measles, chicken pox, tetanus, pertussis and, more recently, pneumonia, diarrhea, meningitis, and diseases caused by Haemophilus influenzae: rotovirus, pneumococcus, and influenza. Paradoxically, chronic disease has increased as much as fourfold due, in part, to the development of life-saving treatments, especially for very low birthweight babies (Perrin, Bloom, & Gortmaker, 2007).

Concurrent with the decrease in acute infectious diseases is the growing recognition that the impact of life experiences and exposures in early childhood are clinically silent during childhood but express themselves as health problems of adults. Stress, neurotoxic and allergic exposures, and poor nutrition, sometimes mediated through the social environment including mothers' health, become embedded in biology resulting in an adverse impact on cardiovascular, metabolic, immunologic, and nervous (brain) systems (Hyman, 2009).

Early exposure and the early social environment affect current provision of pediatric care. The increasing prevalence of chronic disease is leading to the development of systems of care in which a medical home connects children to needed services (American Academy of Pediatrics Medical Home Initiatives for Children with Special Needs Project Advisory Committee,

2002; Antonelli, McAllister, & Popp, 2009). The new knowledge of early childhood antecedents of adult disease will likely add preventing adult diseases to preventing childhood diseases as a goal of pediatrics and child policy. Focusing on mothers' health or two-generation care will be integral to this effort. Developmental science and services will contribute significantly. The goal of this chapter is to explore the nature and scope of direct and indirect linkages between poverty, parental health and child and adult health, and the implications for clinical, public health, and policy-based interventions linked to developmental services.

Childhood Antecedents of Adult Disease

The growing evidence that many important adult diseases have their origins in childhood is captured by the term "health development" (Halfon & Hochstein, 2002). As our understanding of the basic etiologies of illness (e.g., hypertension, diabetes, obesity, and cardiovascular disease) has deepened, there has been a growing appreciation of the role of early social and biologic processes in influencing the onset and severity of these adult diseases. These advances in basic science and epidemiology have underscored the potential that the purposeful modulation of these early processes through health and development intervention and public policy in childhood could alter the timing and severity of adult-onset disease.

Although there appear to be a variety of pathways by which early life events can influence adult health, there are likely three primary mechanisms of how these early events become embedded in biology. First, there may be genetic influences early in life that only express themselves in the face of some external exposures. These gene–environment interactions or epigenetics alter the development of molecular structures or functional processes that determine the risk for specific diseases later in life. For example, there is considerable evidence that a variety of genetic predispositions can influence brain functioning and risk of mental health problems as well as obesity, lipid and glucose metabolism, and other risks for adult-onset cardiovascular disease problems (Guttmacher & Collins, 2002). Second, nongenetic biologic processes, many of which may reside in fetal and infant experiences, may also convey important risks for diseases later in life. For example, a growing series of long-term epidemiologic studies have suggested that low birthweight due to maternal nutrition and/or health is associated with coronary heart disease, hypertension, noninsulin-dependent diabetes, and other metabolic problems five or six decades later (Barker, Eriksson, Forsen, & Osmond, 2002). Similar studies document the impact of early childhood adversity on a similar range of adult health (Shonkoff, Boyce, & McEwen, 2009). Third, the development of important health-related behaviors, such as eating preferences, exercise patterns, and tobacco use early in life may extend into adulthood and affect the risk for a variety of adult-onset diseases.

Together, these three general mechanisms not only outline the linkage of childhood and adult health but also inform the potential opportunities to interrupt this conveyance of risk across the lifespan. A key factor underlying most mechanisms, whether genetic, nongenetic, biological, or health behaviors, is poverty (Conroy, Sandel, & Zuckerman, 2010). Poverty exerts direct and indirect transmission through parents, especially mothers, which become biologically embedded and can lead to health problems after a long latency.

Genetic Influences

New insights into the genetic influences on adult disease have highlighted the potential of identifying individuals at genetic risk early in life and mounting an ameliorative response. Illnesses such as type 2 diabetes, cardiovascular disease, some cancers, hypertension, and mental health problems are among the most important adult conditions with recognized genetic components. These genetically influenced diseases that depend heavily on environmental interactions early in life will become important inquiries of scientific investigation and worthy of special consideration. While the utility of genetic screening early in life for disorders with complex etiologies is relatively unexplored, there exists a tension already between prevention strategies directed at individuals at risk and those promoting healthful environments for all individuals.

For example, recent evidence has suggested important gene–environment interactions in the etiology of low birthweight and prematurity. While cigarette smoking is well known to contribute to low birthweight, its impact on low birthweight may be elevated for women who possess polymorphisms that express reduced levels of those enzymes that metabolize cigarette smoke (Wang et al., 2002). However, this genetic predisposition may only be expressed when women smoke in pregnancy, a behavior that is harmful for everyone. Another example involves intergenerational violence given the well-documented observation that being abused as a child enhances the risk of becoming an abuser as an adult. However, it has long been recognized that not all or even most abused children become perpetrators. For children who are abused, there is some evidence that homozygosity for genes that encode certain enzymes that metabolize common neurotransmitters reduces the likelihood that these children will victimize others later in life. Similarly, stress has its biggest impact in the individuals who are genetically vulnerable (Caspi et al., 2002). It appears that children who are abused and polymorphic for this gene are highly likely to suffer conduct disorders. However, the prevention of smoking-related low birthweight, child abuse, or depression cannot be confined only to children with this apparent genetic predisposition for later antisocial behavior.

Nongenetic Biological Influences

Biological events early in life but without direct genetic association can also lead to lifelong elevations in risk for adult disease. Because gestation and early life are defined by intense developmental processes, events during these periods could have far-reaching "programming" effects on health and disease later in life. Environmental impact on birthweight and brain development provides two examples.

Low Birthweight

A growing body of evidence has called attention to the impact of the intrauterine environment on adult patterns of disease. Initial observation of the association of low birthweight and low weight at 1 year and subsequent coronary heart disease was made in England 15 years ago among men then in their 60's and 70's who were born in the early part of the 20th century (Barker, Winter, Osmond, Margetts, & Simmonds, 1989; Barker et al., 1993). This finding was replicated and expanded in multiple studies indicating low birthweight, not weight at 1 year, being the strongest and most consistent predictor to cardiovascular disease among adults even after confounding variables such as smoking, employment, alcohol consumption, exercise, and social class were controlled. Though the replication from different samples and different countries of the relationship among low birthweight, poor *in utero* nutrition, and cardiovascular disease has been remarkable, there remain methodological concerns with these studies, including failure to control for the life persistence of socioeconomic circumstances and the potential modifying role of health and nutrition during childhood.

Studies of the impact of low birthweight or *in utero* undernutrition on specific organs support these epidemiologic findings and suggest potential mechanisms linking low birthweight and coronary artery disease. For example, fetal undernutrition and/or lower birthweight leads to fewer beta cells within the pancreas at birth and higher concentrations of insulin and glucose concentrations (Hales & Barker, 1992).

Low birthweight is also associated with increased blood pressure as adults (Gennser, Rymark, & Isberg, 1988). The highest blood pressures are found in adults who were small at birth but became overweight as adults. Reduced birthweight or even protein restriction in animal models is associated with reduced number of nephrons in the kidneys (Manalich, Reyes, Herrera, Melendi, & Fundora, 2000). Individuals with few nephrons compensate with a higher glomular filtration rate potentially leading to glomular injury and hypertension. Whether low birthweight is ultimately singularly or in combination with genes or other factors explaining the development of all or some essential hypertension, remains to be seen.

Brain Development

Childhood poverty impairs neurocognitive development that can impair learning (Farah et al., 2006). Learning and memory, in turn, affect school readiness and ultimately educational attainment, which in turn is associated with adult morbidity and mortality. New technologies have provided an understanding of brain development in children that emphasizes, to a degree not previously recognized by many, the importance of experiences in the first decade of life. Studies (e.g., positron emission tomography [PET] scans, magnetic resonance imagings [MRIs], counting synaptic density in pathological specimens) have demonstrated that the full complement of neurons (about 100 billion) is formed before the third trimester of gestation. Synapses, on the other hand, form largely after birth and are the result of an exquisitely complex interaction of genetic controls and environmental input. To some extent, environmental factors promoting both the development and "pruning" of synaptic location and density have been previously underestimated. Equally important, emerging research has also outlined how cortisol in response to stress modifies neural connections needed for memory and learning capacity. Parents and other caregivers ensure appropriate stimulation for learning and buffer the impact from excessive stress on children that impairs memory or learning (McEwen, 2007). School readiness is an early indicator that reflects the appropriate early childhood environment on brain development for cognitive and social–emotional development.

Early infancy is exquisitely sensitive to interactions with caregiving adults, which becomes biologically embedded. Infants and children experiencing chronic stress or social deprivation demonstrate specific patterns of neurotransmitter release, leading to structural alterations in the brain development. These alterations ultimately affect memory (Brunson, Grigoriadis, Lorang, & Baram, 2002), educational attainment, and ability to cope with subsequent stressors (McEwen, 2007).

Specific physiological alterations caused by stress during early childhood highlight how the social environment becomes biologically subsumed. Rat pups not groomed frequently by their mothers in infancy elicit epigenetic programming that increases activation of the hypothalamic–pituitary–adrenal axis in response to stresses (Weaver et al., 2004; Meaney, 2001). Studies indicate that this is due to methylation of the gene encoding for expression of the glucocorticoid receptor, which ultimately participates in feedback inhibition of the stress response. Those groomed show less methylation, express more glucocorticoid receptor, and then have greater feedback inhibition of the stress response and subsequent lower hypothalamic–pituitary–adrenal axis responses to stresses in adulthood (Hyman, 2009). Notably, methylation is found to be a stable response not altered in adulthood (Weaver et al., 2004). The same epigenetic control of the stress response is also described in humans: those abused in early childhood have been shown to have methylation at a key promoter site encoding the gene for the glucocorticoid receptor (McGowan et al., 2009). Fewer glucocorticoid receptors in the hippocampus reduces feedback inhibition as adults, leading to greater hypothalamic–pituitary–adrenal responses to stresses than their nonabused peers.

Prolonged cortisol release in response to stress is thought to result in hippocampal neuron damage and loss by increasing vulnerability to calcium and glutamate (Weaver et al., 2004; Gunnar & Vasquez, 2006), thus causing neural damage and death. This mechanism may explain the finding that increased cortisol levels are detrimental for learning and memory (Brunson et al., 2002; Gunnar & Quevedo, 2007). In support of this explanation are magnetic resonance imaging scans showing atrophy of the hippocampus with stress-related conditions, including recurrent depression and posttraumatic stress disorder (PTSD) arising from severe childhood physical and sexual abuse (Bremner et al., 1995).

Exposure to stress at a young age has consequences, outside of the central nervous system, that impact adult health. Low SES has been linked to long-term increased inflammatory markers, particularly C-reactive protein, fibrinogen, and white blood cells (Danese et al., 2008; Pollitt et al., 2007; Taylor, Lehman, Kiefe, & Seeman, 2006). These may be additional factors on the causal pathway between low socioeconomic status (SES) in childhood and adult cardiovascular disease (Pollitt et al., 2007; Taylor et al., 2006).

Behavioral Influences

Children who experience abuse or neglect in the early social environment also display more high-risk health behaviors, such as cigarette smoking, alcohol abuse, and multiple sexual partners (Hillis, Anda, Felitti, Nordenberg, & Marchbanks, 2000; Anda et al., 1999, 2002). These high-risk behaviors are associated with alcoholism, sexually transmitted disease, unintended pregnancy, and suicide (Hillis et al., 2000; Dietz et al., 1999; Dube et al., 2001). This relationship was found to be graded: those who had experienced more adverse experiences or household dysfunction displayed more high-risk behaviors as adults.

There is strong evidence that health-related behaviors have their roots in childhood. Attitudes and habits regarding eating and exercise patterns, self-care, and the health care system play an important role in determining the emergence and impact of adult-onset disease. Accordingly, a variety of policies and programs have been implemented to address these issues. However, there is an increasing body of information suggesting that these behavioral patterns begin in childhood and are associated with social class and many may, in fact, be difficult to change once adulthood has been reached (Conroy et al., 2010).

Behaviors beginning in childhood including overeating, physical inactivity, and cigarette smoking lead to health problems among adults, resulting in approximately 50% of all adult mortality in the United States (McGinnis & Foege, 1993). Diet and physical activity in childhood contribute to childhood obesity, which is strongly associated with obesity in adulthood (Deckelbaum & Williams, 2001). Eating behaviors early in life are strongly influenced by parental behavior; the choice a parent makes regarding a child's diet starting with whether to breast feed strongly shapes a child's experience with food and tendency toward obesity. While not definitive, data continue to accumulate that children who are breast fed are less likely to be obese (Centers for Disease Control and Prevention, 2007).

The Material Environment: Poverty

Addressing childhood antecedents of adult disease has implications not only for improving personal health but for reducing disparities in health outcomes for groups at risk for poor health due to low income or race. Poverty during childhood has a long and well-documented negative effect on child health. Children living in poverty are more likely to experience low birthweight, learning disabilities, mental health problems, iron-deficiency anemia, asthma, burns and injuries, obesity, and hospitalization than their more affluent peers (Meyers et al., 2005; Sandel, Phelan, Wright, Hynes, & Lanphear, 2004; Dowswell, Towner, Simpson, & Jarvis, 1996; Call, Smith, Morris, Chapman, & Platts-Mills, 1992; Gergen et al., 1999). However, the significance of childhood poverty is likely to be underestimated if health outcomes are measured only during childhood; poverty during childhood also appears to be an important predictor of adult health even with improved social class as an adult.

The individual's physical environment mediates exposure to toxins, infectious disease, and inadequate nutrition. For example, among low-income families, poor housing conditions may increase exposure to toxins and allergens, leading to lower IQ (Needleman & Gatsonis, 1990) or lost school days due to increased asthma (Call et al., 1992). The surrounding social environment brings varying degrees of lessened stimulation, both in terms of amount contingent to child's verbal efforts resulting in less exposure to words and reduced verbal acquisition and readiness for school (Walberg & Marjorikbanks, 1976). Finally, community and social structure influence the quality of and access to health care and education that leads to poor health, poor education, and inadequate social capital.

Social marginalization is also a breeding ground for community violence, a risk factor for serious injuries, PTSD (Glaser, 2000), and other sequelae of mental illness.

The impact of women's health on the health of their children is not limited to birth outcomes; maternal health conditions and behaviors continue to mediate the link between social factors and child outcomes well after delivery. The vulnerability of child behavioral and developmental outcomes to maternal depression has been increasingly recognized. The prevalence of maternal depression shows a strong social gradient, correlating with educational attainment, housing, marital relationship, work role, and stressful life events (Weissman & Olfson, 1995; Zuckerman & Beardslee, 1987). Cognitive outcomes for young children have been clearly linked to early maternal depression. These effects appear to persist through ages 4 to 5 (Cooper & Murray, 1998). Three-year-old children whose mothers were depressed had worse reading skills at age 8 (Richman, Stevenson, & Graham, 1982). Depressive symptoms in a mother appear to lead to diminished maternal–infant attachment, less spontaneous interaction with the child (Zuckerman & Beardslee, 1987), and increases in children's cortisol responses to adverse family environment (Ashman, Dawson, Panagiotides, Yamada, & Wilkins, 2002). Recent work suggests that these children exhibit significantly reduced activity in a region of the brain specialized for expression of positive emotions (Dawson, Frey, Panagiotides, Osterling, & Hess, 1997). Effective treatment of a mothers' depression has been shown to have a beneficial effect on their children (Weissman et al., 2006). This suggests a causal link and opportunity "twofer" by treating the mother.

Child abuse and neglect have been the focus of considerable public attention, but less well recognized is the impact of witnessing violence on child health and development (Taylor, Zuckerman, Harik, & Groves, 1994; Zuckerman, Augustyn, Groves, & Parker, 1995). A 1985 survey reported that more than 3.3 million children per year witnessed physical abuse between their parents (Strauss & Gelles, 1986). Children who witness domestic violence are at risk for a range of sequelae, from mild behavioral and emotional problems to PTSD (Kilpatrick, Litt, & Williams, 1997). Of note, Bremner et al. (1997) found atrophy in the hippocampal region of the brain in adults with PTSD associated with childhood abuse; other studies have identified similar findings in Vietnam veterans with PTSD (Bremner et al., 1995; Gurvits et al., 1996). Domestic violence is reported to be more prevalent among women who are younger and less educated (Centers for Disease Control and Prevention, 1994). Children who are poor are more likely to witness violence in their community; thus, it is likely that cumulative violence exposure is socially stratified. Much work remains to be done to delineate the long-term consequences for children; nevertheless, early evidence suggests that violence against women has substantial ripple effects on the health of children.

A study looking at both mothers' depression and exposure to violence shows that these co-occur often and when they do they have an adverse impact on children's learning and behavior in school that is not additive but rather synergistic (Silverstein, Augustyn, Young, & Zuckerman, 2009). The co-occurrence of this problem may explain the lack of effectiveness of some maternal depression intervention studies. In such interventions the exposure to violence may also have to be addressed.

The Impact of Cumulative Stress

Multiple social and family risk factors combine to increase the risk for poor child outcomes (Parker, Greer, & Zuckerman, 1988; Sameroff, Seifer, Baldwin, & Baldwin, 1993; Sameroff, Seifer, Barocas, Zax, & Greenspan, 1987; Zuckerman et al., 1989). One theory of how physical and social environments become biologically embedded emphasizes the cumulative effects of multiple experiences. Evidence of this theory is the finding that while low-SES children recover as well from early health insults as higher-SES children, they suffer more health insults over time, which leads to poorer health in adolescence and adulthood (Keating & Hertzman, 1999). The impact of multiple stressors on "allostatic load" results in a process of reestablishing equilibrium after a stressor. Each time the body goes through allostasis it pays a small price to reestablish equilibrium; the cumulative cost to the individual of managing stressors is allostatic load. Increased allostatic load is associated with poor health outcomes (McEwen, 2007) suggesting that some of the impact of low SES may become incorporated over time.

Cumulative effects of SES on health has also been called the "pathways" model because the experiences of individuals that are damaging to their health appear to form "a pathway or chain of risk" (Ben-Schlomo & Kuh, 2002; Power & Hertzman, 1997). For example, consider a hypothetical child born at 34 weeks' gestation to a single mother living in poverty who received minimal prenatal care. Following a 3-week hospitalization, the infant is mildly hypotonic and has difficulty maintaining an alert state. The mother feels overwhelmed and depressed. The child's passivity exacerbates the mother's feelings of inadequacy, resulting in a worsening of her depression. Positive interactions with her child are rare. The child does not look to the environment for his or her stimulation, nor does he or she vocalize much. This further heightens the mother's feelings of inadequacy and depression. The child's neurological development is further challenged by mild iron-deficiency anemia and a modest lead burden. By 2 years the child will be clearly delayed in language and cognitive development. The cause of his or her developmental delay is the biologic vulnerability secondary to prematurity and anemia, exacerbated by maternal depression, inadequate environmental stimulation, and insufficient social support. In fact, all these factors operate together to shape the child's outcome. Each factor modifies and potentiates the other. Together, they weave a complex pattern that cannot be fully understood by examining the thread of only a single risk (Parker et al., 1988).

Both child outcomes (such as prematurity, iron deficiency, asthma, and developmental delay) and women's health status (e.g., bacterial vaginosis, poor nutrition, smoking, and depression) are strongly linked to each other and to upstream social factors. Not surprisingly, the few studies of social factors associated with child outcomes have found sizeable effects for women's health (usually depression) as a potential mediator of social factors (Duncan, Brooks-Gunn, & Klebanov, 1994; Korenman, Miller, & Sjaastad, 1994; Miller, 1998). Yet analytically, women's health has been approached as a series of distinct risk factors posing threats to specific child outcomes. Lost has been the breadth and depth of the influence of women's physical and mental health on child health, both as a mediator of social forces and as an independent determinant of child health. Many intervention and policy opportunities have been missed as a result of the failure to recognize that many child health disparities have their origins farther upstream in the general health of women.

Implications for Child Care

Child care providers have a special opportunity to complement parents' efforts to promote children's health. Basic activities include providing healthy foods for meals and snacks, ensuring a physically safe environment, providing opportunities for active play and limiting television watching to less than 1 hour a day for children 2 to 5 years and no television for children under 2 years, helping children brush their teeth after meals, and ensuring adequate sleep during naptime. Child care providers promote children's mental health by supporting relationships and providing responsive caretaking. This is most likely to happen when child care providers are supported and nurtured by others in the organization or community groups. Providing information about available play groups or community festivals and celebrations further broadens support for parents. Children with special health care needs like asthma, sickle cell anemia, autism spectrum disorder, cerebral palsy, and so on may require special adaptations and communication among doctors, developmental services, and child care providers. Doctors may want to know about children's behavior, appetite, energy level, and so forth. Child care staff may need to know about new medication expected effects or side effects. While parents can be sources of information to doctors and child care staff, a better system would be three-way communication. Pediatric practices are developing medical homes to enhance communication, especially for children with special problems.

Women's Health: A Two-Generation Approach to Child Health

To promote child and adult health, much greater attention must be paid to women's health and health services. As discussed earlier, these wide-ranging conditions usually exist prior to conception, and their impact often begins well before any effective prenatal care intervention can be put in place. Many of these problems continue to have a negative impact long after delivery. Effective treatments for such problems as domestic violence, depression, poor nutrition, cigarette smoking, drug and alcohol use, and infections require timely and prolonged therapies that are not well served by prenatal care that starts long after conception and often ends with a single postpartum visit. Traditional strategies that emphasize reproductive health, and specifically prenatal care, are unlikely to address adequately the women's and children's conditions outlined here.

Effective clinical interventions for such problems as depression (Katon et al., 1995), smoking (Hurt et al., 1997), drug addiction (National Consensus Development Panel on Effective Medical Treatment of Opiate Addiction, 1998), and emergency and nonemergency contraception (Glasier, 1997) increase the need to reevaluate existing systems of care for women. The goal must be improving the capacity to engage women in comprehensive health care before, during, and after pregnancy so that they have timely access to these treatments.

Even those women who enter the health care system face substantial fragmentation of their health services (Weisman, 1996). Obstetrician-gynecologists tend to be more thorough in the provision of Pap smears, breast examinations, and mammography, whereas other adult care providers are more likely to offer cholesterol screening, smoking-cessation aids, and screening and initial treatment for depression. The likelihood that a woman sees both a gynecologist and an internist increases with higher income and more years of education. A second contributing factor has been the splintering of reproductive health care services, such as family planning and abortion, from mainstream medicine (Gottlieb, 1995).

For the 50% of births that are second or more, child care and developmental services staff have an opportunity to engage mothers and provide information and encouragement to obtain services and care. An approach that is limited to women who already have children does not ultimately address those health behaviors and conditions that affect first pregnancies. A more universal approach to health care information to improve the general health status of young women is needed. Moreover, medical insurance to cover traditional health services is only part of the access problem.

The social patterns around inadequate use of folate, incorrect positioning of infants for sleep, limited access to over-the-counter smoking-cessation aids, barriers to the marketing of emergency contraception, and inadequate provisions for women subject to domestic violence need to be confronted. Public health strategies must be developed to target messages for selected groups of mothers at high risk because of low literacy, limited English proficiency, and social or cultural marginalization. Public health messages should also highlight the mutual benefits for women and their children of breast feeding, folic acid supplementation, protection against domestic violence, treatment of depression, and particularly, smoking cessation should be explored.

Committing Child-Focused Professionals to the Health of Women

Since attention to the well-being of her child is often the best way to engage a mother concerning her own health needs, professionals and programs involved with young children are important gateways to comprehensive health care for women, especially those with unmet needs. Although the fragmentation of health and social services makes it difficult to link the health of women and their children, there are several strategies that might effectively move us toward a comprehensive, two-generational approach to child health.

Practitioners and programs that serve children from conception through the earliest years of life can no longer afford to miss opportunities to improve children's health by enhancing the health, safety, and well-being of their mothers. Using child health, early care and education, and early intervention settings as the gateway to comprehensive women's health care holds promise as a sustainable, generalizable approach to a two-generational health care strategy. Unfortunately, traditional child health, early child care and education, and early intervention services have no regular mechanisms in place to reach out to women, assess their health care needs, and connect them to appropriate care.

Community-based program staff in a wide range of settings can help to reintegrate fragmented health and social services, beginning with the mothers and children they serve in their own settings. They can identify clinicians in their community who are interested in addressing the health needs of women comprehensively, including nutrition, gynecological care, and behavioral health. Special attributes, such as consultation in languages other than English, should be noted. Practitioners can then make a list of adult health care providers in the community who are available to program participants. In addition, they can help mothers make appointments with adult health practitioners and monitor referrals to ensure that they "take."

Assuming that confidentiality in a setting is ensured, nurses, family advocates, social workers, and others who have developed a relationship with a mother can help her assess her health care needs and suggest appropriate services. A "women's wellness record" could be developed to record their health history, including illnesses and hospitalizations, prenatal history, medications, allergies, and preventive screening results is one approach under investigation. The record would contain self-help information and information on health promotion and disease prevention, especially in connection with domestic violence, depression, and other mental health problems, diet, family planning, exercise, cigarette smoking, alcohol use, and other issues. Like a child health and development record, the woman's wellness record would belong to the woman. Its purpose would be to help her take ownership of her health problems and to serve as a complete record of health information that she could share with different health providers. Although a woman could fill out the record herself, a staff member who already has a relationship with her might spend time with her completing the initial information to identify potential health issues and suggest needed services.

Innovative Programs to Improve Early Child Outcomes

Healthy Steps

Despite the range of home visitation models, most have remained largely unconnected to clinical care for children. One evidenced-based effort, Healthy Steps, demonstrated the potential of integrating home visiting into traditional pediatric primary care (Zuckerman, Parker, Kaplan-Sanoff, Augustyn, & Barth, 2004). An early childhood specialist who sees patients during well-child visits and in their home is added to the pediatric team. Following the time with the doctor or nurse at well-child visits, the early childhood specialist then spends additional time providing developmental screening, identifying and addressing special temperaments that may require adjustments of parents expectations and behavior, providing advice and support to promote all aspects of children's development, and ensuring linkages to community resources, and so on. In addition, identification of maternal depression, violence in the home, cigarette smoking, and referrals to community resources is important. Healthy Steps provides the time and special expertise of the early childhood specialist to address these and other important issues as part of expanded pediatric care.

The evaluation of Healthy Steps shows that families were more likely than control families to practice safer and more responsive parenting, avoid harsh disciplinary tactics, and openly discuss feelings of sadness with a health care professional. The study also reported that Healthy Steps children received regular developmental screenings and were more likely to have current immunizations (Minkovitz et al., 2003). At age 5 Healthy Steps parents continued to use more appropriate disciplinary methods and to remain more sensitive to the child's behavioral cues. Parents tended to remain in Healthy Steps practices, ensuring continuity of care (Minkovitz et al., 2007).

Medical–Legal Partnership

Material hardships associated with poverty that impact child and family health include hunger, safety, utility shutoffs, and substandard housing. Over the past several decades, Congress, state governments, and federal agencies have enacted laws and regulations to address many of these. These social problems generally constitute legal needs and are themselves barriers to good health (Shin et al., 2010). Legal needs are adverse social conditions with legal remedies that reside in laws, regulations, or policies (Washington State Supreme Court, Taskforce on Equal Civil Justice Funding, 2003).

Studies show that low-income households have an average of one to three unmet civil legal needs related to income, housing problems, employment, and family issues such as guardianship or domestic violence (Houseman, 2010). Fewer than one in five legal problems experienced by the poor are addressed with help from a private or legal aid lawyer, and most problems are left unresolved (Legal Services Corporation, 2007). Medical–legal partnerships are an innovation in health care delivery to improve access to legal benefits and protections, which in turn will improve health (Zuckerman, Sandel, Lawton, & Morton, 2008; Sandel et al., 2010). At this time, one medical–legal partnership is working with a large Head Start program in Kansas City (*www.medical-legalpartnership.org/*).

Medical–legal partnership was formally developed in the Department of Pediatrics at Boston Medical Center and the Boston University School of Medicine in 1993 and has three components. The first is providing legal advice and assistance to patients, with a focus on the early detection of legal problems and the prevention of legal crises and health consequences. The second core activity of medical–legal partnership teams is to create internal systems improvement within health care to improve access to a range of government services for patients, including the Supplemental Nutrition Assistance Program and Supplemental Security Income (Legal Services Corporation, 2007). Third, medical–legal partnerships encourage the enactment or amendment of laws and regulations to benefit vulnerable children and families. This includes working with coalitions, developing specific policy initiatives, and creating health impact assessments in response to policy proposals.

Promoting Early Literacy

Low-income families are less likely to read to their children compared to their more well-to-do peers. They face such hurdles as lack of books, poor access to bookstores, language barriers, and sometimes a cultural context where parents do not read to their children. Two strategies for promoting early literacy development opportunities are reopening closed neighborhood libraries and instituting mobile library vans for remote areas where libraries are not available. Early childhood settings, such as child care, family support programs, and pediatric practices are other potential sites to accomplish such a goal. For example, an intervention designed and offered by pediatricians called Reach Out and Read provides age-appropriate books at each well-child visit for low-income children between 6 months and 5 years, as well as advice to parents about age-appropriate literacy-promoting activities. An initial evaluation of this effort demonstrated that mothers were four times more likely—and mothers on welfare were eight times more likely—to read to their children compared to mothers not in the program (Needlman, Fried, Morley, Taylor, & Zuckerman, 1991). Subsequent studies have replicated these findings and extended the documented benefits to include more books in the home and enhanced language development (Golova, Alario, Vivier, Rodriguez, & High, 1999; High, Hopmann, LaGasse, & Linn, 1998). Parallel efforts to ensure that age-appropriate books and literacy activities are available in all child care settings should be evaluated in terms of outcomes and costs. Child care staff and home visitors should help parents with dialogic reading, which has been shown to be effective in promoting children's language development.

Another strategy to enhancing the development of child literacy is to promote parental literacy and literacy-related activities. Messages about the importance of reading to children can be disseminated through posters on the walls of child care centers, pediatrician offices, and supermarkets, or through print and television media. Messages should be tailored to meet the specific cultural and linguistic needs of minorities. More fundamentally, these efforts should promote parental literacy and English as a second language (ESL). Presently, most adult literacy and ESL programs have long waiting lists because they are underfunded. Parents who are themselves proficient are in a better position to promote child literacy activities. Policies that support adult literacy offer an opportunity to improve family health outcomes as well. When parents have difficulty understanding information on prescription bottles, patient education materials, discharge instructions, and appointment slips, there are well-documented health consequences (Ad Hoc Committee on Health Literacy for the Council on Scientific Affairs, 1999).

Conclusion

We have emphasized the importance of social environment on maternal health as a part of the causal pathway between social disadvantage and health. The critical role of women's health (broadly defined) in mediating these influences is not as well recognized nor addressed as it should be. The genomic revolution will actually focus more attention on ways to modify the environment because it is environmental factors that will trigger the timing and severity of health problems. The linkage of child outcomes to brain development and to women's health has several important policy and programmatic implications. Specifically, though all aspects of child development need to be supported, promoting early literacy, reducing or buffering stress, and ensuring basic needs are met increases the likelihood of later school success and health. To further improve children's health, women need access to comprehensive health care that can address their own unmet health needs before, during, and after pregnancy. This needs to be accompanied by public health strategies that engage and support women around such difficult issues as domestic violence, depression, and substance abuse.

REFERENCES

Ad Hoc Committee on Health Literacy for the Council on Scientific Affairs. (1999). Health literacy: Report of the Council on Scientific Affairs. *Journal of the American Medical Association, 281,* 552–557.

American Academy of Pediatrics Medical Home Initiatives for Children with Special Needs Project Advisory Committee. (2002). The medical home. *Pediatrics, 110,* 184–186.

Anda, R. F., Croft, J. B., Felitti, V. J., Nordenberg, D., Giles, W. H., Williamson, D. F., et al. (1999). Adverse childhood experiences and smoking during adolescence and adulthood. *Journal of the American Medical Association, 282,* 1652–1658.

Anda, R. F., Whitfield, C. L., Felitti, V. J., Chapman, D., Edwards, V. J., Dube, S. R., et al. (2002). Adverse childhood experiences, alcoholic parents, and later risk of alcoholism and depression. *Psychiatric Services, 53,* 1001–1009.

Antonelli, R., McAllister, J. W., & Popp, J. (2009). *Making care coordination a critical component of the pediatric health system: A multidisciplinary framework.* New York: Commonwealth Fund.

Ashman, S. B., Dawson, G., Panagiotides, H., Yamada, E., & Wilkins, C. W. (2002). Stress hormone levels of children of depressed mothers. *Development and Psychopathology, 14,* 333–349.

Barker, D. J., Eriksson, J. G., Forsen, T., & Osmond, C. (2002). Fetal origins of adult disease: Strength of effects and biological basis. *International Journal of Epidemiology, 31,* 1235–1239.

Barker, D. J., Gluckman, P. D., Godfrey, K. M., Harding, J. E., Owens, J. A., &

Robinson, J. S. (1993). Fetal nutrition and cardiovascular disease in adult life. *Lancet, 341*, 938–941.

Barker, D. J., Winter, P. D., Osmond, C., Margetts, B., & Simmonds, S. J. (1989). Weight in infancy and death from ischaemic heart disease. *Lancet, 334*(8663), 577–580.

Ben-Shlomo, Y., & Kuh, D. (2002). A life course approach to chronic disease epidemiology: Conceptual models, empirical challenges and interdisciplinary perspectives. *International Journal of Epidemiology, 31*, 285–293.

Bremner, J. D., Randall, P., Scott, T. M., Bronen, R. A., Delaney, R. C., Seibyl, J. P., et al. (1995). MRI-based measurement of hippocampal volume in patients with combat-related posttraumatic stress disorder. *American Journal of Psychiatry, 152*, 973–981.

Bremner, J. D., Randall, P., Vermetten, E., Staib, L., Bronen, R. A., Mazure, C., et al. (1997). Magnetic resonance imaging-based measurement of hippocampal volume in post-traumatic stress disorder related to childhood physical and sexual abuse: A preliminary report. *Biological Psychiatry, 41*(1), 23–32.

Brunson, K. L., Grigoriadis, D. E., Lorang, M. T., & Baram, T. Z. (2002). Corticotropin-releasing hormone (CRH) downregulates the function of its receptor (CRF_1) and induces CRF1 expression in hippocampal and cortical regions of the immature rat brain. *Experimental Neurology, 176*(1), 75–86.

Call, R. S., Smith, T. F., Morris, E., Chapman, M. D., & Platts-Mills, T. A. (1992). Risk factors for asthma in inner city children. *Journal of Pediatrics, 121*, 862–866.

Caspi, A., McClay, J., Moffitt, T. E., Mill, J., Martin, J., Craig, I. W., et al. (2002). Role of genotype in the cycle of violence in maltreated children. *Science, 297*, 851–854.

Centers for Disease Control and Prevention. (1994). Physical violence during the twelve months preceding childbirth: Alaska, Maine, Oklahoma, and West Virginia, 1990–1991. *Morbidity and Mortality Weekly Report, 43*, 132–137.

Centers for Disease Control and Prevention. (2007). Does breastfeeding reduce the risk of pediatric overweight? *Research to Practice Series 7*. Available at *www.cdc.gov/nccdphp/dnpa/nutrition/pdf/breastfeeding_r2p.pdf*.

Conroy, K., Sandel, M., & Zuckerman, B. (2010). Poverty grown up: How childhood socioeconomic status impacts adult health. *Journal of Developmental and Behavioral Pediatrics, 31*, 154–160.

Cooper, P. J., & Murray, L. (1998). Postnatal depression. *British Medical Journal, 316*(7148), 1884–1886.

Danese, A., Moffitt, T. E., Pariante, C. M., Ambler, A., Poulton, R., & Caspi, A. (2008). Elevated inflammation levels in depressed adults with a history of childhood maltreatment. *Archives of General Psychiatry, 65*, 409–415.

Dawson, G., Frey, K., Panagiotides, H., Osterling, J., & Hess, D. (1997). Infants of depressed mothers exhibit atypical frontal brain activity: A replication and extension of previous findings. *Journal of Child Psychology and Psychiatry and Allied Disciplines, 38*(4), 179–186.

Deckelbaum, R. J., & Williams, C. L. (2001). Childhood obesity: The health issue. *Obesity Research, 9*, S239–S243.

Dietz, P. M., Spitz, A. M., Anda, R. F., Williamson, D. F., McMahon, P. M.,

Santelli, J. S., et al. (1999). Unintended pregnancy among adult women exposed to abuse or household dysfunction during their childhood. *Journal of the American Medical Association, 282,* 1359–1364.

Dowswell, T., Towner, E. M., Simpson, G., & Jarvis, S. N. (1996). Preventing childhood unintentional injuries—What works? A literature review. *Injury Prevention, 2,* 140–149.

Dube, S. R., Anda, R. F., Felitti, V. J., Chapman, D. P., Williamson, D. F., Giles, W. H. (2001). Childhood abuse, household dysfunction, and the risk of attempted suicide throughout the life span: Findings from the Adverse Childhood Experiences Study. *Journal of the American Medical Association, 286,* 3089–3096.

Duncan, G., Brooks-Gunn, J., & Klebanov, P. K. (1994). Economic deprivation and early childhood development. *Child Development, 65*(2), 296–318.

Farah, M. J., Shera, D. M., Savage, J. H., Betancourt, L., Giannetta, J. M., Brodsky, N. L., et al. (2006). Childhood poverty: Specific associations and neurocognitive development. *Brain Research, 1110*(1), 166–174.

Gennser, G., Rymark, P., & Isberg, P. E. (1988). Low birth weight and risk of high blood pressure in adulthood. *British Medical Journal (Clinical Research Ed.), 296,* 1498–1500.

Gergen, P. J., Mortimer, K. M., Eggleston, P. A., Rosenstreich, D., Mitchell, H., Ownby, D., et al. (1999). Results of the National Cooperative Inner-City Asthma Study (NCICAS) environmental intervention to reduce cockroach allergen exposure in inner-city homes. *Journal of Allergy and Clinical Immunology, 103*(3 Pt. 1), 501–506.

Glaser, D. (2000) Child abuse and neglect and the brain—A review. *Journal of Child Psychology and Psychiatry, 41,* 97–116.

Glasier, A. (1997). Emergency postcoital contraception. *New England Journal of Medicine, 337*(2), 1058–1064.

Golova, N., Alario, A. J., Vivier, P. M., Rodriguez, M., & High, P. C. (1999). Literacy promotion for Hispanic families in a primary care setting: A randomized, controlled trial. *Pediatrics, 103,* 993–997.

Gottlieb, B. R. (1995). Abortion–1995. *New England Journal of Medicine, 332,* 532–533.

Gunnar, M., & Quevedo, K. (2007). The neurobiology of stress and development. *Annual Review of Psychology, 58,* 145–173.

Gunnar, M., & Vasquez, D. M. (2006). Stress neurobiology and developmental psychopathology. In D. Cicchetti & D. Cohen (Eds.), *Developmental psychopathology: Vol. 2. Developmental neuroscience* (2nd. ed., pp. 533–577). New York: Wiley.

Gurvits, T. V., Shenton, M. E., Hokama, H., Ohta, H., Lasko, N. B., Gilbertson, M. W., et al. (1996). Magnetic resonance imaging study of hippocampal volume in chronic, combat-related post-traumatic stress disorder. *Biological Psychiatry, 40*(11), 1091–1099.

Guttmacher, A., & Collins, F. (2002). Genomic medicine—A primer. *New England Journal of Medicine, 347,* 996–997.

Hales, C. N., & Barker, D. J. (1992). Type 2 (non-insulin-dependent) diabetes mellitus: The thrifty phenotype hypothesis. *Diabetologia, 35,* 595–601.

Halfon, N., & Hochstein, M. (2002). Life course health development: An integrated framework for developing health, policy, and research. *Milbank Quarterly, 80*(3), 433–479, iii.

High, P., Hopmann, M., LaGasse, L., & Linn, H. (1998). Evaluation of a clinic-based program to promote book sharing and bedtime routines among low-income urban families with young children. *Archive of Pediatrics and Adolescent Medicine, 152,* 459–465.

Hillis, S. D., Anda, R. F., Felitti, V. J., Nordenberg, D., & Marchbanks, P. A. (2000). Adverse childhood experiences and sexually transmitted diseases in men and women: A retrospective study. *Pediatrics, 106,* E11.

Houseman, A. W. (2010). *Civil legal aid in the United States: An update for 2009.* Washington, DC: Center for Law and Social Policy. Retrieved January 3, 2010, from *http://s242739747.onlinehome.us/publications/civillegalaid2009.pdf.*

Hurt, R., Sachs, D., Glover, E., Offord, K. P., Johnston, J. A., Dale, L. C., et al. (1997). A comparison of sustained-release bupropion and placebo for smoking cessation. *New England Journal of Medicine, 337,* 1195–1202.

Hyman, S. E. (2009). How adversity gets under the skin. *Nature Neuroscience, 12,* 241–243.

Katon, W., VonKorff, M., Lin, E., Walker, E., Simon, G. E., Bush, T., et al. (1995). Collaborative management to achieve treatment guidelines: Impact on depression in primary care. *Journal of the American Medical Association, 273,* 1026–1031.

Keating, D., & Hertzman, C. (1999). Modernity's paradox. In D. P. Keating & C. Herztman (Eds.), *Developmental health and the wealth of nations* (pp. 1–17). New York: Guilford Press.

Kilpatrick, K., Litt, M., & Williams, L. M. (1997). Post traumatic stress disorder in child witnesses to violence. *American Journal of Orthopsychiatry, 67*(4), 639–644.

Korenman, S., Miller, J., & Sjaastad, J. E. (1994). Long-term poverty and child development in the United States: Results from the NLSY: DP 1044–1094. Madison, WI: Institute for Research on Poverty.

Legal Services Corporation. (2007). Documenting the justice gap in America. Washington, DC: Author. Available at *www.lsc.gov/justicegap.pdf.*

Manalich, R., Reyes, L., Herrera, M., Melendi, C., & Fundora, I. (2000). Relationship between weight at birth and the number and size of renal glomeruli in humans: A histomorphometric study. *Kidney International, 58,* 770–773.

McEwen, B. S. (2007). Physiology and neurobiology of stress and adaptation: Central role of the brain. *Physiological Reviews, 87,* 873–904.

McGinnis, J. M., & Foege, W. H. (1993). Actual cause of death in the United States. *Journal of the American Medical Association, 270,* 2207–2212.

McGowan, P. O., Sasaki, A., D'Alessio, A. C., Dymov, S., Labonte, B., Szyf, M., et al. (2009). Epigenetic regulation of the glucocorticoid receptor in human brain associates with childhood abuse. *Nature Neuroscience, 12,* 342–348.

Meaney, M. J. (2001). Maternal care, gene expression, and the transmission of individual differences in stress reactivity across generations. *Annual Review of Neuroscience, 24,* 1161–1192.

Meyers, A. F., Cutts, D. B., Frank, D. A., Levenson, S. M., Skalicky, A., Heeren, T., et al. (2005). Subsidized housing and children's nutritional status: Data from a multisite surveillance study. *Archives of Pediatrics and Adolescent Medicine, 159,* 551–556.

Miller, J. E. (1998). Developmental screening scores among preschool-aged children: The roles of poverty and child health. *Journal of Urban Health, 75,* 135–152.

Minkovitz, C. S., Hughart, N., Strobino, D., Scharfstein, D., Grason, H., Hou, W., et al. (2003). A practice-based intervention to enhance quality of care in the first 3 years of life: Results from the Healthy Steps for Young Children Program. *Journal of the American Medical Association, 290*(23), 3081–3091.

Minkovitz, C. S., Strobino, D., Mistry, K. B., Scharfstein, D. O., Grason, H., Hou, W., et al. (2007). Healthy Steps for young children: Sustained results at 5.5 years. *Pediatrics, 120*(3), e658–e668.

National Consensus Development Panel on Effective Medical Treatment of Opiate Addiction. (1998). Effective medical treatment of opiate addiction. *Journal of the American Medical Association, 280,* 1936–1943.

Needleman, H. L., & Gatsonis, C. A. (1990). Low-level lead exposure and the IQ of children. A meta-analysis of modern studies. *Journal of the American Medical Association, 263,* 673–678.

Needlman, R., Fried, L. E., Morley, D. S., Taylor, S., & Zuckerman, B. (1991). Clinic-based intervention to promote literacy: A pilot study. *American Journal of Diseases of Children, 145,* 881–884.

Parker, S., Greer, S., & Zuckerman, B. (1988). Double jeopardy: The impact of poverty on early child development. *Pediatric Clinics of North America, 35,* 1227–1240.

Perrin, J. M., Bloom, S. R., & Gortmaker, S. L. (2007). The increase of childhood chronic conditions in the United States. *Journal of the American Medical Association, 297*(24), 2755–2759.

Pollitt, R. A., Kaufman, J. S., Rose, K. M., Diez-Roux, A. V., Zeng, D., & Heiss, G. (2007). Early-life and adult socioeconomic status and inflammatory risk markers in adulthood. *European Journal of Epidemiology, 22,* 55–66.

Power, C., & Hertzman, C. (1997). Social and biological pathways linking early life and adult disease. *British Medical Bulletin, 53,* 210–221.

Richman, N., Stevenson, J., & Graham, P. (1982). *Preschool to school: A behavioral study.* New York: Academic Press.

Sameroff, A. J., Seifer, R., Baldwin, A., & Baldwin, C. (1993). Stability of intelligence from preschool to adolescence: The influence of social and family risk factors. *Child Development, 64*(1), 80–97.

Sameroff, A. J., Seifer, R., Barocas, R., Zax, M., & Greenspan, S. (1987). Intelligence quotient scores of four-year-old children: Social–environmental risk factors. *Pediatrics, 79,* 343–350.

Sandel, M., Hansen, M., Kahn, R., Lawton, E., Paul, E., Parker, V., et al. (2010). Medical–legal partnerships: Transforming primary care by addressing the legal needs of vulnerable populations. *Health Affairs, 29*(9), 1697–1705.

Sandel, M., Phelan, K., Wright, R., Hynes, H. P., & Lanphear, B. P. (2004). The effects of housing interventions on child health. *Pediatric Annals, 33*(7), 474–481.

Shin, P., Byrne, F. R., Jones, E., Teitelbaum, J., Repasch, L., & Rosenbaum, S.

(2010). Medical–legal partnerships: Addressing the unmet legal needs of health center patients. Washington, DC: Geiger Gibson/RCHN Community Health Foundation Research Collaborative, School of Public Health and Health Services, George Washington University. Available at *www.rchnfoundation.org/images/FE/chain207siteType8/site176/client/mlpfinal%20may4-2.pdf*.

Shonkoff, J. P., Boyce, W. T., & McEwen, B. S. (2009). Neuroscience, molecular biology, and the childhood roots of health disparities: Building a new framework for health promotion and disease prevention. *Journal of the American Medical Association, 301,* 2252–2259.

Silverstein, M., Augustyn, M., Young, R., & Zuckerman, B. (2009). The relationship between maternal depression, in-home violence and use of physical punishment: What is the role of child behaviour? *Archives of Disease in Childhood, 94*(2), 138–143.

Strauss, M. A., & Gelles, R. J. (1986). Societal change and change in family violence from 1975 to 1985 as revealed by two national surveys. *Journal of Marriage and Family, 48,* 465–479.

Taylor, L., Zuckerman, Z., Harik, V., & Groves, B. M. (1994). Witnessing violence by young children and their mothers. *Journal of Developmental and Behavioral Pediatrics, 15*(2), 120–123.

Taylor, S. E., Lehman, B. J., Kiefe, C. I., & Seeman, T. E. (2006). Relationship of early life stress and psychological functioning to adult C-reactive protein in the coronary artery risk development in young adults study. *Biological Psychiatry, 60,* 819–824.

Walberg, H., & Marjorikbanks, K. (1976). Family environment and cognitive development. *Review of Educational Research, 46,* 49–62.

Wang, X., Zuckerman, B., Pearson, C., Kaufman, G., Chen, C., Wang, G., et al. (2002). Maternal cigarette smoking, metabolic gene polymorphism, and infant birth weight. *Journal of the American Medical Association, 287*(2), 195–202.

Washington State Supreme Court, Taskforce on Equal Civil Justice Funding. (2003). The Washington State Civil Legal Needs Study: Executive summary. Seattle, WA: Author. Available at *www.courts.wa.gov/newsinfo/content/taskforce/legalneedsexecsummary.pdf*.

Weaver, I., Cervoni, N., Champagne, F. A., D'Alessio, A. C., Sharma, S., Seckl, J. R., et al. (2004). Epigentic programming by maternal behavior. *Nature Neuroscience, 7*(8), 847–854.

Weisman, C. (1996). Women's use of health care. In M. M. Falik & K. S. Collins (Eds.), *Women's health: The Commonwealth Fund Survey* (pp. 19–48). Baltimore: Johns Hopkins University Press.

Weissman, M. M., & Olfson, M. (1995). Depression in women: Implication for health care research. *Science, 269,* 799–801.

Weissman, M. M., Pilowsky, D. J., Wickramaratne, P. J., Talati, A., Wisniewski, S. R., Fava, M., et al. (2006). Remissions in maternal depression and child psychopathology: A STAR*D-child report. *Journal of the American Medical Association, 295*(12), 1389–1398.

Zuckerman, B., Augustyn, M., Groves, B. M., & Parker, S. (1995). Silent victims revisited: The special case of domestic violence. *Pediatrics, 96*(3), 511–513.

Zuckerman, B., & Beardslee, W. R. (1987). Maternal depression: A concern for pediatricians. *Pediatrics, 79,* 110–117.

Zuckerman, B., Frank, D. A., Hingson, R., Amaro, H., Levenson, S. M., Kayne, H., et al. (1989). Effects of maternal marijuana and cocaine use on fetal growth. *New England Journal of Medicine, 320*(12), 762–768.

Zuckerman, B., Parker, S., Kaplan-Sanoff, M., Augustyn, M., & Barth, M. (2004). Healthy steps: A case study of innovation in pediatric practice. *Pediatrics, 114*(3), 820–826.

Zuckerman, B., Sandel, M., Lawton, E., & Morton, S. (2008). Medical–legal partnerships: Transforming healthcare. *Lancet, 372,* 1615–1617.

PART V

IMPLICATIONS FOR FAMILIES

CHAPTER 11

An Ecological View of the Socialization Process of Latino Children

Natasha J. Cabrera

Despite scholars' contention that young Latino children constitute "an urgent demographic imperative" because they are the largest and the poorest ethnic group in the United States, little is known about how their cultural and home environment promote social competencies in the first 5 years of life (Garcia & Jensen, 2009). A robust body of work shows that young children's social competencies (e.g., self-control, interpersonal skills, internalizing and externalizing problem behaviors) contribute to their social adaptation and cognitive learning at school (Galindo & Fuller, 2010). Research to date has found great heterogeneity in the levels of cognitive and social competencies, including social behaviors valued by teachers, that Latino children exhibit at kindergarten entry (Portes & Rumbaut, 2001). Although some studies show that Latino children perform poorly on achievement tests and are not socially ready for kindergarten, others have shown that some children in immigrant families perform well on achievement and cognitive tests and exhibit social competencies at school entry (Crosnoe, 2007; Galindo & Fuller, 2010).

The reason why some young Latino children succeed in school and others do not is unclear. Most salient is the fact that the bulk of the research on Latino children's adaptation has been dominated by studies on the immigration experiences (mostly of mothers), as well as children's vulnerability to the stresses of migration (Bashir, 1993). Consequently, there is relatively little information on how family or individual factors promote child adjustment in a cultural context. Specifically, the ways in which Latino mothers *and* fathers contribute to the development of their children, in particular infants and toddlers, have been neglected. Given that most Latino children live in two-parent families, it is imperative to understand the role of the father in these families. Moreover, insights from recent qualitative and small-scale studies suggest that grandparents and siblings are also important sources of socialization. A couple of caveats are in order. In this chapter I use the term "Latino" to refer to people who come from South and Central America and the Spanish-speaking Caribbean countries who may be native born or immigrants. Although I recognize that there are important interethnic differences that need to be noted, most studies to date do not consider the ethnicity or immigration status of the sample.

In this chapter, I take an ecocultural approach, which emphasizes that every cultural community provides developmental pathways for children within a culturally and linguistically bounded setting, to review the extant literature on the socialization processes of Latino children (Weisner, 2002). Accordingly, I focus on how each member of the family engages in practices and behaviors that are linked to children's social competencies. I first discuss children's social competencies, including both normative and nonnormative outcomes; second, I review studies that show that the socialization context of Latino children include both developmental and acculturative processes; third, I use ecocultural and family system approaches to review literature on the unique influences of mothers, fathers, siblings, and grandparents on the development of children's social competences; and fourth, I conclude with implications for the development of a model for infant/toddler care for low-income children and families.

Children's Positive Social Development: Normative and Non-Normative Social Competences

Children's socialization process begins in the family through parent–child interactions. The importance of early parent–child interactions is embedded in many theoretical frameworks such as attachment (Ainsworth & Bowlby, 1991), family system theories (Cox & Paley, 1997), and ecocultural theories (Weisner, 2002). Parents socialize their children to adapt the culturally appropriate values and behaviors that enable them to be socially competent and act as members of a social group. Typically, researchers define social competence as the ability to integrate thoughts, feelings and emotions, and behaviors to achieve interpersonal goals valued within a particular social/cultural context while at the same time maintaining personal relationships with others (Rubin & Rose-Krasnor, 1992). Children who are socially competent display particular behaviors that suggest a *certain set of values* (e.g., social justice, responsibility), *positive self-identity* (e.g., sense of competence, worth), *interpersonal skills* (e.g., maintains friendly relation-ships, resolves conflicts, expresses emotions), *self-regulation* (e.g., controls impulses, delays gratification), *planning and decision making* (e.g., follows directions, makes choices), and display *cultural competence* (e.g., ability to interact effectively with people of varying ethnic backgrounds; McCay & Keyes, 2002).

Although there are differences across cultural groups in terms of the social competence skills that are emphasized (e.g., cooperation vs. inde-pendence) and in the ways values are reflected in particular behaviors (e.g., words and actions that signal respect), there is considerable agreement that many of these behaviors are universal. In the United States, research suggests that children who are socially competent are independent versus suggestible, responsible rather than irresponsible, cooperative instead of resistive, purposeful rather than aimless, friendly rather than hostile, and self-controlled rather than impulsive (Landy, 2002). In short, the socially competent child exhibits social skills (e.g., has positive interactions with others, expresses emotions effectively), is able to establish peer relationships (e.g., accepted by other children), and has certain individual attributes (e.g., shows capacity to empathize, has coping skills).

The most striking finding of the research on the social adaptation of Latino children is that it is largely atheoretical, with few notable exceptions (Halgunseth, Ispa, & Rudy, 2006). One of the challenges for researchers has been to incorporate into their designs the culture and unique experi-ences of Latino children, including acculturation and enculturation. There is a dearth of theories that can account for immigrant children's success-ful adaptation under at-risk conditions (Knight, Roosa, & Umaña-Taylor, 2009). Consequently, extant research has not examined the factors that influence parenting in a cultural and dynamic context and the mechanisms that link these factors to child social development, especially in early child-hood. Moreover, this research is plagued by methodological and measure-ment shortcomings such as using measures that are often not validated for use with the Latino population (Knight et al., 2009).

Not surprisingly, findings on the social competencies skills of Latino children are inconsistent. For example, although the majority of Latino children participating in a national study were rated by their teachers as not being ready for school (eager to learn, pay attention to a task; West, Denton, & Reaney, 2001), they were also found to exhibit similar levels of internalizing problems as European American children (Crosnoe, 2007). But, no such differences were found when analyses controlled for back-ground factors. In a small-scale study, PreK teachers rated Latino toddlers as having positive social skills (Zucker & Howes, 2009).

Similarly, when analyses are conducted by generational status, find-ings are different. Based on a large sample of 4-year-olds (Central and South American, Cubans, and Caribbean) enrolled in prekindergarten in

Miami, Florida, De Feyter and Winsler (2009) found that although first- and second-generation immigrants lagged behind children in nonimmigrant families in cognitive and language skills, they excelled in socioemotional skills and behavior. Moreover, first-generation immigrant children showed higher social skills than second generation, a finding the authors view as evidence for the *immigrant advantage*. They found no significant group differences in socioemotional factors or behavior according to country of origin. Children with immigrant parents from all countries showed high socioemotional protective factors and low behavior concerns when compared to children with native-born parents. In contrast, Galindo and Fuller (2010) using a nationally representative sample found that although first-generation Latino kindergartners displayed slightly weaker social competencies than did second-generation children, poor Latino children exhibited weaker social competencies compared to middle-class Latinos and European American children. Social competencies, especially approaches to learning, were significantly associated with cognitive growth.

Other factors that might account for some of the inconsistencies found in social skills among Latino children include the nature of the immigration experience. For example, a study of native-born and immigrant Latino families from Central America and Mexico found a normal range of externalizing behaviors among preschool children but higher frequency of internalizing problems (Weiss, Goebel, Page, Wilson, & Warda, 1999). Parents' immigration status and the family's use of coping strategies (e.g., passive appraisal) were linked to children's internalizing problems. However, immigration from Central America was more predictive of externalizing behaviors than was immigration from Mexico. Weiss and colleagues suggest that perhaps Central Americans' immigration to the United States was more fraught with physical and/or emotional trauma than the more voluntary immigration of Mexicans leading to parental stress, which may have long-term impact on their interactions with their children. These findings suggest that the factors that predict adaptation are multiple and systemic and that future research needs to carefully disentangle the effects of contextual, socioeconomic status (SES), and cultural factors on children's outcomes.

The reciprocal association between culture and adaptation has prompted researchers to argue that while normative outcomes are important indicators of children's success in school and other settings, there may be other *non-normative* outcomes that may capture other aspects of well-being and adaptation among children who grow up in disadvantaged neighborhoods. Sternberg's (2002) research on nontraditional learning settings suggests that being smart in everyday life situations means making the most of the skills and information one has. Sternberg underlies the importance of nonverbal communication, creativity, and practical application of information, which he calls ordinary common sense or "street smarts." Children growing up in poor neighborhoods with limited adult supervision, for example, might develop a set of important skills or "street smarts" that enable them to adapt and succeed in that environment. Research based on African American youth samples shows that they often talk about a "revised American dream," commitment to religious and spiritual activities, and kin-care responsibilities that are also related to families' expectations regarding their children's behaviors (Burton & Jarrett, 2000). There is no comparable research with Latino families, but this research has implications for how programs can help Latino parents/ of infants/toddlers foster coping skills that would enable them, as they get older, to adapt and thrive in disadvantaged neighborhoods.

Although there is more research on the influence of neighborhoods on African American children than on Latinos, there are important findings worth pointing out. Research conducted during the 1990s showed that although most inner-city Mexicans were first-generation immigrants, their neighborhoods were less poor than those of Chicago's inner-city African American population. Inner-city Latino immigrants were more likely to live in areas of moderate poverty, in ethnic enclaves, surrounded by small businesses, many owned and operated by Latinos and, consequently, were less isolated from jobs and from employed neighbors than were African Americans (Wilson, 1996). These conditions may set up different expectations for Latinos and thus result in different non-normative outcomes for children. We are in the dark regarding the types of culture-specific and social or "street" skills that Latino children living in bicultural, and often poor communities, might develop over time, beginning in infancy. We need to focus on non-normative outcomes to get away from a deficit view of Latino children's adaptation. It might be worth our efforts to understand the type of neighborhood-specific social skills that infants and toddlers learn as they become socialized into their communities.

Development and Acculturation as Contexts for Socialization

Ecoculturally based research suggests that children develop social competencies by participating in routine activities (e.g., chores, taking care of siblings) and family rituals (e.g., watching television, or going to church; Weisner, 2002). These activities are shared with and initiated by parents, siblings, and grandparents and unfold within the home, which is structured by cultural and linguistic practices, expectations, and behaviors (Rogoff, 2003). In this context, young children interact with their mothers, fathers, siblings, and grandparents, who teach them implicitly or explicitly, to acquire appropriate social behaviors, adapt to expected norms, and learn linguistic conventions and cognitive skills (Sameroff & Fiese, 2000). Cultural theorists' focus is then on understanding the origins of social competencies in particular settings and then determining whether it transfers to other settings such as school. In short, Latino children, as do all children, develop and grow in a cultural context that is dynamic *and* changes over time due to normative sources of developmental change as well as to the acculturation process.

Although the term "acculturation" has been defined in multiple ways, there is consensus that it refers to a process of reciprocal adaptation between immigrants and the host culture. For children, this process is more complex because as they acculturate, they also undergo rapid maturational change. From a developmental perspective, younger children adapt to new situations easier than do older children. From an acculturation perspective, the longer one stays in the host country the higher the likelihood of learning social skills such as acquisition of language. Scholars have argued that while age-related changes in cognitive and social development arise from the dynamic interaction between biological maturational processes and environmental learning experiences, change due to acculturation is a function of learning adaptive and functional coping skills (Sam & Berry, 2006). That is, acculturation is a process whereby adaptation includes both learning and maturation. In this sense, acculturation is embedded in development, which confounds acculturation (Phinney, Berry, Vedder, & Liebkind, 2006). Therefore, as immigrant children develop and acculturate simultaneously, this process is intermingled and difficult to disentangle (Sam & Berry, 2006).

The ways in which the acculturative gap manifests between parents and infants and toddlers are unknown. There is some preliminary evidence that discipline might arouse conflict or tension between parents and their young children. Findings from an ongoing focus group study reveal that Central American mothers and fathers whose children are enrolled in a Head Start center worry about disciplining for fear their children will call the police if parents use physical punishment (Cabrera, Aldoney, & Sidorowicz, 2010). Because parents are informed that Head Start staff must report to child service agencies any physical abuse, parents are fearful and uncertain how to discipline their children. These findings suggest that programs aimed at infants/toddlers need to offer parenting classes that include culturally and developmentally appropriate strategies for disciplining children.

Cultural theorists have argued that in addition to learning about a new culture, immigrants who maintain and retain their culture of origin, or enculturate, exhibit more adaptive behaviors than those who do not. Although most of the research on cultural adaption has focused on acculturation, the extant research on how families enculturate reveals that a strong sense of identity and ethnic identification is strongly linked to positive outcomes for children (Phinney et al., 2006). Some have argued that Mexican Americans are the immigrant group that has most successfully retained their culture and language in the United States (Holmes & Holmes, 1995). In a study of urban preschoolers of four ethnicities (i.e., Latino, black, European American, Asian), researchers found that families that were bicultural, or had indicated high levels of ethnic *and* U.S. identity had children with positive social, academic, and emotional functioning (Calzada, Brotman, Huang, Bat-Chava, & Kingston, 2009). Thus programs that promote and encourage children to maintain their cultural heritage as well as adapt to the host society might best provide children with adaptive skills to function in two cultures.

Systemic View of Family as a Context for Development: Mothers, Fathers, Siblings, and Grandparents

Although the family is considered to be the most important environmental influence on children's learning and development, research has focused almost exclusively on mothers as the central influence on children's lives, and has paid less attention to fathers, siblings, and grandparents. There are virtually no studies of the Latino family as a system. Consequently, we have a partial understanding of how the family system influences children's development and of the mechanism that might explain it. This lack of attention to the role of family in Latino children's development is particularly salient given the cultural importance of the family among Latinos. In this section, I discuss select research on the influence of families on children by highlighting the separate and unique contributions of mothers and fathers, grandparents, and siblings, whenever possible. Given the sparse research on Latino families, I also draw from the larger literature on minority families to highlight similar processes that might be relevant for Latino families.

Maternal Influence: Beliefs and Responsive Parenting

Mothers' beliefs about child rearing reflect the norms, expectations, and value systems of the cultural groups in which they are embedded and are important mechanisms for propagating "systems of cultural priorities" (Kagitcibasi, 1996). Parents transmit values, rules, and standards about ways of thinking and acting, and provide an interpretive lens through which children view social relationships and structures (Super & Harkness, 2002). The *socialization strategies* parents adopt emphasize the development of particular instrumental competencies. Parenting beliefs and practices are transmitted to children via parent–child interactions and activities and routines structured by parents and others (Harwood, Miller, & Irizarry, 1995).

Maternal Beliefs

Research on mothers' beliefs among Latino families suggests that the value of interdependence, for example, is manifested in three important goals or beliefs parents use to socialize their children: *familism, educación,* and *respeto.*

Perhaps the most commonly held belief about Latinos is their connections to their families, or their embracing of *familism.* Familism is conceptualized as feelings of closeness and mutuality with family members as well as the notion that the self is an extension of the family (Gonzalez-Ramos, Zayas, & Cohen, 1998). Studies have shown Latinos tend to report higher levels of family cohesion than European Americans and that some aspects of *familism* decline over generations, whereas others remain stable across generations (Rumbaut, 2005).

The ways in which infants and toddlers are taught allegiance to the family and whether *familism* is linked to positive outcomes for young children are unclear. Through family routines and rituals children learn to put families first, respect family members, and be less independent (García Coll & Pachter, 2002). There is evidence suggesting that this family centrism may be both a protective and a risk factor. Children might be expected to obey their elders even when they don't agree with the elders' views/values, creating tension and conflict. And although family members may rely on each other for social and economic support (e.g., providing child care), they may also share crowded living quarters and provide unsolicited advice on issues ranging from child rearing to food choices, which can lead to stress and conflict.

On the positive side, having a strong sense of family obligation and duty might teach children that the family unit is there to support and protect them. One study found that when siblings reported a strong value of *familism,* perceived differential treatment by their parents was not linked to measures of well-being. For siblings who reported weaker values of *familism,* fewer perceived favorable treatment was correlated with poorer well-being (McHale, Updegraff, Shanahan, Crouter, & Killoren, 2005). Concern for the family may make children less inclined toward social comparisons with their siblings and less likely to perceive unequal treatment as a sign that they are unloved or less valued by their parents. These findings are consistent with attachment-based research showing that children who feel valued and loved by their parents and who display empathy and concern for others are generally able to get along with others, have close relationships with peers, and function adaptively in school.

Educación, unlike the English translation of the word, includes basic beliefs about right and wrong, and school achievement (Greenfield, Quiroz, & Raeff, 2000). It refers to the goal of rearing a moral, responsible, and socially competent child, who will become *una persona de bien* (a good person) who is *bien educado* (has manners and is well brought up), respectful of adults, and is on *el buen camino* (following the good path; Reese, 2001).

Despite parents' strong belief in *educación*, there may be structural and personal barriers preventing them from fully realizing this goal. Although early studies have found that *educación* is an important indicator of Latino children's achievement, especially for young children (Suárez-Orozco & Suárez-Orozco, 2002), later studies have shown that the path might not be so linear. A small study of Latino immigrants and their kindergarteners found that Latino parents' educational aspirations (i.e., hope: "How far do you want your child to go in his or her formal schooling?") are high throughout the elementary school years, but *expectations* (i.e., actual beliefs: "How far do you think your child will go in his or her formal schooling?"), which may be influenced by child's performance, fluctuate (Goldenberg, Gallimore, Reese, & Garnier, 2001). The influence of *educación* on actual children's language and social skills may also depend on the degree to which the home environment, including parenting, practices are structured (Farver, Lonigan,Weisner, Lieber, & Davis, 2004). For example, low-income Latino mothers, on average, read with their young children less frequently than do European American mothers (Bradley, Corwyn, McAdoo, & Coll, 2001). Because reading is a strong indicator of children's cognitive skills, the lack of maternal reading places Latino children at risk for language and cognitive delays as well as behavior problems.

Other personal preferences and beliefs about child rearing may be incompatible with the strong belief on *educación* among Latino mothers who must balance work and family in unfamiliar ways. For example, the use of child care, which can promote child literacy, is varied among Latino families. Overall, Latino children are underrepresented in early childhood programs. Studies show that working Latino mothers, even those who are born in the United States and have more education, prefer to leave their preschool-age children, including infants, in the care of a spouse or relative and rely less on formal child care arrangements than other mothers (Buriel & Hurtado-Ortiz, 2000). However, foreign-born Latino mothers report the lowest rate of availability of relatives to help with child care. Latino mothers' preference for relative care over formal care, especially for infants and toddlers, may reflect their strong sense of family; lack of trust in non-Spanish-speaking caregivers; lack of knowledge about the benefits of quality center-based care; and, cost, accessibility, and availability of child care (Cabrera, Hutchins, & Peters, 2006).

Another important belilef is *respeto*. Latino families raise their children to be bien educados, that is, to be respectful and obey the decisions of parents and elders in the community. This orientation to the lager group is viewed as essential for group harmony and the foundation of children's development (Calzada, Fernandez, & Cortes, 2010). In one study, Puerto Rican mothers described ideal children as those who were obedient to elders, calm in order to attend to the needs of others, and polite and kind compared to European American mothers who emphasized qualities that highlighted self-maximization (Harwood et al., 1995). Another study found that by the age of 4, Latino children were taught the verbal and nonverbal rules of respect such as politely greeting elders, not challenging an elder's point of view, and not interrupting conversations between adults (Valdés, 1996). There is little research on how Latino mothers socialize infants/toddlers to be social and respectful. However, based on these findings, it is reasonable to assume that Latino mothers might first encourage dependence by assisting their infants/toddlers with basic self-care such as feeding, dressing, and so on, but at the same time foster sociability and respect for others as soon as they are able to talk.

The emphasis on good manners and respect for others are important skills that encourage social competence in various settings, including school, and hence can be an important aspect of Latino children's academic success. However, these culturally valued skills that make Latino children socially competent at home might be at odds with values such as participating in class, being assertive, and asking challenging questions, which are emphasized by teachers in the classroom. If Latino children are taught to be obedient and not to challenge authority figures, they might also be less likely to be assertive in the classroom. The lack of fit between social skills taught at home and those encouraged at school might be one source of variation in Latino children's academic outcomes. This calls for increased teacher training to be culturally competent and aware of cultural differences in skills that parents teach their children.

Maternal Sensitivity and Responsiveness

Parents' responsiveness and nurturance have been directly linked to child well-being in European American and minority families (Cabrera, Shannon, West, & Brooks-Gunn, 2006). A small-scale study of low-income Mexican American and European American families showed that mothers with high levels of warmth and acceptance, consistent use of discipline and enforcing rules, and low levels of conflict and hostility had children with fewer conduct problems than the comparison group (Hill, Bush, & Rosa, 2003). A small-scale study found that Mexican American children with a more secure mother–child attachment relationship also had more concurrent complex play and more rapid growth of complex play (Howes, Wishard Guerra, & Zucker, 2008). Using a nationally representative sample of Latino infants born in 2001, Cabrera, Shannon, and her colleagues (2006) found that Mexican American infants had lower mother–infant interaction scores than did the other Latino infants, with differences not being accounted for by SES differences between the two groups (the Mexican American parents were younger, less educated, poorer, and more likely to be unemployed). The differences between Mexican mothers and other Latino mothers were associated with differences in maternal and paternal English proficiency. Moreover, they also found that after controlling for SES, acculturation, and levels of depression, mother–infant interactions (but not paternal engagement) were positively related to infant cognition.

Physical and Psychological Control

Latino families use physical and psychological control to foster goals of *familism* and *respeto* (Carlson & Harwood, 2003). Cross-cultural studies of young children reveal that Mexican American and Puerto Rican parents are more controlling (and perhaps intrusive) than European American mothers, regardless of level of acculturation or SES, but are also warm and sensitive toward their children (Ispa et al., 2004). The use of physical and verbal punishment, regardless of child age, in Latino families, however, is strongly linked to SES (Halgunseth et al., 2006). Although the effects of punishment on infants/toddlers' well-being is understudied, there is evidence that for older children these forms of punishment are linked with negative child outcomes (Hill et al., 2003).

However, other studies have not found Latino mothers' controlling behaviors to be linked to children's behavior problems in expected ways. Research with Latino mothers has found that despite Latino mothers being more intrusive and physically controlling than European American mothers, Latino children did not always exhibit negative outcomes (Carlson & Harwood, 2003). For example, several studies have shown that maternal physical control, even with 14-month-olds, predicted secure attachment and child engagement in Puerto Rican, Dominican, and Mexican infants and toddlers (Halgunseth et al., 2006). In the context of low parental stress, children may perceive parental controlling behaviors as a form of caring. These findings suggest that parenting must be understood in a cultural context to shed light on what behaviors are normative for that ethnic group, the emotional connotation of certain behaviors as well as the meaning that individuals attribute to those behaviors (Grusec, Rudy, & Martini, 1997).

Latino families have also been found to use other cultural strategies such as using *dichos* (proverbs) or *consejos* (advice) to control their children. It is unclear whether these are a form of psychological control or if they are merely ways to teach by example (Azmitia & Brown, 2002). Whether the use of *consejos* is effective in shaping children's behaviors in expected ways is an empirical question that has not been addressed. Similarly, the use of *dichos*, unique to the Latino culture, is consistent with a strong oral tradition, and seems to be important in the socialization of even young children (Burciaga, Christensen, & Christensen, 1997). The use of *dichos* (e.g., *"Dime con quién andas, y te diré quién eres"*—Tell me who your friends are and I will tell you who you are) is commonly used by parents in efforts to monitor their children's friendships. As with the use of *consejos,* the impact of the use of *dichos* on children's behavior is unknown.

Fathers' Influence

Research on the role of the father on children's development has surged over the last two decades, but there is still a dearth of data on the impact of Latino fathers on their children's development (Cabrera & Garcia Coll, 2004). In contrast to research on mothers, research on fathers has not examined traditional areas of parenting, such as beliefs. Early research on fathers focused on the effects of father absence on children. More recently, studies have paid attention to the nuanced and multiple ways in which fathers can be involved with their children, the factors that explain variation in involvement and its impact on children's development.

The role of the father in Latino families needs to be considered in a unique demographic and cultural context. In contrast to African American children, most Latino children live in two-parent families. This means that, unlike other minorities in the United States, most Latino children do not have the added stress of living in single-headed households. Despite the paucity of research on the ways Latino fathers are engaged with their children, there are studies that show that Latino fathers are actively engaged with their children (Cabrera, Hofferth, & Chae, 2011). Recent research has challenged the traditional stereotypes of Latino fathers as being authoritarian and emotionally uninvolved with their children. A study found that Mexican American fathers used parenting strategies associated with authoritative parenting, endorsed coaching on emotions, and were observed to be supportive and responsive to their children (Gamble, Ramakumar, & Diaz, 2007). Another study using a qualitative approach found that Latino fathers placed a high value on their role as a teacher and role model for their children and also saw themselves as educators (Raikes, Summers, & Roggman, 2005). In another study, Mexican fathers from both sides of the border reported that the main values they hope to give to their children are the importance of education, a strong work ethic, and having respect for themselves and others (Taylor & Behnke, 2005). Finally, a recent analysis showed that Latino fathers are as involved in caregiving and physical activities with their infants as are African American and European American fathers (Cabrera et al., 2011).

Research on the factors that explain variation in father involvement in Latino families is limited. Studies of determinants of fathering have shown that the father's human capital (education, income), and family processes, including relationship to the child's mother, as well as the father's relationship to his family at the transition to parenthood are important predictors of father engagement in low-income families (Coley & Hernandez, 2006). Fathers' education and income are uniquely associated with child measures and fathers' education consistently predicted the quality of mother–child engagement (Tamis-LeMonda, Shannon, Cabrera, & Lamb, 2004). A study of Mexican American mothers' and fathers' pregnancy intentions revealed that when mothers wanted the pregnancy, fathers engaged in more activities with the baby (e.g., literacy and caregiving activities) than when mothers did not want the pregnancy. Moreover, the effects of parents' wanting the pregnancy on mother–infant interactions and fathers' engagement were moderated by the quality of the couple relationship (Cabrera, Shannon, Mitchell, & West, 2009).

Other studies have focused on how other aspects of family functioning such as the coparenting relationship is related to father involvement. A study of Mexican American fathers and mothers found that couples who reported marital conflict also reported conflict over child-rearing responsibilities, which had a significant and negative effect on mother–infant interaction and father engagement. That is, when couples disagree over child issues, fathers and mothers are more likely to withdraw from their children than when they agree. They also found that when there is high coparenting conflict, more acculturated fathers engaged in more caregiving than less acculturated fathers (Cabrera, Shannon, & La Taillade, 2009).

In recent years, scholars have focused on how fathers *matter* for their children's development (Lamb, 2010). Although most of this emerging research has not been conducted with Latino samples or with infants/toddlers, valuable insights can be gained from these studies (Cabrera & Garcia Coll, 2004). Studies have shown that fathers who exhibited high levels of positive physical play, allowed for mutual exchanges and followed partners' suggestions, displayed patience, and used less directive or coercive tactics during play had children who were rated as popular and less aggressive, more competent, and better liked by their peers (McDowell & Parke, 2009). These findings suggest that programs need to encourage and promote positive father–child play as an important vehicle of children's socialization.

Other studies have shown links between fathers' behaviors and children's outcomes. For example, a study of the degree to which parenting attitudes and behavior (self-reported warmth, restrictiveness, and behavioral sensitivity as assessed during a free-play session) were related to toddlers' development found that fathers' restrictive attitude was negatively related to social and cognitive development, whereas paternal sensitivity was positively related to aspects of social development that are less dependent on language skills (e.g., motor and daily living skills; Kelley, Smith, Green, Berndt, & Rogers, 1998).

Another study of low-income fathers, including Latinos, and their toddlers assessed the quality of father–child interactions using 14 Likert ratings of fathers (e.g., responsiveness, language quality, and intrusiveness) and 12 of children (e.g., play, participation, emotional regulation, and communication; Shannon, Tamis-LeMonda, London, & Cabrera, 2002). They found that fathers who were responsive to their children during play were nearly five times more likely to have children within the normal range on a cognitive measure than were fathers who were not as responsive. A longitudinal study of observed father–child and mother–child engagements in a sample of toddlers enrolled in the Early Head Start National Evaluation Study found that fathers' and mothers' supportive parenting independently predicted children's outcomes after covarying significant demographic factors (Tamis-LeMonda et al., 2004).

Other studies have focused on the impact of father–child interactions on children's peer relationships. Youngblade and Belsky (1992) found that a positive father–child relationship at age 3 was associated with less negative friendships at age 5, whereas more negative father–child relationships forecast less satisfactory friendships. Studies with older children have shown that fathers influence children's peer relationships through the lessons children learn in the context of the father–child relationship, fathers' direct advice concerning peer relationships, and fathers' regulation of access to peers and peer-related activities (McDowell & Parke, 2009).

Recent studies have sought to understand the mechanism by which father–child interactions are linked to children's social behaviors. Studies by Flanders and his colleagues (2010) show that the influence of fathers' physical play (rough-and-tumble) on children's social behaviors with peers is moderated by the quality of the father–child interactions. Rough-and-tumble play was associated with more aggressive behavior only when fathers were less dominant and only when fathers were unable to maintain an authoritative position in the play interactions. In the context of play, dominant fathers who set up boundaries and communicate to their child that crossing those boundaries is unacceptable are more able to regulate their children's actions than low-dominant, possibly permissive or uninvolved, dads (Flanders et al., 2010).

There is also exploratory research suggesting that increased father involvement is not always better, especially when fathers report being stressed about their parenting role. In a study of African American fathers and their toddlers, researchers found that fathers reported moderate levels of parenting stress, but found no evidence of a direct effect of stress on children's social development. However, parenting stress predicted more engagement in management activities, which predicted children's increased problem behavior (Mitchell & Cabrera, 2009).

The Role of Siblings and Grandparents

It is estimated that Latino children spend around 17 hours a week in shared activities with siblings compared to 10 hours for European Americans (Tucker, 2004). Thus, older siblings are an important source of socialization for Latino infants/toddlers. Siblings are more likely to take on caregiving and parenting roles when there is a lack of economic resources and social support (Walsh, Shulman, Bar-On, & Tsur, 2006). The emphasis on contributing to the collective interest of the family suggests that siblings help maintain ethnic values, provide access to cultural traditions, act as cultural brokers for the family, and function as emotional support (Zayas & Solari, 1994). Moreover, because children typically overcome linguistic and cultural barriers quicker than adults, siblings may also serve as cultural brokers for less acculturated younger siblings and parents. The research on the influence of siblings on children's linguistic and social competencies is just emerging, so it is difficult to draw major conclusions. One study found that warm sibling relationships are associated with better behavioral, emotional, and peer adjustment. The companionship and guidance offered by older siblings may also enhance motivation and achievement for younger children in the family (Gamble & Modry-Mandell, 2008).

As with research on siblings, research on the role of grandparents on Latino children's socialization is just emerging. Grandparents' caregiving in Latino communities reflects the value of *familism* and the strong emphasis on the extended family and intergenerational ties in Latino culture. Findings show that a relatively large proportion of Latino grandparents raise their grandchildren (Fields, 2003). However, the prevalence of grandparental caregiving is consistently higher among the more disadvantaged Mexican Americans than others (Fuller-Thomson & Minkler, 2007). These data support the idea that Latino grandparents play an extensive caregiving role for their grandchildren (Cox, Brooks, & Valcarcel, 2000). Grandparent involvement may benefit young grandchildren directly through interactions with responsive and committed adults, or indirectly by providing support and material resources to foster positive parenting (Pittman & Boswell, 2007). However, given the demographic characteristics of this population, it is unclear how grandparent care impacts children's well-being.

Implications

The literature reviewed in this chapter paints a complex picture of the ways in which low-income Latino families support their children's development. Though the research base is weak on some areas, there is enough evidence to suggest that despite the harrowing conditions and economic hardships Latinos face, many display strengths, which they use to teach children the necessary skills to be competent members of social groups be it at home or at school. In this section, based on the research on these families, I outline a set of potential implications for the development of a model for infant/toddler care for children and families who are poor.

1. Providers and teachers must be trained to view the families and children they serve from a perspective of strengths rather than deficits. We must acknowledge that this is difficult to do in light of the underlying belief that children from poor families suffer a range of difficulties because they are "at risk." To change teachers' and providers' expectations and beliefs, they must learn the sources of strength in this population. First, children who are learning a second language should be valued and praised for learning a second language rather than devalued for not speaking English (Farver, Xu, Eppea, & Lonigan, 2005). Second, most Latino children live in two-parent families that are very invested in their children and spend time providing and caring for them (Goldenberg et al., 2001). Third, most Latinos have a strong work ethic that they transmit to their children (Dinan, 2006). In addition to building on these skills, providers should validate what families do well and acknowledge the difficulties they experience in navigating in the new culture. Fourth, Latino mothers engage in healthy prenatal practices and give birth to robust healthy newborns (García Coll et al., 2009).

2. The core elements of Latino socialization stress good behavior and respectful communication with adults (*bien education, respeto*), cooperation and caring for peers (*carino*), and the child's contribution to the family well-being (*familism*; Garcia Coll & Pachter, 2002). These socialization practices suggest that many Latino children may enter school with social competencies—self-control, interpersonal communication, and low levels of aggressiveness behaviors—that may not be recognized within classrooms (La Paro & Pianta, 2000). These social skills, however, are not necessarily at odds with behaviors valued by teachers such as self-control, communication, and avoidance of external problems (Hair, Halle, Terry-Humen, Lavelle, & Calkins, 2006). When children are taught to respect adults and not pose questions, not asking questions or raising one's hand in the classroom is viewed as risky because it does not fit with the highly verbal norms of many early childhood education classrooms. The problem might be lack of goodness of fit between the home and the school. If teachers do not recognize these strengths and interpret them instead as lack of interest or passivity or that children do not understand the language, then children's behaviors are likely to be misinterpreted.

3. We must question the assumption that *poor* parents do not teach their children appropriate social skills or that the cultural-specific competencies nurtured by Latino families may not be useful in the classroom. Teachers must be trained to recognize that children are situated in particular cultural contexts that promote particular social skills and behaviors. Latino children's humility or respect for authority should not be interpreted as lack of interest; instead providers and teachers need to be trained to respect cultural differences and promote bicultural knowledge.

4. The Latino family is extended and large. Whenever possible, fathers, siblings, and grandparents should be included in program activities. One Head Start center in Washington, D.C., invites fathers (and mothers) to a yard clean-up activity at the beginning of the spring and summer (Cabrera et al., 2010). Fathers are also invited to help out in minor carpentry tasks, depending on fathers' level of skill and interest. Helping fathers engage in literacy activities with their infants and toddlers is very important especially because some fathers believe that very young children don't understand and therefore reading is not useful. An event such as "daddy time" that encourages fathers to sing songs, tell stories, and even read to infants in a developmentally appropriate manner is an effective way to promote literacy.

5. Programs serving Latino families need to recognize the heterogeneity of families, while at the same time recognizing the similarities due to language and traditions, and developmental period of children. This tremendous variation means that some families may need more resources and intervention than others. For example, parents' immigration history is an important influence on parenting behaviors and children's outcomes. Parents who flee oppressive and brutal regimes in their country of origin suffer from mental health issues, anxiety, and stress, which can have a negative effect on their parenting skills (Weiss et al., 1999). Immigration status may be both a protective and a risk factor. Immigrant parents' optimism and encouragement as well as warmth and sensitive parenting may be protective factors resulting in positive educational outcomes among second-generation children compared to others. On the other hand, the limited economic resources and parental education of some immigrant parents may place them at a higher risk for further hardship. Thus, programs must recognize that the health and well-being of children depends to a larger extent on the health and well-being of the family.

6. Most mothers and fathers report that they are willing to do everything they can for their children. Their belief that teachers (as authority figures) need to be looked up to and respected are important elements of a positive parent–teacher relationship. Teachers and providers must be respectful of this trust but also use it as a platform from which parents can be engaged in positive and meaningful ways in the schooling of their children.

7. Children are active participants in their own upbringing. Through temperament and other characteristics, children can direct resources toward themselves and influence the way adults interact and relate to them. Acknowledging individual differences among Latino children can help them to master appropriate classroom-relevant skills and behaviors while at the same time valuing and encouraging concern for the group. It is possible

for teachers to help children develop strong individual and ethnic identities. Fostering children's curiosity, motivation, and interest in intellectual activities are important investments because studies have shown that these explain how children's early experiences result in later gains (Farver et al., 2005).

    8. Promote biculturalism. Maintaining one's cultural heritage as well as learning and adapting the cultural norms of the host society is the best model for healthy development of Latino children. Latino immigrant children, unlike nonimmigrant children, develop in a bi-cultural context that places many, often competing, demands on them. The task of learning two languages and cultural-specific social competencies can be taxing. Teachers and providers need to be aware of these tasks and through activities and lessons promote and support this development.

Conclusion

In this chapter I highlighted research that focused on how Latino children's developmental niche, with particular attention to family, influences their social development. The bulk of the research on Latino children's socialization has focused mainly on mothers and less so on fathers, siblings, or grandparents who may also exert influence on their children's development. This has resulted in an incomplete view of Latino children's adaptation and a lack of understanding on the positive pathways that families influence children. More research is needed to understand how fathers, siblings, and grandparents socialize Latino children.

    Theoreticians have argued that to fully understand the adaptation of immigrant children, theoretical models need to include acculturation/enculturation and developmental theories into their models. Extant research has focused mainly on how children and families adapt to two often opposing cultures and the challenges they face at home and within the larger society rather than on normative developmental processes. The challenge is to conduct scientifically rigorous studies that capture the fact that immigrant children develop and grow in a cultural context that is dynamic and changes over time due to normative sources of change as well as to the acculturation process. This type of research is needed to capitalize on the finding that Latino children's social skills as reported by teachers and parents are positive and adaptive. Latino children are more likely to follow directions, listen to teachers' instruction, and develop positive relationships with peers. If social skills are important for academic performance, the question is why are Latino children still falling behind their peers in academic achievement? This type of research is urgently needed if we are going to mount interventions during the early years to improve learning opportunities and outcomes for all Latino children.

REFERENCES

Ainsworth, M. D. S., & Bowlby, J. (1991). An ethological approach to personality development. *American Psychologist, 46*(4), 333–341.

Azmitia, M., & Brown, J. R. (2002). Latino immigrant parents' beliefs about the "path of life" of their adolescent children. In J. M. Contreras, K. A. Kerns, & A. M. Neal-Barnett (Eds.), *Latino children and families in the United States: Current research and future directions* (pp. 77–105). Westport, CT: Greenwood.

Bashir, M. R. (1993). Issues of immigration for the health and adjustment of young people. *Journal of Pediatrics and Child Health, 29* (Suppl. 1), 42–45.

Bradley, R. H., Corwyn, R. F., McAdoo, H. P., & Coll, C. G. (2001). The home environments of children in the United States: Part 1. Variations by age, ethnicity, and poverty status. *Child Development, 72*(6), 1844–1867.

Burciaga, J. A., Christensen, C., & Christensen, T. (1997). *In few words: A compendium of Latino folk wit and wisdom: A bilingual collection.* San Francisco: Mercury House.

Buriel, R., & Hurtado-Ortiz, M. T. (2000). Child care practices and preferences of native- and foreign-born Latina mothers and Euro-American mothers. *Hispanic Journal of Behavioral Sciences, 22*(3), 314–331.

Burton, L. M., & Jarrett, R. L. (2000). In the mix, yet on the margins: The place of families in urban neighborhood and child development research. *Journal of Marriage and the Family, 62,* 444–465.

Cabrera, N., Aldoney, D., & Sidorowicz, K. (2010). *Latino mothers, fathers, and their children.* Paper presented at the Family Lab Involvement, University of Maryland.

Cabrera, N. J., & Garcia Coll, C. (2004). Latino fathers: Uncharted territory in need of much exploration. In M. E. Lamb (Ed.), *The role of father in child development* (4th ed., pp. 417–452). Mahwah, NJ: Erlbaum.

Cabrera, N., Hofferth, S., & Chae, S. (2011). Patterns and predictors of father–infant engagement across race/ethnic groups. *Early Childhood Research Quarterly, 26,* 365–375.

Cabrera, N., Hutchins, R., & Peters, E. (Eds.), (2006). *From welfare to child care: What happens to children when mothers exchange welfare for work.* Mahwah, NJ: Erlbaum.

Cabrera, N., Shannon, J., & LaTaillade, J. (2009). Predictors of co-parenting in Mexican American families and direct effects on parenting and child social emotional development. *Infant Mental Health Journal, 30*(2), 523–548.

Cabrera, N., Shannon, J., Mitchell, S., & West, J. (2009). Mexican American mothers' and fathers' prenatal attitudes and father prenatal involvement: Links to mother–infant interaction and father engagement. *Journal of Sex Roles, 60,* 510–526.

Cabrera, N., Shannon, J., West, J., & Brooks-Gunn, J. (2006). Parental interactions with Latino infants: Variation by country of origin and English proficiency. *Child Development, 74,* 1190–1207.

Calzada, E., Brotman, L. M., Huang, K., Bat-Chava, J., & Kingston, S. (2009). Parent cultural adaptation and child functioning in culturally diverse, urban families of preschoolers. *Journal of Applied Developmental Psychology, 30,* 515–524.

Calzada, E. J., Fernandez, Y., & Cortes, D. E. (2010). Incorporating the cultural value of *respeto* into a framework of Latino parenting. *Cultural Diversity and Ethnic Minority Psychology,* 16(1), 77–86.

Carlson, V. J., & Harwood, R. L. (2003). Attachment, culture, and the caregiving system: The cultural patterning of everyday experiences among Anglo and Puerto Rican mother–infant pairs, *Infant Mental Health Journal, 24,* 53–73.

Coley, R. L., & Hernandez, D. C. (2006). Predictors of paternal involvement for resident and nonresident low-income fathers. *Developmental Psychology, 42,* 1041–1056.

Cox, C. B., Brooks, L. R., & Valcarcel, C. (2000). Culture and caregiving: A study of Latino grandparents. In C. B. Cox (Ed.), *To grandmother's house we go and stay: Perspectives on custodial grandparents* (pp. 218–232). New York: Springer.

Cox, M. J., & Paley, B. (1997). Families as systems. *Annual Review of Psychology, 48,* 243–267.

Crosnoe, R. (2007). Early child care and the school readiness of children from Mexican immigrant families. *International Migration Review,* 41(1), 152–181.

De Feyter, J. J., & Winsler, A. (2009). The early developmental competencies and school readiness of low-income, immigrant children: Influences of generation, race/ethnicity, and national origins. *Early Childhood Research Quarterly,* 24(4), 411–431.

Dinan, G. K. A. (2006). *Young children in immigrant families: The role of philanthropy.* New York: Natonal Center for Children in Poverty.

Farver, J. M., Lonigan, C. J., Weisner, T., Lieber, E., & Davis, H. (2004). *Helping parents support their children's pre-literacy skills.* Symposium conducted at the meeting of National Association for the Education of Young Children, Anaheim, CA.

Farver J. M., Xu, Y., Eppea, S., & Lonigan, C. J. (2005). Home environments and young Latino children's school readiness. *Early Childhood Research Quarterly,* 21(2), 196–212.

Fields, J. (2003). *Children's living arrangements and characteristics: March 2002* (Current Population Reports, Report No. P20-547). Washington, DC: U.S. Census Bureau.

Flanders, J. L., Simard, M., Paquette, D., Parent, S., Vitaro, F., Pihl, R. O., et al. (2010). Rough-and-tumble play and the development of physical aggression and emotion regulation: A five-year follow-up study. *Journal of Family Violence, 25,* 357–367.

Fuller-Thompson, E., & Minkler, M. (2007). Central American grandparents raising grandchildren. *Hispanic Journal of Behavioral Sciences,* 29(1), 5–18.

Galindo, C., & Fuller, B. (2010). The social competence of Latino kindergartners and growth in mathematical understanding. *Developmental Psychology,* 46(3), 579–592.

Gamble, W. C., & Modry-Mandell, K. (2008). Family relations and the adjustment of young children of Mexican descent: Do family cultural values moderate these associations? *Social Development,* 17(2), 358–379.

Gamble, W. C., Ramakumar, S., & Diaz, A. (2007). Maternal and paternal similarities and differences in parenting: An examination of Mexican-American parents of young children. *Early Childhood Research Quarterly, 22*(1), 72–88.

García, E., & Jensen, B. (2009). Early educational opportunities for children of Hispanic origins. *Social Policy Report, 23*(2), 3–11.

García Coll, C., Marks, A., Patton, F., & Slama, S. (2009, April). *A longitudinal study of adolescent immigrant paradox in education.* Paper presented at the meeting of Society for Research in Child Development, Denver, CO.

García Coll, C., & Pachter, L. M. (2002). Ethnic and minority parenting. In M. H. Bornstein (Ed.), *Handbook of parenting* (Vol. 4, 2nd ed., pp. 1–20). Mahwah, NJ: Erlbaum.

Goldenberg, C. N., Gallimore, R., Reese, L. J., & Garnier, H. (2001). Cause or effect? A longitudinal study of immigrant Latino parents' aspirations and expectations and their children's school performance. *American Educational Research Journal, 38*(3), 547–582.

Gonzalez-Ramos, G., Zayas, L. H., & Cohen, E. V. (1998). Child-rearing values of low-income, urban Puerto Rican mothers of preschool children. *Professional Psychology: Research and Practice, 29*(4), 377–382.

Greenfield, P., Quiroz, B., & Raeff, C. (2000). Cross-cultural conflict and harmony in the social construction of the child. In S. Harkness, C. Raeff, & C. M. Super (Eds.), *Variability in the social construction of the child. New directions in child and adolescent development* (Vol. 87, pp. 93–108). San Francisco: Jossey-Bass.

Grusec, J. E., Rudy, D., & Martini, T. (1997). Parenting cognition and child outcomes: An overview and implications for children's internalization of values. In J. E. Grusec & L. Kuczynski (Eds.), *Parenting and children's internalization of values: A handbook of contemporary theory* (pp. 259–282). New York: Wiley.

Hair, E., Halle, T., Terry-Humen, E., Lavelle, B., & Calkins, J. (2006). Children's school readiness in the ECLS-K: Predictions to academic, health, and social outcomes in first grade. *Early Childhood Research Quarterly, 21*(4), 431–454.

Halgunseth, L., Ispa, J. M., & Rudy, D. (2006). Parental control in Latino families: An integrated review of the literature. *Child Development, 77*(5), 1282–1297.

Harwood, R. L., Miller, J. G., & Irizarry, N. L. (1995). *Culture and attachment: Perceptions of the child in context.* New York: Guilford Press.

Hill, N. E, Bush, K. R., & Rosa, M. W. (2003). Parenting and family socialization strategies and children's mental health: Low-income Mexican-American and Euro-American mothers and children. *Child Development, 74*(1), 189–204.

Holmes, E. R., & Holmes, L. D. (1995). *Other cultures, elder years.* Thousand Oaks, CA: Sage.

Howes, C., Wishard Guerra, A., & Zucker, E. (2008). Migrating from Mexico and sharing pretend with peers in the United States. *Merrill-Palmer Quarterly, 54*(2), 256–288.

Ispa, J. M., Fine, M. A., Halgunseth, L. C., Harper, S., Robinson, J., Boyce, L., et al. (2004). Maternal intrusiveness, maternal warmth, and mother–toddler relationship outcomes: Variations across low-income ethnic and acculturation groups. *Child Development, 75*(6), 1613–1631.

Kagitcibasi, C. (1996). *Family and human development across cultures: A view from the other side.* Mahwah, NJ: Erlbaum.

Kelley, M. L., Smith, T. S., Green, A. P., Berndt, A. E., & Rogers, M. C. (1998). Importance of fathers' parenting to African-American toddlers' social and cognitive development. *Infant Behavior and Development, 21*(4), 733–744.

Knight, G. P., Roosa, M. W., & Umaña-Taylor, A. J. (2009). *Studying ethnic minority and economically disadvantaged populations.* Washington, DC: American Psychological Association.

Lamb, M. E. (Ed.). (2010). *The role of the father in child development* (5th ed.). Hoboken, NJ: Wiley.

Landy, S. (2002). *Pathways to competence: Encouraging healthy social and emotional development in young children.* Baltimore: Brookes.

La Paro, K. M., & Pianta, R. C. (2000). Predicting children's competence in the early school years: A meta-analytic review. *Review of Educational Research, 70*(4), 443–484.

McCay, L. O., & Keyes, D. W. (2002). Developing social competence in the inclusive primary classroom. *Childhood Education, 78*(2), 70–78.

McDowell, D. J., & Parke, R. D. (2009). Parental correlates of children's peer relations: An empirical test of a tripartite model. *Developmental Psychology, 45,* 224–235.

McHale, S. M., Updegraff, K. A., Shanahan, L., Crouter, A. C., & Killoren, S. E. (2005). Siblings' differential treatment in Mexican American families. *Journal of Marriage and Family, 67*(5), 1259–1274.

Mitchell, S., & Cabrera, N. (2009). An exploratory study of fathers' parenting stress and toddlers' social development in low-income African American families. *Fathering, 7*(3), 201–225.

Phinney, J. S., Berry, J. W., Vedder, P., & Liebkind, K. (2006). The acculturation experience: Attitudes, identities and behaviors of immigrant youth. In J. W. Berry, J. S. Phinney, D. L. Sam, & P. Vedder (Eds.), *Immigrant youth in cultural transition: Acculturation, identify, and adaptation across national contexts* (pp. 71–116). Mahwah, NJ: Erlbaum.

Pittman, L. D., & Boswell, M. K. (2007). The role of grandmothers in the lives of preschoolers growing up in urban poverty. *Applied Developmental Science, 11*(1), 20–42.

Portes, A., & Rumbaut, R. G. (2001). *Legacies: The story of the immigrant second generation.* Berkeley: University of California Press.

Raikes, H., Summers, J. A., & Roggman, L. A. (2005). Father involvement in Early Head Start programs. *Fathering, 3,* 29–58.

Reese, L. (2001). Morality and identity in Mexican immigrant parents' visions of the future. *Journal of Ethnic and Migration Studies, 27*(3), 455–472.

Rogoff, B. (2003). *The cultural nature of human development.* New York: Oxford University Press.

Rubin, K. H., & Rose-Krasnor, L. R. (1992). Interpersonal problem solving and social competence in children. In V. B. van Hasslet & M. Hersen (Eds.), *Handbook of social development: A lifespan perspective.* New York: Plenum Press.

Rumbaut, R. G. (2005). Sites of belonging: Acculturation, discrimination, and ethnic identity among children of immigrants. In T. S. Weisner (Ed.), *Discovering successful pathways in children's development: Mixed methods in the study of childhood and family life* (pp. 111–162). Chicago: University of Chicago Press.

Sam, D. L., & Berry, J. W. (2006). Introduction to psychology of acculturation. In D. L. Sam & J. Berry (Eds.), *Cambridge handbook of acculturation psychology* (pp. 1–7). Cambridge, UK: Cambridge University Press.

Sameroff, A. J., & Fiese, B. H. (2000). Transactional regulation: The developmental ecology of early intervention. In J. P. Schonkoff & S. J. Meisels (Eds.), *Handbook of early childhood intervention* (Vol. 2, pp. 135–159). New York: Cambridge University Press.

Shannon, J., Tamis-LeMonda, C., London, B., & Cabrera, N. (2002). Beyond rough and tumble: Low-income fathers' interactions and children's cognitive development at 24 months. *Parenting Science and Practice, 2*(2), 77–104.

Sternberg, R. J. (2002). What does it mean to be smart? *California Journal of Science Education, II*(2), 99–109.

Suárez-Orozco, C., & Suárez-Orozco, M. M. (2002). *Children of immigrants*. Cambridge, MA: Harvard University Press.

Super, C. M., & Harkness, S. (2002). Culture structures the environment for development. *Human Development, 45*, 270–274.

Tamis-LeMonda, C. S., Shannon, J. D., Cabrera, N. J., & Lamb, M. E. (2004). Fathers and mothers at play with their 2- and 3-year-olds: Contributions to language and cognitive development. *Child Development, 75*(6), 1806–1820.

Taylor, B., & Behnke, A. O. (2005). Fathering across the border: Latino fathers in Mexico and the United States. *Fathering: A journal of theory, research, and practice about men as fathers, 3*(2), 99–120.

Tucker, C. J. (2004, March). *Sibling shared time: An important context for adolescent well-being*. Poster session presented at the biennial meeting of the Society for Research on Adolescence, Baltimore.

Valdés, G. (1996). *Con respeto: Bridging the distances between culturally diverse families and schools. An ethnographic portrait*. New York: Teachers College Press.

Walsh, S., Shulman, S., Bar-On, Z., & Tsur, A. (2006). The role of parentification and family climate in adaptation among immigrant adolescents in Israel. *Journal of Research on Adolescence, 16*(2), 321–350.

Weisner, T. (2002). Ecocultural understanding of children's developmental pathways. *Human Development, 45*, 275–281.

Weiss, S. J., Goebel, P., Page, A., Wilson, P., & Warda, M. (1999). The impact of cultural and familial context on behavioral and emotional problems of preschool Latino children. *Child Psychiatry and Human Development, 29*(4), 287–301.

West, J., Denton, K., & Reaney, L. M. (2001). *The kindergarten year: Findings from the Early Childhood Longitudinal Study, Kindergarten Class of 1998–99*. Washington, DC: U.S. Department of Education and National Center for Education Statistics.

Wilson, W. J. (1996). *When work disappears: The world of the new urban poor*. New York: Knopf.

Youngblade, L. M., & Belsky, J. (1992). Parent–child antecedents of 5-year-olds' close friendships: A longitudinal analysis. *Developmental Psychology, 28,* 700–713.

Zayas, L. H., & Solari, F. (1994). Early childhood socialization in Hispanic families: Context, culture, and practice implications. *Professional Psychology: Research and Practice, 25*(3), 200–206.

Zucker, E., & Howes, C. (2009). Respectful relationships: Socialization goals and practices among Mexican mothers. *Infant Mental Health Journal, 30,* 501–522.

CHAPTER 12

Infant/Toddler Care and High-Risk Families
Quality Services for "Omitted" Children

Brenda Jones Harden, Colleen Monahan, and Meryl Yoches

The disparities between the environmental experiences and developmental outcomes of children reared in poverty and nonpoverty contexts are substantial and persistent. Poverty is a major risk factor for maladaptive outcomes, with larger associations documented with cognition and academic achievement than behavior, mental health, and physical health (Ackerman, Brown, & Izard, 2004; Evans, 2004). The greatest impacts of poverty appear for children at the lower end of the low socioeconomic status (SES) continuum (i.e., less than 50% of the poverty threshold; Aber, Jones, & Raver, 2007; Duncan & Brooks-Gunn, 1997). Further, poverty in early childhood seems to have larger effects on development than poverty in adolescence (Knitzer & Perry, 2009), with adverse outcomes evident as early as the infancy period (Halle et al., 2009).

Recent research has painted a more complex picture of the link between poverty and child and adult outcomes (Aber et al., 2007; Mayer, 2010). In their study on the relation between early childhood poverty and adult outcomes, Duncan, Ziol-Guest, and Kalil (2010) ask to what extent is poverty itself the cause of negative child outcomes. They emphasize addressing "omitted variable bias," in other words, considering the risk factors that are associated with poverty, such as demographic variables (e.g., family structure, race/ethnicity), prenatal factors (e.g., low birthweight, prematurity), and larger ecological factors (e.g., child care/school experience, neighborhood disadvantage). In their study, the impact of early childhood poverty on later outcomes was substantially reduced after controlling for a rich set of "omitted variables."

Although Duncan et al. (2010) do not focus on "omitted variables" that pertain to individual parent and family functioning, the thesis of this chapter is that these parent and family risk factors are also important to consider. These risk factors characterize the various ecological environments that a significant portion of children from impoverished backgrounds experience (Ackerman et al., 2004; Evans, 2004). Further, these risk factors may represent the mechanisms by which poverty affects children, and may be more influential on child outcomes than poverty per se (Gassman-Pines & Yoshikawa, 2006; Mayer, 2010).

In fact, Shonkoff, Boyce, and McEwen (2009) argue that the accumulation of such risk factors in early childhood may be at the root of socioeconomic and racial/ethnic disparities in adult physical and mental health. These authors assert that young children who are exposed to poverty, maltreatment, depression, substance abuse, and family violence are at high risk for "toxic stress." In their view, toxic stress pertains to a physiologic response to environmental risks that adversely affects brain structure and processes, and leads to poor health, cognitive, and mental health outcomes throughout childhood and adulthood.

An ecological context that may compensate for some of the ecological risks that lead to toxic stress may be the early care and education program. There is some evidence that high-quality infant/toddler care, which has been linked to a variety of positive outcomes for children (Love et al., 2003; NICHD Early Child Care and Research Network, 2005), may be particularly beneficial for children who are reared in impoverished circumstances (Votruba-Drzal, Coley, & Chase-Lansdale, 2004; Burchinal, Roberts, Zeisel, Hennon, & Hooper, 2006). Such evidence has led to a proliferation of early care and education programs for young children reared in poverty, including the federal Early Head Start program.

That poverty is a major risk factor for negative child outcomes is indisputable. However, there are resilient children who do not evidence these outcomes, as well as children who show particularly pernicious effects of poverty (Luthar, 2003; Wadsworth & Santiago, 2008). The variability in the functioning and experiences of young children in poverty begs the question of whether early intervention programs are similarly beneficial for all children in poverty. For example, the Early Head Start Research and Evaluation Project (see Chapter 13 by Love and colleagues, in this volume; Administration for Children and Families, 2002) examined risk indices that reflect some combination of demographic, child, family, and environmental risks (e.g., being a single parent, receiving public assistance, being neither employed nor in school or in job training, being a teenage parent, and lacking a high school diploma or general equivalency diploma). Twenty-six percent of the families enrolled in Early Head Start experienced four or more of these risk factors and did not benefit from the program in the same way that other families did. No impacts were found for families in the highest-risk group (i.e., families with 4–5 demographic risk factors).

Further, limited research has explicitly examined program effects in the context of the "omitted variables" that are experienced by children from impoverished backgrounds. For example, few studies have explored the benefits of early childhood programs for specific racial/ethnic groups that are more likely to live in poverty. The available literature suggests an advantage of participating in high-quality programs for African American children and families (see Burchinal, Peisner-Feinberg, Bryant, & Clifford, 2000; Jones Harden, Sandstrom, & Chazan-Cohen, in press), but there is little evidence specific to children and families of other minority groups. Also, we know little about the range of impacts of quality early childhood settings for children who may have experienced perinatal insults or ecological risks beyond poverty. In particular, there is scant evidence about the effects of early care and education programs on families in whom parents exhibit psychological vulnerability and impaired parenting.

This chapter considers the outcomes of children from impoverished backgrounds who experience multiple ecological risks, and the implications of these experiences for early childhood care and education contexts. Specifically, we explore conceptualizations of poverty-related risk that have implications for the design of programs that serve families in poverty, in order to provide a framework for understanding the risks and outcomes young children in these families experience. Then, we summarize the knowledge on the impact of poverty and specific ecological risks on young children. Finally, we explore the implications of this knowledge for the design of quality early childhood settings that have the potential to benefit infants and toddlers who are from impoverished, high-risk backgrounds.

Conceptualization of Risk in the Context of Poverty

Risk has been broadly defined as exposure to the biological and environmental conditions that increase the likelihood of negative developmental outcomes (Brooks-Gunn, 1990; Nelson, 1994). Biological risk factors center on the characteristics of the individual that negatively affect development, such as prematurity, low birthweight, and perinatal complications (Adams, Hillman, & Gaydos, 1994). Environmental risk factors include low SES, adverse neighborhoods, and family factors that are associated with poverty such as parental psychopathology (Laucht et al., 2000). In their recent study, Halle et al. (2009) identified risk factors, such as minority race/ethnicity, home language other than English, and low maternal education, as contributors to the cognitive, social, behavioral, and health disparities among infants and toddlers from high- and low-risk backgrounds.

Children and families from impoverished backgrounds rarely experience one risk factor in isolation; more often, multiple risks are experienced at once. These risks include parental psychopathology, harsh or insensitive parenting, low family income, low maternal educational attainment, racial/ethnic minority status, single parenthood, stressful life events, and large family size (Aber et al., 2007). To conceptualize the effects of these risk factors on children, several theoretical models have emerged.

The *additive risk model* assumes that each risk factor contributes independently to developmental outcomes, and addresses how contextual adversity translates into child adjustment difficulties by examining the unique effects of multiple risk factors (Ackerman, Izard, Schoff, Youngstrom, & Kogos, 1999). Additionally, the model isolates qualitatively distinct sources of risk that are concealed when only the number of risk factors, rather than the specific nature of each risk, is considered (Jones, Forehand, Brody, & Armistead, 2002). The *ecological risk model* (Bronfenbrenner, 1979) emphasizes the multiple, interdependent ecologies in which children develop. This theory maintains that it is essential for children to experience protective and nurturing caregiving environments (i.e., microsystem) in order to achieve optimal developmental outcomes.

The *family stress model* extends ecological systems theory and examines the effects of poverty on children's socioemotional well-being (Conger & Donnellan, 2007; McLoyd, 1990). The model suggests that chronic stressors such as single parenthood, life stress, financial worries, and the constant struggle to make ends meet take a toll on parents' mental health, which diminishes their capacity to be sensitive and supportive parents (Mistry, Vandewater, Huston, & McLoyd, 2002). Similarly, models that emphasize *mediators of risk* assume that the influence of larger ecological variables on child outcomes is mediated by proximal process variables, such as parent psychological distress (Mistry, Biesanz, Taylor, Burchinal, & Cox, 2004), parenting behaviors (Ackerman et al., 1999), and child care quality (Burchinal et al., 2006).

Following the *transactional risk model* (Sameroff , 2009), the development of the child is a product of the continuous dynamic interactions of the child and the experience provided by his or her family and social context. The transactional model emphasizes the plasticity of environments and individuals as they actively participate in their own development, and as such provides a comprehensive view of how nature and nurture work together (Sameroff, 2009). The *cumulative risk model,* originally developed by Rutter (1979), rests on the assumption that it is not just any one risk factor or type of risk that matters for child outcomes, but rather an accumulation of risk factors that can adversely affect the course of child development (Rutter, 1979; Sameroff, Bartko, Baldwin, Baldwin, & Seifer, 1998). In this model, the action of risk factors is cumulative in the sense that the presence of more risk factors is related to a higher certainty of negative outcomes (Seifer, Sameroff, Baldwin, & Baldwin, 1992).

Finally, the recent hypothesis pertaining to children's *differential susceptibility to risk* holds that children with biologic risk are more vulnerable to the effects of environmental risk, and that children with specific risk factors may be more amenable to positive environmental experiences (Belsky, Bakermans-Kranenburg, & van IJzendoorn, 2007; Power, Jefferies, Manor, & Hertzman, 2006). Specific to the thesis herein, child care quality has been found to be more consequential for the long-term cognitive–academic and social–emotional developmental outcomes of temperamentally difficult infants (Pluess & Belsky, 2010) and to lead to greater benefits for children from impoverished backgrounds (e.g., Burchinal et al., 2006).

In sum, there are several models that have been applied to research on children in poverty. Although each has merit in and of itself, the evolution of these models shows that the later frameworks have built on features of prior conceptualizations. In the main, the confluence of risk factors that characterize the experiences of young children in poverty requires the utilization of models that underscore the complexity of relationships between these various risk factors. As such, our understanding of the developmental consequences of poverty-related risks is informed by mediation models that allow for a consideration of the mechanisms by which poverty and other larger ecological risks affect young children. Specifically, we are interested in parent functioning and parenting as mediators of these ecological risks, as well as the potential impact of processes within the child care environment. From the perspective of the differential susceptibility framework, we are interested in how children who experience poverty and other related risk factors may be more likely to benefit from the early care and education experience.

Poverty-Related Risks and Developmental Outcomes for Young Children

The design of infant/toddler programs to serve high-risk families must be informed by the knowledge about the developmental functioning of the children these programs serve. Thus, an understanding of poverty's impact on children is critical, as well as of the consequences of exposure to poverty-related risk factors. In this section, we briefly explore the developmental effects of poverty, and quickly turn to a consideration of the developmental consequences of specific risk factors. Although we acknowledge that there are many other biological and environmental risk factors that children may face, we focus herein on the ecological factors often linked with early childhood poverty (Gassman-Pines & Yoshikawa, 2006) that precipitate extremely adverse outcomes in young children, such as parental mental illness and substance abuse, child maltreatment, and exposure to violence.

A substantial body of research links poverty with lower levels of child well-being. These linkages are particularly strong for children whose families experience deep poverty, are poor during early childhood, and are trapped in poverty for a long time (Anderson Moore, Redd, Burkhauser, Mbwana, & Collins, 2009). Poverty places children at risk beginning at conception, due to the mothers' lack of prenatal care, inadequate nutritional intake, and increased likelihood of psychological vulnerability (Halpern, 2000). Poverty significantly heightens the risk of physical health problems such as asthma, malnutrition, obesity, elevated lead levels, HIV seropositivity, and dental decay (Klerman, 1991; Hernandez, Montana, & Clarke, 2010). Physical effects of poverty also include stunted brain growth and central nervous system disorders, delayed physical growth, delayed motor skills, higher rates of infant mortality, prematurity, low birthweight, and higher rates of injuries (Power et al., 2006).

When compared to children from more affluent families, children reared in poverty are more likely to have deficits in cognitive development and academic achievement (Najman et al., 2009). Higher rates of early developmental and language delays, and lack of readiness for formal schooling have also been documented among children from impoverished backgrounds (Rouse & Fantuzzo, 2009). Recent research has suggested that these deficits may be at least partially attributable to altered brain processes in these children, which affect their executive functioning and cognitive self-regulation (Buckner, Mezzacappa, & Beardslee, 2009; Evans & Rosenbaum, 2008). These early cognitive and academic deficits are linked to later academic difficulties, such as poor reading and math skills, as well as higher rates of special education placement and school dropout (Evans & Rosenbaum, 2008; Power et al., 2006).

Finally, poverty affects children's functioning in the socioemotional domain. Core socioemotional processes that may be affected by poverty include prosocial skills, peer relationships, and affective regulation (Eamon, 2001). Additionally, higher rates of internalizing and externalizing behavior problems, and other mental health difficulties have been documented among children in poverty (Gyamfi, 2004).

There are multiple contextual risks that have been linked to poverty and increased child vulnerability, including parental psychopathology, compromised parenting, and exposure to violence. Specifically, higher rates of depression and other mental illness have been documented among persons living in poverty, particularly women of childbearing age (Chazan-Cohen et al., 2007; Rafferty, Griffin, & Robokos, 2010). Although substance abuse crosses socioeconomic status, the use of certain substances, which have severe implications for caregiving of children (e.g., cocaine, methamphetamine), is more likely among women of childbearing age who live in impoverished circumstances (Gardner, Barajas, & Brooks-Gunn, 2010).

The link between poverty and child maltreatment has been consistently documented, with a particularly large association between poverty and child neglect, the most common form of maltreatment (Sedlak et al., 2010). Despite the fact that intimate partner violence (IPV) occurs across socioeconomic groups, there is evidence that IPV is more common among impoverished families (Benson, Fox, DeMaris, & Van Wyk, 2003). Finally, the relation between poverty and community violence has been well established (Morenoff, Sampson, & Raudenbush, 2001). As Shonkoff et al. (2009) assert, these risk factors have deleterious outcomes for young children in particular, leading to their experience of "toxic stress." In the following sections, we briefly address each of these risk factors with respect to their consequences for affected children's developmental outcomes.

Parental Mental Illness

Parents' mental health status has a major influence on their capacity to parent (Seifer & Dickstein, 2000; Windham et al., 2004) and the associated outcomes for their children. Although there are many forms of mental illness found among parents from impoverished backgrounds, depression stands out as a particularly pernicious problem (Chazan-Cohen et al., 2007). Young children who are reared in poverty and exposed to maternal depression seem to be at heightened risk for adverse outcomes (Patterson & Albers, 2001). Prenatal exposure to parental mental health difficulties has been linked to adverse delivery and infant developmental outcomes such as premature birth, low birthweight, failure to thrive, compromised cognitive development (King & Laplante, 2005), and asymmetric frontal lobe activity (Field, Fox, Pickens, & Nawrocki, 1995).

　　Children exposed to parental mental illness have elevated risk of cognitive problems (Murray, Hipwell, Hooper, Stein, & Cooper, 1996), deficits in their regulatory and representational skills (Ashman, Dawson, & Panagiotides, 2008), insecure attachments and less optimal interactions with their mothers (Carter, Garrity-Rokous, Chazan-Cohen, Little, & Briggs-Gowan, 2001), and social cognitive deficits such as a less developed theory of mind (Rohrer, Cicchetti, Rogosch, Toth, & Maughan, 2011). Parental mental illness has also been associated with a wide range of emotional difficulties and neurointegrative deficits, such as distractibility, hypersensitivity to stimuli, emotional lability, restricted range of emotion expression, negative responses to emotionally salient events, and higher rates of internalizing and externalizing behavior problems such as inattentiveness, aggression, and impulsivity (Campbell, Shaw, & Gilliom, 2000; Hay, Pawlby, Waters, Perra, & Sharp, 2010).

Maternal Substance Abuse

Parental substance abuse is a major public health problem affecting millions of children in the United States (Substance Abuse and Mental Health Services Administration, 2009). Alcohol use during pregnancy is one of the top preventable causes of birth defects and developmental disabilities, and may lead to miscarriage, stillbirth, and fetal alcohol spectrum disorders that affect children's organs such as the heart and brain, and their intellectual development (Centers for Disease Control and Prevention, 2010). Babies born to mothers who smoke during pregnancy and beyond are more likely to be born prematurely and with low birthweight (increasing their risk for illness or death), to die of sudden infant death syndrome and have respiratory difficulties and deficits in their self-regulatory skills (Centers for Disease Control and Prevention, 2009).

The full extent of the consequences of prenatal illicit drug exposure on a child is not known, as the impact is often dependent on complex factors such as the timing of use, the dosage, level of prenatal care, the type of drug used, and the caregiving a child receives. Despite these caveats, studies show that various drugs may result in premature birth, miscarriage, low birthweight, and a variety of health problems, developmental and language delays, and a variety of emotional difficulties including neurobehavioral deficits, affective dysregulation, attentional deficits, hyperactivity, impulsivity, and aggression (Lester et al., 2009).

Experience of Child Maltreatment

Very young children are the primary victims of maltreatment (i.e., child abuse and neglect) within this country (Administration for Children and Families, 2011; Kolko, 2001) and are also more likely to die as a result of maltreatment (Administration for Children and Families, 2011). Physical sequelae of physical abuse include bruises, cuts and permanent physical disabilities (Christian & Block, 2009), and abusive head trauma that may lead to brain damage, motor and intellectual deficiencies, impaired physical growth, and visual loss and/or blindness (Chiesa & Duhaime, 2009). Maltreated infants and toddlers are also more likely to develop failure-to-thrive (Batchelor, 2008) and have an increased rate of childhood diseases including ear infections, respiratory problems, and lead exposure. Exposure to maltreatment alters young children's developing brains (Fiske & Hall, 2008), which increases the likelihood of academic problems when they enter school as well as language and communication difficulties (De Bellis, Hooper, & Sapia, 2005; Kolko, 2001).

Young maltreated children are also at higher risk for insecure attachments with their parents (Barnett, Ganiban, & Cicchetti, 1999), traumatic stress-like symptoms (Kolko, 2001; Margolin & Gordis, 2000) including hyperarousal (being extremely vigilant and conscious of their surroundings) or dissociation (detaching themselves from the abusive event; Twardosz & Lutzker, 2010), and internalizing problems such as depression and anxiety (Van Voorhees & Scarpa, 2004). They also exhibit less independent play (Valentino, Cicchetti, Toth, & Rogosch, 2006), difficulties in their peer relationships (Fantuzzo & Mohr, 1999), attention-deficit/hyperactivity disorder (ADHD; Margolin & Gordis, 2000), and increased levels of aggression, noncompliance, negative emotion, and externalizing behaviors (Kaufmann, 2008).

Exposure to Intimate Partner Violence

The majority of children indirectly victimized by violence experience it within their own homes in the form of interpersonal violence between adults—usually their parents (Finkelhor, Turner, Ormond, & Hamby, 2009). Children exposed to family violence experience more developmental difficulties than children living in nonviolent homes (Wolfe, Crooks, Lee, McIntyre-Smith, & Jaffe, 2003), and those exposed to community violence, because the violence experienced at home is proximal and the victim and perpetrator are familiar (Bogat, DeJonghe, Levendosky, Davidson, & von Eye, 2006). These children are also at greater risk of being physically injured during these confrontations (Margolin & Gordis, 2000) and of being physically abused and neglected (Osofky, 1999).

Young children may show emotional distress, illness, and immature behavior including a regression in toileting and language skills (Osofsky, 2003). Children exposed to family violence may have future academic problems and lower verbal abilities than other children (Osofsky, 2003), and exhibit symptoms of traumatic stress, including eating and sleeping problems and hypervigilance, as well as a loss of developmental milestones (Osofsky, 2003; Carpenter & Stacks, 2009; Wolfe et al., 2003). They may also display symptoms of depression and anxiety (Litrownik, Newton, Hunter, English, & Everson, 2003), emotional intensity or emotional overreaction to events (DeJonghe, Bogat, Levendosky, von Eye, & Davidson, 2005), externalizing behaviors, including aggression (Gewirtz & Edleson, 2007), and insecure attachments with their parents (Carpenter & Stacks, 2009).

Exposure to Community Violence

Community violence exposure, broadly defined as being victimized or witnessing violence outside of the home but within the neighborhood, committed by people who are not known or related to the children (National Center for Children Exposed to Violence, 2006), is common for some children in the United States, including very young children (Finkelhor et al., 2009). Although exposure to community violence is linked with exposure to other risk factors, it has a unique impact on young children's development (Overstreet & Mazza, 2003). Infants and toddlers exposed to community violence often show physical changes and increased behavioral problems including bed-wetting and toileting problems (Berkowitz, 2003), sleep and eating problems (McAlister Groves, 2005), compromised motor skills, and the loss of developmental milestones (Berkowitz, 2003). Children may also exhibit intellectual difficulties and language problems (Sampson, Sharkey, & Raudenbush, 2008), concentration problems (Margolin & Gordis, 2000), and generalized developmental delays (Osofsky, 1999).

Young children may experience severe socioemotional consequences from their exposure to community violence including symptoms of traumatic stress (Fowler, Tompsett, Braciszewski, Jacques-Tiura, & Baltes, 2009) such as reexperiencing a witnessed event, avoiding situations or locations of the event, and increased arousal and anxiety (McAlister Groves, 2005), symptoms of depression (Lynch, 2003), aggression (Fowler et al., 2009), irritability (Osofsky, 1999), emotional distress and intensity (Lorion, Brodsky, & Cooley-Quille, 1998), fear of being left alone (Osofsky, 1999; Overstreet, 2000), mistrust of adults, and difficulty feeling safe (Overstreet, 2000).

Implications for Infant/Toddler Early Care and Education Programs

Early care and education programs are primary preventive interventions that have the potential to improve the developmental outcomes of children in poverty. Consistent with a prevention science approach (National Research Council and Institute of Medicine, 2009), these programs are designed to alleviate the risk factors (e.g., understimulating and unstable environments) and promote the protective factors (e.g., children's inherent capacity to develop, parents' investment in young children) that are linked to adaptation (Groark, Mehaffie, McCall, & Greenberg, 2007). Further, these programs attempt to intervene with young children and their families prior to the manifestation of the effects of risk factors that affect them (Reynolds, Rolnick, Englund, & Temple, 2010).

Benefits of High-Quality Care for Children from Impoverished Backgrounds

Although the extant literature suggests that neighborhood social disadvantage is related to lower child care quality (McCartney, Dearing, Taylor, & Bub, 2007; Votruba-Drzal et al., 2004), publicly funded programs (e.g., Head Start), which are typically of higher quality, are more likely to be situated in impoverished neighborhoods (Burchinal, Nelson, Carlson, & Brooks-Gunn, 2008). There is a growing body of evidence that high-quality care may protect socioeconomically disadvantaged children from the environmental risk factors that affect their developmental functioning.

In several studies, impoverished children had better cognitive outcomes if they had been in high-quality care (Magnuson & Waldfogel, 2005). Additionally, low-income children participating in high-quality child care have been found to have higher expressive and receptive language than those who did not experience these contexts (McCartney et al., 2007). These authors noted that sensitive care and cognitive stimulation were the pathways through which child care quality led to better child outcomes. Further, higher-quality care during infancy and early childhood has been found to enhance low-income children's school readiness, which in turn improves their math and reading skills in elementary school (Dearing, McCartney, & Taylor, 2009; McCartney et al., 2007).

There is some evidence that the type of program the child attends has an impact on the magnitude of their improvement in school-readiness skills. For example, low-income children in PreK programs in public schools made greater gains relative to their cognitive and language skills than those in center-based programs in the community (Winsler et al., 2008). Whereas more gains are noted for highly intensive child care and preschool interventions (Campbell, Pungello, Miller-Johnson, Burchinal, & Ramey, 2001), modest improvements in children's language, literacy, and preacademic skills are found in less intensive programs such as Head Start and high-quality child care settings (Duncan & Brooks-Gunn, 1997; Burchinal et al., 2000).

Benefits of high-quality care and education for children from impoverished backgrounds have also been reported in other domains. For example, children enrolled in Head Start were more likely to be up-to-date on their immunizations and were reported to have better health habits (e.g., hand washing) than non-Head Start participants (Abbott-Schim, Lambert, & McCarty, 2003). In a study of low-income 3-year-olds, Votruba-Drzal et al. (2004) found that the quality of child care was related to children's internalizing and externalizing behavior. Sustained effects of higher-quality child care on reducing children's behavior problems have been found for children from at-risk and minority backgrounds (Burchinal et al., 2006; Administration for Children and Families, 2002).

Care for Children from High-Risk Backgrounds

Despite the documented benefit of early care and education programs for children in poverty, some children and families may not be amenable to the primary prevention approach that these programs undertake. Families at high risk have been found to be more challenging to engage into early care and education programs (Roggman, Cook, Peterson, & Raikes, 2008), which may translate into more sporadic attendance of their infants and toddlers to center-based programs. Moreover, high-risk children and families who participate may not evidence the improved outcomes that are found with other program participants. For example, Burchinal et al. (2006) documented limited support for the benefits of high-quality care for low-income children experiencing social risks. Similarly, as documented by the Early Head Start Research and Evaluation Project, there were no benefits of Early Head Start for high-risk families (Administration for Children and Families, 2002). Thus, there is a need to identify what types of early childhood care and education programs can promote the developmental outcomes of infants and toddlers from high-risk backgrounds.

The conceptualizations of risk that were provided in a previous section of this chapter have important implications for the design of infant/toddler programs serving children from high-risk backgrounds. First, they highlight the importance of understanding and identifying the various risks that participant children and families experience at program entry and throughout their tenure with the program. These risk factors may be individual or environmental, and/or biological or ecological, and are likely to co-occur. Evidence from studies in this vein indicates that poverty-specific indicators (e.g., family income) are but one component of the risks that families face (Gassman-Pines & Yoshikawa, 2006). Second, these conceptualizations underscore that children and families who experience higher levels of risk may require a different set of environmental experiences in order to achieve more positive outcomes. An understanding of the protective mechanisms that are relevant for specific developmental outcomes, as well as the strategies to address specific risk factors is essential.

Most important, such conceptualizations suggest that high-quality early care and education settings have the potential to offset the negative consequences that are more likely for young children who are reared in risky environments, if they are delivered in a way that addresses the risk factors that participant families manifest. High-quality early care and education has been touted as a compensatory mechanism for young children being reared in high-risk environments (Watamura, Phillips, Morrissey, McCartney, & Bub, 2011). Specifically, quality early care and education may protect children from the effects of the risks that emanate from experiences of maternal depression (Papero, 2005), child maltreatment (Reynolds, Mathieson, & Topitzes, 2009), foster care (Corrrington & Phillips, 2009), and violence (Osofsky & Fenichel, 2000). Following are specific recommendations for the delivery of early care and education services for infant and toddlers from high-risk backgrounds.

High-Quality Child Care

Given the data on the import of child care quality for the developmental outcomes of children from impoverished circumstances, at the very least children from high-risk backgrounds should experience child care that meets the field's standards for high quality. Specifically, child care environments should have small group sizes (e.g., fewer than three infants in a room) and appropriate staff:child ratios (e.g., one caregiver to three infants; Cassidy, Lower, Kintner, & Hestenes, 2009). Although the evidence is ambiguous with respect to teacher education (Early et al., 2007), it appears that caregiver training (e.g., inservice workshops), especially on early childhood issues, seems to be linked to child care quality (Torquati, Raikes, & Huddleston-Casas, 2007).

Beyond these structural variables, certain process variables, which pertain to less tangible characteristics of the early childhood setting, are perceived as reflective of quality (Zaslow et al., 2006). Sensitive caregiving represents one facet of child care quality that is associated with child outcomes. Specifically, positive teacher–child relationships and interactions have been linked to later academic and social outcomes among preschool children, and seem to be particularly beneficial for children from low-income and other high-risk backgrounds (Pianta et al., 2005). In a study comparing relationship-based (i.e., continuous, primary caregiver–child relationships) and nonrelationship-based-focused programs, higher levels of child compliance and better caregiver–parent relationships were documented in the relationship-based programs, particularly for African American children (Owen, Klausli, Mata-Otero, & Caughy, 2008).

Experiences that allow for cognitive stimulation of children reflect another global aspect of high-quality child care programs. Early childhood programs and classrooms with an emphasis on curricular content and academic instruction tend to have better child outcomes, particularly regarding cognition and language (Downer & Pianta, 2006; Love, Tarullo, Raikes, & Chazan-Cohen, 2006). Although the evidence is limited, research suggests that early childhood teachers often have difficulty integrating academic content (e.g., preliteracy, numeracy) into children's experiences and often do not follow curricula with fidelity (Lieber et al., 2009).

In an extension of this line of research, scholars have found that the focus of teacher–child interactions affects the types of program benefits, with interactions focusing on concept development leading to children's cognitive and language gains and those focusing on emotional support promoting child social competence (Curby et al., 2009). Further, research has underscored the relation between structural and process characteristics of child care programs. For example, the National Institute of Child Health and Human Development (NICHD) Study of Early Child Care found a link between lower staff:child ratios and caregivers who were more stimulating and responsive to children's needs, and also documented that caregivers were more responsive and less controlling when group sizes were small (NICHD Early Child Care Research Network, 2005).

Comprehensive Approach

The variability in the needs and experiences of families from impoverished and high-risk backgrounds argues for a wide range of services within the early care and education service sector. Consistent with Head Start and other similar preschool initiatives, these programs must address the needs of both parents and children across developmental domains. Many scholars have underscored the benefit of two-generation programs—interventions that serve young children as well as their parents. For example, the Early Head Start Research and Evaluation Project documented changes in parental functioning as a mediator for the long-term outcomes for children that emerged in the area of school readiness (Chazan-Cohen et al., 2009). Additionally, the evaluation of the Infant Health and Development Program yielded findings that indicated that enhanced parenting mediated the program's effects on children's IQ and problem behaviors at age 3 (Bradley et al., 1994), though these findings did not hold 15 years postintervention (Martin, Brooks-Gunn, Klebanov, Buka, & McCormick, 2008). Further, an examination of the 5-year outcomes of the New Hope intervention, an employment and income support program for families in poverty, suggested that participating parents created enhanced out-of-home experiences for their children (i.e., child care and out-of-schooltime activities), which may be the pathway through which the program produced improved school performance and social behavior in children (Casey, Ripke, & Huston, 2005). Taken together, these findings underscore the importance of intervening with parents as well as children. Parent intervention is a component of the design of many early care and education programs such as Early Head Start. For community-based child care programs that do not have the resources for intensive parent intervention, a formal collaboration with a family support program may accomplish this goal.

Early care and education programs should also undertake a comprehensive approach with respect to addressing the needs of children. In their discussion of the evaluation of Head Start programs, Raver and Zigler (1997) advocate for early childhood care and education that focuses on the needs of the whole child. In other words, programs should not only provide custodial care of children, but should attend to their developmental needs across domains, including their physical and dental health, cognitive and language development, and their social–emotional functioning and mental health. Early Head Start and similarly designed programs are mandated to address all these areas, and show enhanced outcomes for children as a result of such services (Administration for Children and Families, 2002).

Community-based child care programs without public subsidies may not have the resources to provide intensive intervention in each of these domains. However, the susceptibility of low-income and other high-risk children to adverse outcomes across domains (Duncan & Brooks-Gunn, 1997; Aber et al., 2007) argues for careful attention to these issues. At the very least, child care staff can be trained to recognize physical health, developmental and mental health vulnerabilities in young children, and refer them to early intervention and other services that can support children's functioning in these domains.

Culture-Specific Programming

Duncan et al. (2010) identify race/ethnicity as one of the variables that have to be examined in the context of early childhood poverty. Multiple studies have documented that race/ethnicity is a risk factor for adverse developmental outcomes, above and beyond poverty (e.g., higher levels of infant mortality and compromised academic achievement among African American children of all SES groups compared to European American children; Hudley, 2009). In consideration of the culture–child care link, scholars and practitioners have underscored the impact of race/ethnicity and culture on children's caregiving experiences and outcomes (Zepeda, Rothstein-Fisch, Gonzalez-Mena, & Trumbull, 2006).

The literature is replete with evidence that culture shapes parents' beliefs and their childrearing practices, particularly in the early years (Ippen, 2009). There is also some evidence that interventions may be more effective if they are grounded in the culture of the families who receive it (e.g., Jones Harden & Nzinga-Johnson, 2006). Thus, early care and education programs may need to adapt their approaches and services to meet the needs of particular cultural groups and to be consistent with the childrearing practices prominent in these groups.

There is some evidence that specific types of programs may be more beneficial for particular racial/ethnic groups. For example, the Early Head Start Impact Study reported more robust, broad, and persistent benefits for African American families than all other groups (Jones Harden et al., in press). In a study comparing relationship-based (i.e., continuous, primary caregiver–child relationships) and nonrelationship-based-focused child care programs, higher levels of child compliance and better caregiver–parent relationships were documented in the relationship-based-programs for African American children, whereas these two outcomes were more pronounced for Latino families in the nonrelationship-based programs (Owen et al., 2008).

Interventions Targeted to Families at Risk

Given the large numbers of families from impoverished backgrounds that contend with various other risk factors, infant/toddler programs should incorporate services designed explicitly for families at environmental risk. Child care and education would remain the primary goal of the program, with the idea that quality care and education represents a critical protective factor for children from high-risk backgrounds (Watamura et al., 2011). However, as was discussed in prior sections of this chapter, parents' physical and mental health, and parenting capacity have important implications for the well-being of their children.

Although it is beyond the scope of early care and education programs to provide mental health intervention to parents, they can develop formal collaborations with community-based mental health providers. Additionally, and perhaps more importantly, early care and education programs can provide parenting interventions in the context of the families' specific needs. For example, parent–child interaction approaches for substance-affected families (Milligan et al., 2010) and parents diagnosed with depression (Compas et al., 2009; Toth, Rogosch, & Cicchetti, 2006) have been created and tested, which could become part of the intervention repertoire of the child care program. Additionally, practitioners and scholars have designed and implemented interventions to improve the responsiveness and child management skills of maltreating parents (e.g., Whitaker, Crimmins, Edwards, & Lutzker, 2008) and foster parents (e.g., Fisher, Chamberlain, & Leve, 2009), interventions that could be delivered within the venue of infant/toddler programs.

Further, the developmental vulnerability of children from high-risk backgrounds may necessitate more intensive developmental interventions that include specialized services (e.g., speech and language therapy, occupational therapy), as well as the developmental stimulation that occurs in the typical infant/toddler group setting. Often, toddlers from these high-risk families manifest behavior problems that may be the result of early vulnerabilities in emotion regulation or their responses to environmental challenges (Fox, 1994). Many evidence-based interventions exist to address the behavior problems of very young children within their family contexts or the early childhood care and education setting (e.g., Connell et al., 2008; Webster-Stratton & Herman, 2010). Such studies also point to the promise of integrating these targeted services into primary prevention settings, such as early care and education programs.

Concluding Remarks

It is evident that high-quality early care and education programs can alter the developmental trajectories of infants and toddlers from impoverished backgrounds. Yet, there are critical groups of this population that may not benefit from traditional programs. These children and families manifest increased vulnerability through their experience of multiple risk factors that are often unattended by early care and education programs. Thus, these families have service needs that are often omitted from the menu of programmatic activities that early childhood care and education settings offer.

The adverse outcomes common for children from these high-risk backgrounds call for early and intensive intervention to alter their developmental trajectories. Such intervention must be informed by an understanding of the comprehensive needs of the children and the families in which they are reared. Evidence-based interventions designed to address specific child and parent risk factors can be integrated into traditional infant/toddler programs, which address risk factors commonly associated with poverty including poor birth outcomes, parental psychopathology, poor parenting, family violence, and racial/ethnic minority status. For programs that do not have the capacity to integrate such services, formal collaborations with appropriate service providers is imperative. Attention to families' specific needs, coupled with the delivery of early childhood programs with the highest quality, holds promise for promoting the positive developmental trajectories of this vulnerable group of young children.

REFERENCES

Abbott-Schim, M., Lambert, R., & McCarty, F. (2003). A comparison of school readiness outcomes for children randomly assigned to Head Start program and the program's wait list. *Journal of Education for Students Placed at Risk, 8*(2), 191–214.

Aber, J., Jones, S., & Raver, C. (2007). Poverty and child development: New perspectives on a defining issue. In J. L. Aber, S. Bishop-Josef, S. Jones, K. McLearn, & D. Phillips (Eds.), *Child development and social policy: Knowledge for action* (pp. 149–166). Washington, DC: American Psychological Association.

Ackerman, B., Brown, E., & Izard, C. (2004). The relations between persistent poverty and contextual risk and children's behavior in elementary school. *Developmental Psychology, 40*(3), 367–377.

Ackerman, B. E., Izard, C. E., Schoff, K., Youngstrom, E. A., & Kogos, J. (1999). Contextual risk, caregiver emotionality, and the problem behaviors of six- and seven-year-old children from economically disadvantaged families. *Child Development, 70*, 1415–1427.

Adams, C. D., Hillman, N., & Gaydos, G. R. (1994). Behavioral difficulties in toddlers: Impact of sociocultural and biological risk factors. *Journal of Clinical Child Psychology, 23*, 373–381.

Administration for Children and Families. (2002). *Making a difference in the lives of infants and toddlers and their families: The impacts of Early Head Start.* Washington, DC: Department of Health and Human Services.

Administration for Children and Families. (2011). *Child maltreatment 2010.* Washington, DC: Author.

Anderson Moore, K., Redd, Z., Burkhauser, M., Mbwana, K., & Collins, A. (2009). *Children in poverty: Trends, consequences, and policy options* (Child Trends Research Brief). Washington, DC: Child Trends.

Ashman, S., Dawson, G., & Panagiotides, H. (2008). Trajectories of maternal depression over 7 years: Relations with child psychophysiology and behavior and role of contextual risks. *Development and Psychopathology, 20*(1), 55–77.

Barnett, D., Ganiban, J., & Cicchetti, D. (1999). Maltreatment, emotional reactivity, and the development of type D attachments from 12- to 24-months of age. In J. Vondra & D. Barnett (Eds.), *Atypical patterns of attachment in* infancy and early childhood among children at developmental risk. *Monographs of the Society for Research in Child Development, 64*(3, Serial No. 258), 97–118.

Batchelor, J. (2008). Failure to thrive revisited. *Child Abuse Review, 17,* 147–159.

Belsky, J., Bakermans-Kranenburg, M., & van IJzendoorn, M. H. (2007). For better and for worse: Differential susceptibility to environmental influences. *Current Directions in Psychological Science, 16*(6), 300–304.

Benson, M., Fox, G., DeMaris, A., & van Wyk, J. (2003). Neighborhood disadvantage, individual economic distress and violence against women in intimate relationships. *Journal of Quantitative Criminology, 19*(3), 207–235.

Berkowitz, S. J. (2003). Children exposed to community violence: The rationale for early intervention. *Clinical Child and Family Psychology Review, 6*(4), 293–302.

Bogat, G. A., DeJonghe, E., Levendosky, A. A., Davidson, W. S., & von Eye, A. (2006). Trauma symptoms among infants exposed to intimate partner violence. *Child Abuse and Neglect, 30,* 109–125.

Bradley, R., Whiteside, L., Mundfrom, D., Casey, P., Kelleher, K., & Pope, S. (1994). Contribution of early intervention and early caregiving experiences to resilience in low-birthweight, premature children living in poverty. *Journal of Clinical Child Psychology, 23*(4), 425–434.

Bronfenbrenner, U. (1979). *The ecology of human development: Experiments by nature and design.* Cambridge, MA: Harvard University Press.

Brooks-Gunn, J. (1990). Identifying the vulnerable young child. In D. E. Rogers & E. Ginzberg (Eds.), *Improving the life chances of children at risk* (pp. 104–124). Boulder, CO: Westview.

Buckner, J., Mezzacappa, E., & Beardslee, W. (2009). Self-regulation and its relations to adaptive functioning in low-income youths. *American Journal of Orthopsychiatry, 79*(1), 19–30.

Burchinal, M., Nelson, L., Carlson, M., & Brooks-Gunn, J. (2008). Neighborhood characteristics and child care type and quality. *Early Education and Development, 19*(5), 702–725.

Burchinal, M., Peisner-Feinberg, E., Bryant, D., & Clifford, R. (2000). Children's social and cognitive development and child-care quality: Testing for differential associations related to poverty, gender, or ethnicity. *Applied Developmental Science, 4*(3), 149–165.

Burchinal, M., Roberts, J. E., Zeisel, S. A., Hennon, E. A., & Hooper, S. (2006). Social risk and protective child, parenting, and child care factors in early elementary school years. *Parenting: Science and Practice, 6,* 79–113.

Campbell, F., Pungello, E., Miller-Johnson, S., Burchinal, M., & Ramey, C. (2001). The development of cognitive and academic abilities: Growth curves from an early educational experiment. *Development Psychology, 37*(2), 231–242.

Campbell, S., Shaw, D., & Gilliom, M. (2000). Early externalizing behavior problems: Toddlers and preschoolers at risk for later maladjustment. *Development and Psychopathology, 12*(3), 467–488.

Carpenter, G. L., & Stacks, A. M. (2009). Developmental effects of exposure to intimate partner violence in early childhood: A review of the literature. *Children and Youth Service Review, 31*(8), 831–839.

Carter, A., Garrity-Rokous, F. E., Chazan-Cohen, R., Little, C., & Briggs-Gowan,

M. (2001). Maternal depression and comorbidity: Predicting early parenting, attachment security, and toddler social-emotional problems and competencies. *Journal of the American Academy of Child and Adolescent Psychiatry, 40*(1), 18–26.

Casey, D., Ripke, M., & Huston, A. (2005). Activity participation and the well-being of children and adolescents in the context of welfare reform. In J. Mahoney, W. R. Larson, & J. Eccles (Eds.), *Organized activities as contexts of development: Extracurricular activities, after-school and community programs* (pp. 65–84). Mahwah, NJ: Erlbaum.

Cassidy, D., Lower, J., Kintner, V., & Hestenes, L. (2009). Teacher ethnicity and variation in context: The implications for classroom quality. *Early Education and Development, 20*(2), 305–320.

Centers for Disease Control and Prevention. (2009). What do we know about tobacco use and pregnancy? Retrieved from *www.cdc.gov/reproductive-health/tobaccousepregnancy/.*

Centers for Disease Control and Prevention. (2010). Fetal alcohol spectrum disorders (FADs). Retrieved from *www.cdc.gov/ncbddd/fasd/alcohol-use.html.*

Chazan-Cohen, R., Ayoub, C., Pan, B., Roggman, L., Raikes, H., McKelvey, L., et al. (2007). It takes time: Impacts of Early Head Start that lead to reductions in depression two years later. *Infant Mental Health Journal, 28*(2), 151–170.

Chazan-Cohen, R., Raikes, H., Brooks-Gunn, J., Ayoub, C., Pan, B., Kisker, E., et al. (2009). Low-income children's school readiness: Parent contributions over the first five years. *Early Education and Development, 20*(6), 958–977.

Chiesa, A., & Duhaime, A. (2009). Abusive head trauma. *Pediatric Clinics of North America, 56*(2), 317–331.

Christian, C., & Block, R. (2009). Abusive head trauma in infants and children. *Pediatrics, 123*(5), 1409–1411.

Compas, B. E., Forehand, R., Keller, G., Champion, J. E., Rakow, A., Reeslund, K. L., et al. (2009). Randomized controlled trial of a family cognitive-behavioral preventive intervention for children of depressed parents. *Journal of Consulting and Clinical Psychology, 77*(6), 1007–1020.

Conger, R. D., & Donnellan, M. B. (2007). An interactionist perspective on the socioeconomic context of human development. *Annual Review of Psychology, 58,* 175–199.

Connell, A., Bullock, B., Dishion, T., Shaw, D., Wilson, M., & Gardner, F. (2008). Family intervention effects on co-occurring early childhood behavioral and emotional problems: A latent transition analysis approach. *Journal of Abnormal Child Psychology, 36*(8), 1211–1225.

Corrington, M. E., & Phillips, D. (2009). *Rethinking the role of early care and education in child abuse and neglect prevention: A developmental perspective on quality child care as a protective factor for foster children.* Paper presented at the Second National Research Conference on Child and Family Programs and Policy, Bridgewater, MA.

Curby, T., LoCasale-Crouch, J., Konold, T., Pianta, R., Howes, C., Burchinal, M., et al. (2009). The relations of observed pre-K classroom quality profiles to children's achievement and social competence. *Early Education and Development, 20*(2), 346–372.

Dearing, E., McCartney, K., & Taylor, B. (2009). Does higher quality early child care promote low-income children's math and reading achievement in middle childhood? *Child Development, 80*(5), 1329–1349.

De Bellis, M. D., Hooper, S. R., & Sapia, J. L. (2005). Early trauma exposure and the brain. In J. J. Vasterling & C. R. Brewin (Eds.), *Neuropsychology of PTSD: Biological, cognitive, and clinical perspectives* (pp. 153–177). New York: Guilford Press.

DeJonghe, E. S., Bogat, G. A., Levendosky, A. A., von Eye, A., & Davidson II, W. S. (2005). Infant exposure to domestic violence predicts heightened sensitivity to adult verbal conflict. *Infant Mental Health Journal, 26*(3), 268–281.

Downer, J., & Pianta, R. (2006). Academic and cognitive functioning in first grade: Associations with earlier home and child care predictors and with concurrent home and classroom experiences. *School Psychology Review, 35*(1), 11–30.

Duncan, G., & Brooks-Gunn, J. (1997). Income effects across the life span: Integration and interpretation. In G. J. Duncan & J. Brooks-Gunn (Eds.), *Consequences of growing up poor* (pp. 596–610). New York: Russell Sage Foundation Press.

Duncan, G., Ziol-Guest, K., & Kalil, A. (2010). Early-childhood poverty and adult attainment, behavior, and health. *Child Development, 81*(1), 306–325.

Eamon, M. (2001). Poverty, parenting, peer and neighborhood influences on young adolescent antisocial behavior. *Journal of Social Service Research, 28*(1), 1–23.

Early, D., Maxwell, K., Burchinal, M., Bender, R., Ebanks, C., Henry, G., et al. (2007). Teachers' education, classroom quality, and young children's academic skills: Results from seven studies of preschool programs. *Child Development, 78*(2), 558–580.

Evans, G. (2004). The environment of childhood poverty. *American Psychologist, 59*(2), 77–92.

Evans, G., & Rosenbaum, J. (2008). Self-regulation and the income achievement gap. *Early Childhood Research Quarterly, 23*(4), 504–514.

Fantuzzo, J. W., & Mohr, W. K. (1999). Prevalence and effects of child exposure to domestic violence. *The Future of Children, 9*(3), 21–32.

Field, T., Fox, N., Pickens, J., & Nawrocki, T. (1995). Relative right frontal EEG activation in 3- to 6-month-old infants of depressed mothers. *Developmental Psychology, 31*(3), 358–363.

Finkelhor, D., Turner, H. A., Ormond, R. K., & Hamby, S. L. (2009). Violence, crime, and exposure in a national sample of children and youth. *Pediatrics, 124*(5), 1411–1423.

Fisher, P., Chamberlain, P., & Leve, L. (2009). Improving the lives of foster children through evidenced-based interventions. *Vulnerable Children and Youth Studies, 4*(2), 122–127.

Fiske, F., & Hall, J. (2008). Inflicted childhood neurotrauma. *Advanced Nursing Trauma, 31*, E1–E8.

Fowler, P. J., Tompsett, C. J., Braciszewski, J. M., Jacques-Tiura, J., & Baltes, B. B. (2009). Community violence: A meta-analysis on the effect of exposure and mental health outcomes of children and adolescents. *Development and Psychopathology, 21*(1), 227–259.

Fox, N. (1994). Dynamic cerebral processes underlying emotion regulation. *Monographs of the Society for Research in Child Development, 59*(2-3), 152–166, 250–283.

Gardner, M., Barajas, R. G., & Brooks-Gunn, J. (2010). Neighborhood influences on substance use etiology: Is where you live important? In L. Scheier (Ed.), *Handbook of drug use etiology: Theory, methods and empirical findings* (pp. 423–441). Washington, DC: American Psychological Association.

Gassman-Pines, A., & Yoshikawa, H. (2006). The effects of antipoverty programs on children's cumulative level of poverty-related risk. *Developmental Psychology, 42*(6), 981–999.

Gewirtz, A., & Edleson, J. (2007). Young children's exposure to intimate partner violence: Towards a developmental risk and resilience framework for research and intervention. *Journal of Family Violence, 22,* 151–163.

Groark, C., Mehaffie, K., McCall, R., & Greenberg, M. (Eds.). (2007). *Evidence-based practices and programs for early childhood care and education.* Thousand Oaks, CA: Corwin Press.

Gyamfi, P. (2004). Children with serious emotional disturbance: The impact of poverty and receipt of public assistance on behavior, functioning, and service use. *Children and Youth Services Review, 26,* 1129–1139.

Halle, T., Forry, N., Hair, E., Perper, K., Wandner, L., Wessel, J., et al. (2009). *Disparities in early learning and development: Lessons from the Early Childhood Longitudinal Study–Birth Cohort (ECLS-B).* Washington, DC: Child Trends.

Halpern, D. F. (2000). Validity, fairness, and group differences: Tough questions for selection testing. *Psychology, Public Policy, and Law, 6,* 56–62.

Hay, D., Pawlby, S.,Waters, C., Perra, O., & Sharp, D. (2010). Mothers' antenatal depression and their children's antisocial outcomes. *Child Development, 81*(1), 149–165.

Hernandez, V., Montana, S., & Clarke, K. (2010). Child health inequality: Framing a social work response. *Health and Social Work, 35*(4), 291–301.

Hudley, C. (2009). Academic motivation and achievement of African American youth. In H. Neville, B. Tynes, & S. Utsey (Eds.), *Handbook of African American psychology* (pp. 187–197). Thousand Oaks, CA: Sage.

Ippen, C. (2009). The sociocultural context of infant mental health: Toward contextually congruent interventions. In C. Zeanah (Ed.), *Handbook of infant mental health* (3rd ed., pp. 104–119). New York: Guilford Press.

Jones, D., Forehand, R., Brody, G., & Armistead, L. (2002). Psychosocial adjustment of African American children in single-mother families: A test of three risk models. *Journal of Marriage and Family, 64,* 105–115.

Jones Harden, B., & Nzinga-Johnson, S. (2006). Young, wounded and black: The maltreatment of African-American children in the early years. In R. L. Hampton & T. P. Gullotta (Eds.), *Interpersonal violence in the African-American community* (pp. 17–46). New York: Springer.

Jones Harden, B., Sandstrom, H., & Chazan-Cohen, R. (in press). Early Head Start and African American families: Impacts and mechanisms of child outcomes. *Early Childhood Research Quarterly.*

Kaufman, J. (2008). Genetic and environmental modifiers of risk and resiliency in maltreated children. In J. J. Hudziak (Ed.), *Developmental psychopathology and wellness: Genetic and environmental influences* (pp. 141–160). Washington, DC: American Psychiatric.

King, S., & Laplante, D. (2005). The effects of prenatal maternal stress on children's cognitive development: Project Ice Storm. *Stress: International Journal on the Biology of Stress, 8*(1), 35–45.

Klerman, L. (1991). The health of poor children: Problems and programs. In A. C. Huston (Ed.), *Children in poverty* (pp. 79–104). New York: Cambridge University Press.

Knitzer, J., & Perry, D. (2009). Poverty and infant and toddler development: Facing the complex challenges. In C. Zeanah (Ed.), *Handbook of infant mental health* (3rd ed., pp. 135–152). New York: Guilford Press.

Kolko, D. J. (2001). Child physical abuse. In J. E. B. Meyers, L. Berliner, J. Briere, C. T. Hendrix, C. Jenny, & T. A. Reid (Eds.), *The APSAC handbook on child maltreatment* (pp. 21–54). Thousand Oaks, CA: Sage.

Laucht, M., Esser, G., Baving, L., Gerhold, M., Hoesch, I., Ihle, W., et al. (2000). Behavioral sequelae of perinatal insults and early family adversity at 8 years of age. *Journal of the American Academy of Child and Adolescent Psychiatry, 39*, 1229–1237.

Lester, B., Bagner, D., Liu, J., LaGasse, L., Seifer, R., Bauer, C., et al. (2009). Infant neurobehavioral dysregulation: Behavior problems in children with prenatal substance exposure. *Pediatrics, 124*(5), 1355–1362.

Lieber, J., Butera, G., Hanson, M., Palmer, S., Horn, E., Czaja, C., et al. (2009). Factors that influence the implementation of a new preschool curriculum: Implications for professional development. *Early Education and Development, 20*(3), 456–481.

Litrownik, A., Newton, R., Hunter, W., English, D., & Everson, M. (2003). Exposure to family violence in young at-risk children: A longitudinal look at the effects of victimization and witnessed physical and psychological aggression. *Journal of Family Violence, 18*(1), 59–73.

Lorion, R., Brodsky, A., & Cooley-Quille, M. (1998). Exposure to urban violence: A framework for conceptualizing risky settings. In D. Biegel & A. Blum (Eds.), *Innovations in practice and service delivery across the lifespan.* New York: Oxford University Press.

Love, J., Harrison, L., Sagi-Schwartz, A., van IJzendoorn, M., Ross, C., Ungerer, J., et al. (2003). Child care quality matters: How conclusions may vary with context. *Child Development, 74*(4), 1021–1033.

Love, J., Tarullo, L., Raikes, H., & Chazan-Cohen, R. (2006). Head Start: What do we know about its effectiveness? What do we need to know? In K. McCartney & D. Phillips (Eds.), *Blackwell handbook of early childhood development* (pp. 550–575). Malden, MA: Blackwell.

Luthar, S. (Ed.). (2003). *Resilience and vulnerability: Adaptation in the context of childhood adversities.* New York: Cambridge University Press.

Lynch, M. (2003). Consequences of children's exposure to community violence. *Clinical Child and Family Psychology Review, 6*(4), 265–274.

Magnuson, K., & Waldfogel, J. (2005). Early childhood care and education: Effects on ethnic and racial gaps in school readiness. *The Future of Children, 15*(1), 169–196.

Margolin, G., & Gordis, E. B. (2000). The effects of family and community violence on children. *Annual Review of Psychology, 51,* 445–479.

Martin, A., Brooks-Gunn, J., Klebanov, P., Buka, S., & McCormick, M. (2008). Long-term maternal effects of early childhood intervention: Findings from the Infant Health and Development Program (IHDP). *Journal of Applied Developmental Psychology, 29*(2), 101–117.

Mayer, S. (2010). Revisiting an old question: How much does parental income affect child outcomes? *Focus, 27*(2), 21–26.

McAlister Groves, B. (2005). Witness to violence. In S. Parker, B. Zuckerman, & M. Augustyn (Eds.), *Developmental and behavioral pediatrics: A handbook for primary care* (pp. 370–375). Philadelphia: Lippincott Williams & Wilkins.

McCartney, K., Dearing, E., Taylor, B., & Bub, K. (2007). Quality child-care supports the achievement of low-income children: Direct and indirect pathways through caregiving and the home environment. *Journal of Applied Developmental Psychology, 28,* 411–426.

McLoyd, V. (1990). The impact of economic hardship on black families and children: Psychological distress, parenting, and social–emotional development. *Child Development, 61,* 311–346.

Milligan, K., Niccols, A., Sword, W., Thabane, L., Henderson, J., Smith, A., et al. (2010). Maternal substance use and integrated treatment programs for women with substance use issues and their children: A meta-analysis. *Substance Abuse Treatment, Prevention, and Policy, 5,* 21.

Mistry, R. S., Biesanz, J. C., Taylor, L. C., Burchinal, M., & Cox, M. J. (2004). Family income and its relation to preschool children's adjustment for families in the NICHD study of early child care. *Developmental Psychology, 40,* 727–745.

Mistry, R. S., Vandewater, E. A., Huston, A. C., & McLoyd, V. C. (2002). Economic well-being and children's social adjustment: The role of family process in an ethnically diverse low-income sample. *Child Development, 73,* 935–951.

Morenoff, J., Sampson, R., & Raudenbush, S. (2001). Neighborhood inequality, collective efficacy, and the spatial dynamics of urban violence. *Criminology, 39,* 517–560.

Murray, L., Hipwell, A., Hooper, R., Stein, A., & Cooper, P. (1996). The cognitive development of 5-year-old children of postnatally depressed mothers. *Journal of Child Psychology and Psychiatry, 37*(8), 927–935.

Najman, J., Hayabakhsh, M., Heron, M., Bor, W., O'Callaghan, M., & Williams, G. (2009). The impact of episodic and chronic poverty on child cognitive development. *Pediatrics, 154*(2), 284–289.

National Center for Children Exposed to Violence. (2006). *Domestic violence.* Available at *www.nccev.org/violence/domestic.html.*

National Research Council and Institute of Medicine. (2009). *Preventing mental, emotional, and behavioral disorders among young people: Progress and possibilities.* Washington, DC: National Academies Press.

Nelson, C. (Ed.). (1994). *Threats to optimal development: Integrating biological, psychological and social risk factors.* Hillsdale, NJ: Erlbaum.

NICHD Early Child Care Research Network. (2005). *Child care and child development: Results of the NICHD Study of Early Child Care and Youth Development.* New York: Guilford Press.

Osofsky, J. D. (1999). The impact of violence on children. *The Future of Children, 9*(3), 33–49.

Osofsky, J. D. (2003). Prevalence of children's exposure to domestic violence and child maltreatment: Implications for prevention and intervention. *Clinical Child and Family Psychology Review, 6*(3), 161–170.

Osofsky, J. D., & Fenichel, E. (Eds.). (2000). *Protecting young children in violent environments.* Washington, DC: Zero to Three.

Overstreet, S. (2000). Exposure to community violence: Defining the problem and understanding the consequences. *Journal of Child and Family Studies, 9*(1), 7–25.

Overstreet, S., & Mazza, J. (2003). An ecological–transactional understanding of community violence: Theoretical perspectives. *School Psychology Quarterly, 18*(1), 66–87.

Owen, M., Klausli, J., Mata-Otero, A., & Caughy, M. (2008). Relationship-focused child care practices: Quality of care and child outcomes for children in poverty. *Early Education and Development, 19*(2), 302–329.

Papero, A. (2005). Is early, high-quality daycare an asset for the children of low-income, depressed mothers? *Developmental Review, 25*(2), 181–211.

Patterson, S., & Albers, A. (2001). Effects of poverty and maternal depression on early child development. *Child Development, 72*(6), 1794–1813.

Pianta, R., Howes, C., Burchinal, M., Bryant, D., Clifford, R., Early, D., et al. (2005). Features of pre-kindergarten programs, classrooms, and teachers: Do they predict observed classroom quality and child–teacher interactions? *Applied Developmental Science, 9*(3), 144–159.

Pluess, M., & Belsky, J. (2010). Differential susceptibility to parenting and quality child care. *Developmental Psychology, 46*(2), 379–390.

Power, C., Jeffries, B., Manor, O., & Hartzman, C. (2006). The influence of birthweight and socioeconomic position on cognitive development. *Journal of Pediatrics, 148*, 54–61.

Rafferty, Y., Griffin, K., & Robokos, D. (2010). Maternal depression and parental distress among families in the Early Head Start Research and Evaluation Project. *Infant Mental Health Journal, 31*(5), 543–569.

Raver, C., & Zigler, E. (1997). Social competence: An untapped dimension in evaluating Head Start's success. *Early Childhood Research Quarterly, 12*(4), 363–385.

Reynolds, A., Mathieson, L., & Topitzes, J. (2009). Do early childhood interventions prevent child maltreatment? A review of the research. *Child Maltreatment, 14*(2), 182–206.

Reynolds, A., Rolnick, A., Englund, M., & Temple, J. (Eds.). (2010). *Childhood practices and programs in the first decade of life: A human capital integration.* New York: Cambridge University Press.

Roggman, L., Cook, G., Peterson, C., & Raikes, H. (2008). Who drops out of Early Head Start home visiting programs? *Early Education and Development, 19*(4), 574–599.

Rohrer, L., Cicchetti, D., Rogosch, F., Toth, S., & Maughan, A. (2011). Effects of maternal negativity and of early and recent recurrent depressive disorder on children's false belief understanding. *Developmental Psychology, 47*(1), 170–181.

Rouse, H., & Fantuzzo, J. (2009). Multiple risks and educational well-being: A population-based investigation of threats to early school success. *Early Childhood Research Quarterly, 24*(1), 1–14.

Rutter, M. (1979). Maternal deprivation, 1972–1978: New findings, new concepts, new approaches. *Child Development, 50*(2), 283–305.

Sameroff, A. J. (Ed.). (2009). *The Transactional Model of Development: How children and contexts shape each other.* Washington, DC: American Psychological Association.

Sameroff, A. J., Bartko, W. T., Baldwin, A., Baldwin, C., & Seifer, R. (1998). Family and social influences on the development of child competence. In C. Feiring & M. Lewis (Eds.), *Families, risk and competence* (pp. 161–185). Mahwah, NJ: Erlbaum.

Sampson, R. J., Sharkey, P., & Raudenbush, S. W. (2008). Durable effects of concentrated disadvantage on verbal ability among African-American children. *Proceedings of the National Academy of Sciences, 105,* 845–852.

Sedlak, A. J., Mettenburg, J., Basena, M., Petta, I., McPherson, K., Greene, A., et al. (2010). *Fourth National Incidence Study of Child Abuse and Neglect (NIS-4): Report to Congress.* Washington, DC: U.S. Department of Health and Human Services; Administration for Children and Families; Office of Planning, Research and Evaluation; and the Children's Bureau.

Seifer, R., & Dickstein, S. (2000). Parental mental illness and infant development. In C. Zeanah (Ed.), *Handbook of infant mental health* (2nd ed., pp. 145–160). New York: Guilford Press.

Seifer, R., Sameroff, A., Baldwin, C., & Baldwin, A. (1992). Child and family factors that ameliorate risk between 4 and 13 years of age. *Journal of the American Academy of Child and Adolescent Psychiatry, 31*(5), 893–903.

Shonkoff, J., Boyce, W. T., & McEwen, B. (2009). Neuroscience, molecular biology, and the childhood roots of health disparities: Building a new framework for health promotion and disease. *Journal of the American Medical Association, 301*(21), 2252–2259.

Substance Abuse and Mental Health Services Administration. (2009). *Results from the 2009 National Survey on Drug Use and Health: National findings.* Retrieved from *http://oas.samhsa.gov/NSDUH/2k9NSDUH/2k9Results.htm.*

Torquati, J., Raikes, H., & Huddleston-Casas, C. (2007). Teacher education, motivation, compensation, workplace support, and links to quality of center-based child care and teachers' intention to stay in the early childhood profession. *Early Childhood Research Quarterly, 22*(2), 261–275.

Toth, S., Rogosca, F., & Cicchetti, D. (2006). The efficacy of toddler–parent psychotherapy to reorganize attachment in the young offspring of mothers with major depressive disorder: A randomized preventive trial. *Journal of Consulting and Clinical Psychology, 74*(6), 1006–1016.

Twardosz, S., & Lutzker, J. R. (2010). Child maltreatment and the developing brain: A review of neuroscience perspectives. *Aggression and Violent Behavior, 15*(1), 59–68.

Valentino, K., Cicchetti, D., Toth, S. L., & Rogosch, F. A. (2006). Mother–child play and emerging social behaviors among infants from maltreating families. *Developmental Psychology, 42*(3), 474–485.

Van Voorhees, E., & Scarpa, A. (2004). The effects of child maltreatment on the hypothalamic–pituitary–adrenal axis. *Trauma, Violence, and Abuse, 5,* 333–352.

Votruba-Drzal, E., Coley, R. L., & Chase-Lansdale, P. L. (2004). Child care and low-income children's development: Direct and moderated effects. *Child Development, 75*(1), 296–312.

Wadsworth, M., & Santiago, C. (2008). Risk and resiliency processes in ethnically diverse families in poverty. *Journal of Family Psychology, 22*(3), 399–410.

Watamura, S., Phillips, D., Morrissey, T., McCartney, K., & Bub, K. (2011). Double jeopardy: Poorer social–emotional outcomes for children in the NICHD SECYD experiencing home and child-care environments that confer risk. *Child Development, 82*(1), 48–65.

Webster-Stratton, C., & Herman, K. (2010). Disseminating the incredible years series early-intervention programs: Integrating and sustaining services between home and school. *Psychology in the Schools, 47*(1), 36–54

Whitaker, D., Crimmins, D., Edwards, A., & Lutzker, J. (2008). Safety training/violence prevention using the SafeCare Parent Training Model. In W. O'Donohue & J. Fisher (Eds.), *Cognitive behavior therapy: Applying empirically supported techniques in your practice* (2nd ed., pp. 473–477). Hoboken, NJ: Wiley.

Windham, A., Rosenberg, L., Fuddy, L., McFarlane, E., Sia, C., & Duggan, A. (2004). Risk of mother-reported child abuse in the first 3 years of life. *Child Abuse and Neglect, 28*(6), 645–667.

Winsler, A., Tran, H., Hartman, S., Madigan, A., Manfra, L., & Bleiker, C. (2008). School readiness gains made by ethnically diverse children in poverty attending center-based childcare and public school pre-kindergarten programs. *Early Childhood Research Quarterly, 23*(3), 314–329.

Wolfe, D., Crooks, C., Lee, V., McIntyre-Smith, A., & Jaffe, P. (2003). The effects of children's exposure to domestic violence. A meta-analysis and critique. *Clinical Child and Family Psychology Review, 6*(3), 171–187.

Zaslow, M., Halle, T., Martin, L., Cabrera, N., Calkins, J., Pitzer, L., et al. (2006). Child outcome measures in the study of child care quality. *Evaluation Review, 30*(5), 577–610.

Zepeda, M., Rothstein-Fisch, C., Gonzalez-Mena, J., & Trumbull, E. (2006). *Bridging cultures in early care and education: A training module.* Mahwah, NJ: Erlbaum.

PART VI

INFANT/TODDLER CARE AND EDUCATION

CHAPTER 13

Beginnings of School Readiness in Infant/Toddler Development
Evidence from Early Head Start

John M. Love, Rachel Chazan-Cohen, Jeanne Brooks-Gunn, Helen Raikes, Cheri A. Vogel, and Ellen Eliason Kisker

Children's development, beginning even before birth, is enhanced by many circumstances and experiences, including sound nutrition and health care, a supportive parent–child relationship, safe neighborhoods and housing, healthy marriages, involved fathers, quality early care and education programs, and many, many other factors (McCartney & Phillips, 2006; Shonkoff & Phillips, 2000). Research from the past several decades indicates: "(1) the importance of early life experiences, as well as the inseparable and highly interactive influences of genetics and environment, on the development of the brain and the unfolding of human behavior; (2) the central role of early relationships as a source of either support and adaptation or risk and dysfunction; (3) the powerful capabilities, complex emotions, and essential social skills that develop during the earliest years of life; and (4) the capacity to increase the odds of favorable developmental outcomes through planned interventions" (Shonkoff & Phillips, 2000, pp. 1–2). A large body of research shows that positive environments can lead to enhanced language, vocabulary, and cognitive skills; positive social–emotional development; self-regulation, impulse control, and task engagement; appropriate body mass index; and healthy attachment with parents (e.g., Heckman, 2006).

Positive and supportive experiences in the first 3 years of life set the stage for lifelong learning and health (Pianta, Cox, & Snow, 2007). In the early years, they prepare children for the beginning of formal schooling, including PreK. Children in low-income families, however, too often are developing in environments that are less supportive in many ways, including being less likely to live in two-parent households, experiencing hunger or food insecurity, facing exposure to environmental risks and toxins, living in homes with parental substance abuse and depression, having access to lower-quality child care, and so forth (Duncan & Magnuson, 2005; Duncan, Brooks-Gunn, & Klebanov, 1994; Leventhal, Dupéré, & Brooks-Gunn, 2009; Magnuson & Waldfogel, 2005). Children in poverty are born at lower birthweights, are more likely to exhibit behavior problems and, when older, commit crimes, are at higher risk of becoming a teen parent, experience more accidents and injuries, suffer higher rates of obesity, have chronic health problems such as asthma and anemia, and lead lives in poverty when they become adults (Brooks-Gunn, Duncan, & Aber, 1997; Duncan, Ziol-Guest, & Kalil, 2010; Moore, Redd, Burkhauser, Mbwana, & Collins, 2009).

These circumstances and their consequences are not trivial for American society. The accompaniments and consequences of poverty affect the 24% of infants and toddlers under the age of 3 who live in families below the federal poverty level (FPL). If one considers 200% of the FPL to indicate low income, this group includes a whopping 46% of children under 3; the latter means that 5.9 million children grow up in circumstances that do not lead to the positive outcomes American society needs for all its children (Chau, Thampi, & Wight, 2010).

Children growing up in poverty have very different outcomes than their more-advantaged peers, resulting in a large achievement gap, even at the outset of schooling (Rouse, Brooks-Gunn, & McLanahan, 2005). From the early 1960s through the mid-1990s, many interventions have been tried, with varying degrees of success, to enhance the developmental trajectories of infants and toddlers in the areas that are most likely to improve their chances for successful entry into kindergarten—and for continuing successful progress through school (Brooks-Gunn & Markman, 2005; Currie, 2001). The familiar list of programs includes the Syracuse Family Development Program (Lally, Mangione, & Honig, 1988), the Ypsilanti–Carnegie Infant Education Project (Lambie, Bond, & Weikart, 1974), Levenstein's Verbal Interaction Project/Parent–Child Home Program (Levenstein, Levenstein, Shiminski, & Stpolzberg, 1998; Levenstein & Levenstein, 2008), the Carolina Abecedarian Project (Campbell & Ramey, 1995), the Comprehensive Child Development Program (St. Pierre, Layzer, Goodson, & Bernstein, 1997), the Infant Health and Development Project (IHDP, Brooks-Gunn, Lebanon, Liaw, & Spiker, 1993; McCormick et al., 2006, Nurse–Family Partnership (e.g., Olds et al., 2007), and Parents as Teachers

(PAT; Drotar, Robinson, Jeavons, & Lester Kirchner, 2009; Wagner, Clayton, Gerlach-Downie, & McElroy, 1999).

But none (except PAT) has been attempted on a scale as large as that of the federal Early Head Start (EHS) program. EHS is a two-generation program designed to provide high-quality child and family development services to low-income pregnant women and families with infants and toddlers. EHS began with 68 programs in 1995, grew steadily through the years, and with recent federal stimulus finds, the program increased in 2011 to about 1,000 programs serving more than 100,000 children. As with Head Start, EHS offers children and families comprehensive child development services through center-based, home-based, and combination program options.

In this chapter, we show how this relatively recent, national intervention has strived to alter the developmental trajectories of thousands of infants and toddlers in low-income families. We show how EHS has the potential for altering the life course of infants and toddlers in poverty in all the areas of development commonly associated with kindergarten readiness. We show how evidence from the EHS national evaluation demonstrates not only significant gains by age 3 when families complete their enrollment in EHS programs but also gains that are maintained 2 years later. We show that, indeed, preparations for school readiness begin during the infant–toddler years, but caution that the continuation of these gains into the school years does not happen automatically. Finally, in summarizing the implications of these findings for delivering effective infant–toddler programs, we show areas in which EHS programs need to be strengthened if they are to have stronger and broader benefits for the children and families they serve.[1]

Early Head Start Effects at Ages 3 and 5

The EHS evaluation began in 1995 when the Administration for Children and Families (ACF) funded the first cohort of 68 programs.[2] By design, ACF selected 17 programs to study from the first two cohorts of programs funded. Each selected program was required to partner with a viable university-based research group. The sites were distributed across the country, including rural and urban sites. Analyses demonstrated that, although the programs were not a statistical representative sample, they did reflect the diverse characteristics of all programs in operation at that time (see Administration for Children and Families, 2001, chapter I). The 17 programs recruited twice as many families as they could serve and Mathematica randomly assigned 3,001 to the treatment and control groups. All families were low income. Thirty-five percent of the sample was African American, 37% Hispanic, and 37% white. At the time of enrollment, 75% of mothers were unmarried, 48% had less than a high school education, 39% were teenage mothers, 55% were not employed or in school or job training, and 35% of the households received Aid to Families with Dependent Children/ Temporary Assistance to Needy Families. This was the first impact evaluation of services for poor pregnant women and families with children under age 3 in which some program sites offered center-based services (with a relatively low level of home visits), others offered only home visiting, while still others provided both center-based care and home visitation. Of the 17 sites, four provided only center-based care, six provided only home-based, and seven programs provided both center- and home-based services.

The EHS evaluation examined impacts for these three types of programs—referred to here as center-based, home-based, and mixed-approach programs—when families were still enrolled in the program (when children were 2 and 3 years of age), and in a PreK follow-up 2 years later. After the original evaluation ended and children left the program (or control condition) to enter whatever programs awaited them between ages 3 and 5, we tracked children's program attendance. Program group children (across all program approaches) were significantly more likely than their control counterparts to enroll in formal preschool programs at ages 3–5 (47% vs. 42%; $p < .05$) and, in particular, more likely to be in Head Start at some time between ages 3 and 5 (55% vs. 49%; $p < .01$).[3] Although the treatment group in this evaluation was significantly more likely to experience formal PreK programs between ages 3 and 5, the control group was catching up in that the differences in program participation rates between the program and control groups in the 2-year postexperiment period were not large, as seen in the preceding percentage differences.

The EHS evaluation also captured in-depth information about all program services required by the then newly released Head Start Program Performance Standards (which had been expanded to include requirements for programs serving pregnant women and families with infants and toddlers). The evaluation team created detailed rating scales for assessing the extent to which programs implemented services that met the requirements laid out in the EHS grant solicitation and Head Start Performance Standards in all areas, including child development, family development, staffing, and program management. Researchers applied the rating scales in a consensus-based process based on qualitative and quantitative data collected during two rounds of site visits. The ratings were validated with program monitoring data. Based on these ratings, it was possible to categorize programs in terms of the timing with which they fully met the standards: early implementers, later implementers, and incomplete implementers (see our report, *Pathways to Quality,* for details; Administration for Children and Families, 2002b). Because multisite trials often (perhaps always) show variability in impacts across sites, it was crucial to document fidelity to the program requirements and standards.

Analytic Approach

We present the impacts of participation in EHS on child and family outcomes as differences in mean outcomes between the program and control groups. To adjust for any differences in the observable characteristics of the two groups due to random sampling and interview nonresponse, we estimated regression-adjusted means for each group, controlling for a large number of covariates measured before random assignment. Each site was weighted equally because EHS services are administered at the site level and differ across programs. In this chapter, we present findings from the experimental analyses using what is often referred to as a "treatment on the treated" (TOT) analysis. That is, we identified the EHS program sample members who received some program services and adjusted the treatment–control comparisons for this reduced sample. The impact per participant in a site was obtained by dividing the impact per eligible applicant in that site by the site's program group participation rate. The estimated global impact per participant across all sites was then calculated as the average of the estimated impacts per participant in each site.

We defined an EHS participant as a program group member who received more than one EHS home visit, met with an EHS case manager more than once, received at least 2 weeks of EHS center-based care, and/or participated in EHS group parent–child socialization activities. More than 91% of those families assigned to EHS participated by this definition, and we found no differences between impact estimates that compared program group "participants" with the control group (TOT), as we report here, and impact estimates that compared the entire program and control groups (intent to treat; see Administration for Children and Families, 2002a, volume II).

Overall Impact Findings

Overall, averaging across all program sites and all children and families in the sample, EHS programs showed significant impacts on a wide range of child and parent outcomes when the children were 3 years old, at the end of the program. These included impacts in cognitive, language, and social–emotional development. (Many of the effects appeared as early as age 2 and were, for the most part, maintained through age 3; see Administration for Children and Families, 2001, 2002a.) Two years later, at age 5, significant impacts continued to be seen in the social–emotional domain and approaches to learning. However, the former EHS group did not continue to show the impacts on vocabulary seen in the earlier years, except for the children who were still tested in Spanish at the PreK follow-up; EHS children did not differ from control group children on measures of school-related achievement. Table 13.1 presents findings for selected child, parenting, and

TABLE 13.1. Impacts on Selected Child and Family Outcomes at Ages 3 and 5: Full Sample

	Program–control differences							
	Age 3				Age 5			
Outcome	Program group participants[a]	Control group[b]	Impact estimate[c]	Effect size[d]	Program group participants[a]	Control group[b]	Impact estimate[c]	Effect size[d]
Child social–emotional development and approaches to learning								
CBCL Aggressive Behavior	10.6	11.3	-0.7*	-0.11	10.6	11.0	-0.4	-0.05
FACES Social Behavior Problems					5.3	5.7	-0.4*	-0.12
Engagement during Play	4.8	4.6	0.2**	0.20	4.7	4.7	-0.0	-0.01
Sustained Attention with Objects during Play	5.0	4.8	0.2**	0.16				
FACES Positive Approaches to Learning					12.2	11.9	0.3**	0.14
Observed Attention					8.6	8.4	0.2+	0.09
Leiter Attention Sustained					10.9	10.9	0.1	0.02
Child language, cognitive, and academic skills								
English Receptive Vocabulary (PPVT)	83.3	81.1	2.1*	0.13	91.9	90.6	1.3	0.09
Spanish Receptive Vocabulary (TVIP)	97.2	94.9	2.3	0.27	90.0	83.0	7.0*	0.29
Average Bayley MDI	91.4	89.9	1.6*	0.12				
Woodcock–Johnson Letter–Word Identification (English)					89.5	90.4	-0.9	-0.06
Woodcock–Johnson Applied Problems					89.8	88.4	1.4	0.07
Parenting and the home environment								
HOME Language and Literacy	10.6	10.4	0.2*	0.10	10.4	10.3	0.1	0.03
Percent Reading Daily	56.8	52.0	4.9*	0.10	34.0	29.3	4.8*	0.10
Percent Spanked Last Week	46.7	53.8	-7.1**	-0.14	35.3	36.6	-1.2	-0.03
Parent Supportiveness during Play	4.0	3.9	0.1**	0.15	4.0	3.9	0.1	0.06

Measure	Age 3: Program group mean [a]	Control group mean [b]	Impact per participant [c]	Effect size [d]	Age 5: Program group mean [a]	Control group mean [b]	Impact per participant [c]	Effect size [d]
Teaching Activities	4.4	4.3	0.1+	0.09	11.3	11.0	0.3*	0.11
Parent Attends Meetings/Open Houses [e]					87.5	79.2	8.3**	0.21
Parent self-sufficiency								
Employed [f]	86.8	83.4	3.4+	0.09	3.6	3.5	0.1	0.04
In School or Job Training [g]	60.0	51.4	8.6**	0.17				
Income (dollars) [h]	16,871.7	17,813.1	−941.4	−0.07	2,337.8	2,258.5	79.3	0.04
Sample sizes								
Parent Interview	1,105	999	2,104		978	1,084	2,062	
Parent–Child Interactions	874	784	1,658		827	890	1,717	
Bayley MDI	879	779	1,658		NA	NA	NA	
Child Assessments	928	832	1,760		836	919	1,755	

Note. Sources are parent interviews, interviewer observations, and assessments of semistructured parent–child interactions conducted when children were age 3 or in their PreK year. HOME, Home Observation for Measurement of the Environment; CBCL, Child Behavior Check List; FACES, Family and Child Experiences Survey; PPVT, Peabody Picture Vocabulary Test; TVIP, Test de Vocabulario de Imagines Peabody. All impact estimates were calculated using regression models in which each site was weighted equally.

[a] A participant is defined as a program group member who received more than one EHS home visit, met with an EHS case manager more than once, received at least 2 weeks of EHS center-based care, and/or participated in EHS group parent–child activities.

[b] The control group mean is the mean for the control group members who would have participated in EHS if they had been assigned to the program group instead. This unobserved mean was estimated as the difference between the program group mean for participants and the impact per participant.

[c] The estimated impact per participant is measured as the estimated impact per eligible applicant divided by the proportion of program group members who participated in EHS services (which varied by site). The estimated impact per eligible applicant is measured as the difference between the regression-adjusted means for all program and control group members.

[d] The effect size was calculated by dividing the estimated impact per participant by the standard deviation of the outcome measure for the control group.

[e] Includes only parents whose children were in a formal program.

[f] At age 3 the time frame for this question is 26 months after random assignment. Sample sizes for this outcome were $N = 440$ and $N = 467$ for program and control groups, respectively, but at age 5 we asked "How much time in the past 6 months have you held a job or jobs in which you worked at least 20 hours per week?" Answers were on a 5-point scale from $1 = never$ to $5 = all$ of the $time$.

[g] At age 3 the time frame for this question is 26 months after random assignment.

[h] At age 3 the time frame for this question is 26 months after random assignment. Amounts are annual income at age 3 and monthly income at age 5.

$+p < .10$; $*p < .05$; $**p < .01$.

family impacts at ages 3 and 5.[4] In our view, impacts on parenting and the home environment were as important as the child impacts, because these are crucial mediators of young children's later development. The program enhanced parental support for children's language and literacy development, daily reading, and teaching activities at age 3 with, for the most part, these effects continuing through age 5. Details of these findings follow.

Child Social–Emotional Outcomes and Approaches to Learning

We found positive impacts on several outcomes in this area. At each age, parent–child dyads were videotaped while engaging in a semistructured play interaction. Both parent and child behaviors were later coded. At age 3, program group children were more engaged and displayed greater attention during play than control group children. The program group children also were rated by their mothers as being less aggressive than the control group children. Group means were not significantly different at age 5 on this same measure. However, at age 5, social behavior problems as measured by the Head Start Family and Child Experiences Survey (FACES) scale, were significantly lower in the program group, indicating a pattern of the EHS intervention reducing aggressive behavior at both ages.

Sustained attention with objects during play was higher in the program group at age 3, and at age 5, the program group showed more positive approaches to learning (this FACES measure also taps attention) and higher observed attention scores on the Leiter (an observation made by assessors during the test administration).

Child Language, Cognitive, and Academic Skills

EHS enhanced children's cognitive skills at age 3, as evidenced by higher Bayley Mental Development Index scores. Vocabulary was positively affected as well—as measured by the Peabody Picture Vocabulary Test (PPVT-III). At age 5, the two groups did not differ in their PPVT-III scores. For those children taking the Spanish version of the PPVT (TVIP; Test de Vocabulario de Imagines Peabody), however, we found no significant differences at age 3, but these became significant at age 5. (The group of children taking the TVIP was small, particularly at age 5.) We found no group differences on the early achievement test scores at age 5 (Woodcock–Johnson Letter–Word Identification and Applied Problems).

Parenting and the Home Environment

When the children were 3 years old, mothers in the program group engaged in more stimulating activities with their children than control group mothers. EHS mothers had higher language scores on the Home Observation for Measurement of the Environment (HOME) measure, were more likely to read daily to their children, initiated more teaching activities, and exhibited higher supportiveness during play. At age 5, these effects were sustained for reading daily and teaching activities, although there were no longer any significant differences for HOME language scores or supportiveness during play. In addition, mothers of the 5-year-olds who had participated in EHS (and who were enrolled in a formal program at that time) were more likely to attend meetings at the child's school. With respect to negative parenting, mothers in the program group were less likely to spank their 3-year-olds than control group parents. This difference was not evident at age 5, however.

Parental Self-Sufficiency

We found a trend for a higher percentage of mothers in the program group to be employed when their children were age 3 but not at age 5. The percentage of employed mothers was high—87% at age 3. Further, EHS mothers were more likely to be in school or to have a job. We found no group differences in income at any age point in the full-group analysis. Given that so many mothers in both groups were employed, this finding is not surprising.

Impact Analyses by Key Subgroups

In many ways, the most important messages about the value of EHS come from understanding what happened in various subgroups. We know that averages don't tell the whole story, especially when considerable variability exists within any group we are studying, and EHS programs and families differ along many dimensions. These include community characteristics (such as urban–rural settings), program characteristics (such as the approaches implemented and patterns of fidelity of implementation), race and ethnicity of families enrolled, extent to which families experience various demographic risk factors, and so forth. We focus here on five key subgroups defined by (1) the type of program implemented, (2) the quality (or fidelity) of program implementation, (3) the families' race/ethnicity, (4) whether the family enrolled during pregnancy, and (5) families' level of risk.

Program Approach

When we focused on the age 3 impacts, the lesson was clear. Across the program sites that implemented a "mixed" approach to providing services (i.e., they enrolled families in either center- or home-based services or both), the impacts on children and families were stronger than the impacts observed for children and families in the home- or center-based programs.[5,6] For example, at age 3, mixed-approach programs had strong impacts on children's vocabulary (effect size [ES] = .23, $p < .05$), children's sustained attention with objects during parent–child play (ES = .31, $p < .01$), and the percentage of parents who reported reading to their child every day (ES = .28, $p < .01$).

One of the more noteworthy findings at the age-5 follow-up was a change in the apparent importance of a particular program approach. Whereas mixed-approach programs had more impacts at age 3, it was the home-based approach that seemed to provide the greatest benefits for children and parents 2 years later. And although we did not observe a large number of impacts for the children from home-based programs at age 5 (impacts included reduction in behavior problems and enhanced approaches to learning), we found several parenting impacts (HOME language and literacy, percentage of parents reading to their child every day, and teaching activities), and perhaps most significant, the only impact on earnings found in this study was seen for Hispanic parents—with a significant treatment–control difference in income of $302 per month.

Quality of Program Implementation

As noted earlier, as part of the EHS implementation study, we measured the extent to which programs met the criteria set forth in the Head Start Program Performance Standards along several dimensions. At the end of program participation (age 3) across the programs that we classified as fully implemented, the impacts for children and families were greater than in the programs that had only incompletely implemented the quality standards within the evaluation time frame (see Love et al., 2005). However, at age 5, differential impacts by pattern of implementation had practically disappeared.

Family Race/Ethnicity

EHS had more-positive impacts on African American children and families than on Hispanic or white families (and with substantially larger ESs than for the overall impacts—often one-third to one-half of a standard deviation; Administration for Children and Families, 2002a). These effects were sustained at age 5 in areas of reduced aggressive behavior problems, positive approaches to learning, attention, and engagement, and receptive vocabulary—but not in the achievement-related outcomes of letter–word identification and applied problems (Administration for Children and

Families, 2002a). Additionally, effects on African American parents were sustained at age 5 in observed supportiveness during play (Administration for Children and Families, 2006). As has been seen in other programs, such as IHDP (Duncan et al., 1994), the African American families in the EHS study were more disadvantaged than the white and Hispanic families. As can be seen from the means for control group members, the African American families had lower levels of positive parenting, reading to their children, and learning activities than the other racial/ethnic control groups. In addition, the African American children in the control group had lower means on cognitive and language outcomes than did the white children in the control group. If a subset of children and mothers have, in the absence of an intervention, lower scores on outcomes being targeted by an intervention, it is possible that they might benefit more from a particular intervention.

Few impacts of EHS were found for Hispanic children at ages 2 and 3, but important ones appeared in PreK, including positive approaches to learning and receptive vocabulary for the Spanish-speaking Hispanic children. Hispanic parents continued to be more likely to read to their children every day at age 5 as they had at age 3 relative to the control group (although the percentage declined). At age 3, Hispanic EHS parents were more likely to be in school or job training compared with their control group counterparts; and when their children were 5, Hispanic parents were somewhat more likely to be employed.

Time of Enrollment

When families enrolled while the mother was pregnant, EHS had stronger impacts than when families enrolled after the child's birth (Administration for Children and Families, 2002a). At age 3, impacts on children's cognitive and social–emotional development, as well as some parenting behaviors, were stronger for those who enrolled during pregnancy. However, at age 5, differential impacts by age of enrollment had mostly disappeared.

Family Risk

One finding that initially surprised us was that the families with the highest risk levels, as defined in this study, showed no positive impacts of the program when children were 3 years old.[7] Effects were more likely to be seen in families with moderate risk levels (Administration for Children and Families, 2002a). At age 5, however, some impacts for the high-risk group emerged—for children (in approaches to learning) and for parenting and home environment outcomes (supportiveness during play and reduction in percentage of families in which someone in the household had an alcohol or drug problem in the past year). However, it was in the higher-risk group that we also found one of the few negative impacts in the EHS study—children in the EHS high-risk group scored significantly lower than high-risk controls on the Woodcock–Johnson Letter–Word Identification test at age 5. In the moderate-risk group a number of impacts remained at age 5, in social–emotional and attention domains, and parenting. At age 5, EHS moderate-risk parents had significantly fewer depressive symptoms than reported by moderate-risk parents in the control group.

Nonexperimental Analyses

The results reviewed so far are from analyses conducted within the framework of the randomized experimental design, looking at experiences in the 0 to 3 age range, which were experimentally controlled. In addition to these impact analyses, the team conducted nonexperimental analyses in an effort to learn about the contributions of children's experiences from birth (or, at times, before birth) to age 3, and after the EHS intervention between ages 3 and 5 to functioning at kindergarten entry, controlling for child and family baseline characteristics. The main message from these analyses is that the children and families who experienced EHS *followed by* center-based formal program enrollment (whether Head Start, preschool, or center child care) in the 3- to 5-year age period demonstrated the most favorable PreK outcomes (Administration for Children and Families, 2006; Love, Chazan-Cohen, Raikes, & Brooks-Gunn, in press). However, these analyses are not based on randomization (i.e., children were not assigned to be in formal programs or not at the end of EHS) and thus are subject to selection bias, although our analyses included multiple controls for selection.

Experiences between Ages 3 and 5

Our tracking data (collected from interviews with families after they left their EHS program) enabled us to distinguish children who experienced formal programs (FPs) in each of the 2 years between the original experiment and the PreK follow-up. Some children enrolled in FPs in both the 3 to 4 and 4 to 5 age periods, some enrolled during only one of those periods, and some never enrolled in an FP. For the EHS program group, 49% were enrolled in an FP at ages 3 to 4, 82% at ages 4 to 5, and 47% at both ages 3 to 4 and 4 to 5. Among control group children, enrollment rates were lower: 44% were in FPs at ages 3 to 4, 82% at ages 4 to 5, and 42% at both ages 3 to 4 and 4 to 5. Fifty-five percent of the program group and 49% of the control group enrolled in Head Start at some point between ages 3 and 5.

Analytic Approach

We conducted analyses with the 2,273 children for whom we had data on whether they participated in center-based program settings at ages 3 to 4 and 4 to 5. Families in both the program and control groups could have enrolled their children in any formal early care and education programs that existed in their communities. Children were not randomly assigned to enter FPs, so families who placed their child in an FP during both preschool years may have differed from those who did not in ways that could also influence child and parenting outcomes. In fact, background characteristics differed based on participation in services during the 3 to 5 age period. Specifically, children who experienced FPs in the 3 to 5 age period were (1) more likely to be African American and less likely to be Hispanic or white, (2) less likely to have lived with two parents at baseline, and (3) more likely to have had mothers with an education beyond high school at baseline. In addition, children who were born premature or at a low birthweight were more likely to attend formal programs or Head Start, but only if they had experienced EHS. To some extent, these observed differences reflect parental choice in selecting early care and education settings for their children, but they may also reflect differences in what was available in different communities as well as eligibility requirements of programs. For instance, some families may not have been able to participate in Head Start because they had incomes above the federal poverty level when their children were 3 to 5 years old. To minimize potential selection bias, we estimated regression models that examined the associations among FP participation during both preschool years, exposure to Head Start, and PreK outcomes, controlling for these and other observed differences between the groups. The regressions controlled for:

- The outcome at age 3 (using the same measure or the closest measure available at that age). To the extent that later outcomes can be predicted by the earlier ones, any fixed observed and unobserved factors that affect outcomes over time would be controlled by the inclusion of the earlier outcome.
- EHS status, to control for any continuing influence of EHS experiences on outcomes.
- Child and family background characteristics that could influence outcomes, such as the child's gender, birthweight, birth order, race/ethnicity, and age at assessment, and the parent's age at the child's birth, highest grade completed, language and cognition skill, work and welfare experience when the child was young, marital status and living arrangements, whether the mother had more children during the first 2 years after entering the study, maternal risk of depression when the child was 3 years old, and site.

Because not all potential differences among the groups of children could be controlled in the analyses, caution must be exercised in interpreting the results. Any differences in outcomes could be due to differences in formal early care and education experiences or to other unmeasured differences that are correlated with the experiences and outcomes. We estimated the models using maximum likelihood estimation methods with the Mplus4 software. The maximum likelihood methods available in Mplus were chosen because they use all available data and produce statistically efficient estimates of the relationships between FP participation and PreK outcomes. In a test of the sensitivity of results for handling missing data, we conducted multiple imputation procedures in SAS software, which yielded results that were very similar to those produced by Mplus. Results are depicted in Table 13.2.

TABLE 13.2. Associations of Formal Program Participation at Both Preschool Ages and Any Head Start Experience with Child and Family Outcomes, in Effect Size Units

	Formal program participation at both preschool ages	Any preschool Head Start experience
Child social–emotional outcomes		
CBCL Aggressive Behavior	0.09*	−0.01
FACES Aggression	0.10*	−0.04
FACES Social Behavior Problems	0.12**	−0.04
FACES Positive Approaches to Learning	−0.04	0.01
Engagement during Play	0.04	0.07
Child academic outcomes		
Woodcock–Johnson-R Letter–Word Identification administered in English (N = 1,751)	0.09*	0.08+
English Receptive Vocabulary (PPVT; N = 1,674)	0.01	0.00
Spanish Receptive Vocabulary (TVIP; N = 170)	0.00	−0.26*
Woodcock–Johnson-R Applied Problems	−0.03	0.08+
Sample sizes (except as noted above)	1,712–2,063	1,712–2,063

$+ p < .10$; $* p < .05$; $** p < .01$.

Results: Associations between FP Participation and PreK Outcomes

Child Social–Emotional Outcomes and Approaches to Learning

Formal early care and education program participation during both preschool years was associated with more-aggressive behavior and greater behavior problems as reported by parents when their children were entering kindergarten. This pattern of findings is consistent across several measures of negative social–emotional outcomes. Controlling for other factors, children with FP participation in both the 3 to 4 and 4 to 5 years exhibited significantly more aggressive behaviors than other children who received no FP experience or FP experience in only 1 year between ages 3 and 5, according to their parents' reports. However, participation in Head Start was not associated with increased aggressive behavior or social behavior problems. Neither FP participation in both preschool years nor Head Start participation was significantly associated with children's positive social–emotional outcomes and approaches to learning.

Child Vocabulary and Academic Skills

FP participation in both preschool years was associated with higher scores on the Woodcock–Johnson-R Letter–Word Identification subtest (i.e., better prereading skills), but was not associated with better vocabulary or math skills. It is notable that any experience in preschool Head Start was associated with more-positive prereading and math skills, but negatively associated with receptive vocabulary for the Spanish-speaking children.

Considering both the experimental and nonexperimental findings, experiences 0 to 3 (EHS vs. no EHS) were related to more-positive social–emotional and parenting outcomes, whereas participation in formal early care and education programs 3 to 5 was associated with more-aggressive behavior and better prereading academic skills. Thus, to maximize positive outcomes across domains when children are entering kindergarten, programs in both age periods may be needed: It appears that EHS should be followed by formal early care and education experiences before children enter kindergarten.

Interpretations and Implications of Findings

Some of the most persistent impacts of EHS were in domains particularly important for later success in school. For example, aggressive behavior problems, which EHS programs significantly reduced at both age points, are predictive of later behavior problems and low school engagement (Caspi, Moffitt, Newman, & Silva, 1996; Dishion, French, & Paterson,

1995). Attention, which EHS also influenced positively at age 5, is linked to school achievement (Duncan et al., 2007). Parent reading to children (and learning stimulation) is also linked to positive academic outcomes later on (Phillips, Brooks-Gunn, Duncan, Klebanov, & Jencks, 1998). Nevertheless, EHS failed to produce clear impacts on academic achievement-related performance at age 5 (in the full-group analyses), even though significant cognitive and language impacts were apparent at age 3.

We now consider a number of factors that are important about the EHS findings: context, quality, impacts for Hispanic children, and continuity.

Context

When we consider that these impacts occurred when averaged across 17 program sites that were among the first 143 programs to be funded in a large-scale, nationwide rollout of a completely new initiative, they really are quite notable, even though the effects are smaller when compared with the common benchmark Abecedarian Project (Campbell, Ramey, Pungello, Sparling, & Miller-Johnson, 2002).

Several contextual issues are apparent, some of which are amenable to further testing, some not. The first has to do with the counterfactual, vis-à-vis what is available in communities and what is needed by parents. With more low-income mothers working than ever before (Moore et al., 2009), child care is necessary; families in the control group who did not receive child care provided by their EHS programs had to find it on their own. Compared to studies of the 1970s, many more of the EHS study control group children were in child care. The more modest effects of EHS could be a function of differences in services available to control group families in the late 1990s and early 2000s compared with those available in the 1970s. Indeed, in a propensity scoring matching procedure used in IHDP, the largest impacts were seen for children who, if not in the treatment group, would have not been in child care (Hill & Reiter, 2006). If the majority of poor mothers are working, then EHS services, as currently implemented, will not be of much help on the child care front (i.e., given the relatively small number of full-time, full-year, center-based care centers in the EHS family of programs).

A second issue has to do with the proximal goals of EHS compared with Abecedarian and IHDP. The two earlier programs focused primarily on child cognitive and language development. In EHS, enhancing child development was the main goal, but programs also focused to varying degrees on improving parenting and family environment as key ways of promoting child development; the latter was especially true in the home-based and mixed-approach programs. The impacts found are consistent with what programs tried to achieve, as confirmed by examining their logic models or theories of change (Administration for Children and Families, 2002b).

A third and related issue has to do with home visiting and center-based education. We are unable to make definitive statements about whether one or the other is most effective (for certain outcomes) or whether a mixed-approach is most beneficial, given the inconsistent impacts for these sub-groups seen at ages 3 and 5.

Focus on Quality Services

Head Start performance standards define quality comprehensively, and include requirements for certain levels of service breadth and intensity. The standards encompass services that include child and family development services, staff development, community building, and program manage-ment; for programs, doing things well means doing as much of the required programmatic activities as possible. The findings from the EHS evaluation show the importance of program quality, as defined through these stan-dards, for achieving program goals. We saw that when programs had not achieved good quality, they generally were unable to produce their intended effects on children and families by the end of the families' enrollment, at least in terms of the age 3 impacts.

Enhancing Impacts for Hispanic Children and Families

At age 5, EHS had an impact on receptive vocabulary for Spanish-speaking children, yet impacts overall for the Hispanic subgroup (including both English- and Spanish-speaking Hispanic children) were not notable. More needs to be done to understand why impacts are smaller for this group of children and families, especially because the same pattern was found in the Head Start Impact Study (Administration for Children and Families, 2010). We recommend experimentation with different intervention models, curricula, and various instructional strategies for dual language learners to identify best practices. (Work in this area is currently being funded by the National Institute of Child Health and Human Development and Adminis-tration for Children and Families.)

With the U.S. Hispanic population growing rapidly, programs like EHS must be ready to serve—and positively impact—these children and parents. This is particularly important in that Hispanic children are significant less likely to be enrolled in programs in the first 5 years of life than white and African American children (Magnuson & Waldfogel, 2005). Differences in enrollment rates may explain part of the test score gap between Hispanic and white children upon entrance to school. We recommend more work to determine why the enrollment rates are so different (supply, information, distrust of programs, concerns about immigration status?). In addition,

we welcome experimental testing of different models for increasing enrollment.

Continuity

The Office of Head Start surely intended for EHS to positively impact cognitive, language, and academic outcomes when children were age 3 and,
with subsequent Head Start and other preschool program experiences, for
the effects to be sustained at least until kindergarten entry. We did not
find overall sustained effects, but we did not find that most of the children
received the intended follow-up services, either. The good news at age 5,
however, was that EHS achieved overall impacts in some facets of development important for school readiness and long-term school outcomes: reducing aggressive behavior and improving positive approaches to learning for
children and enhancing their home environments. In addition, the program
produced vocabulary gains for African American children and Hispanic
Spanish-speaking children.

Most important, it appears that those EHS children and families whose
EHS enrollment was followed by FPs in the 3- to 5-year age period fared
the best overall. They experienced benefits in social–emotional, parenting,
and home environment from EHS along with some benefits in achievement-
oriented outcomes from their formal preschool program participation during ages 3 to 5. Finally, EHS seems to be especially effective for families that
enroll during pregnancy. Thus, it appears to us that following a prenatal-
to-3 program like EHS with formal preschool programs in the 3- to 5-year
age period creates the greatest opportunity for ensuring that children from
low-income families will begin formal schooling on a more positive foot-
ing. This finding is important because few programs have attempted a full
birth to age 5 intervention within a single program—the notable exceptions
are the Abecedarian Project (Campbell & Ramey, 1995) and the Comprehensive Child Development Program (St. Pierre et al., 1997). However, the
fact that links are seen with the robust set of control variables we used in
EHS leads us to speculate that larger impacts would be seen if continuity
of services were provided, beginning during pregnancy and following EHS
through the preschool years for all children. Our findings echo the call
made by many (including Heckman & Masterov, 2004; Reynolds, Wang,
& Walberg, 2003) that early intervention should be followed by continued
supportive services. It would be useful to be able to document where children go when they leave EHS—and/or create plans (much like an individualized education plan) for the services they should receive after graduating
from EHS. It would be useful to test various models for providing this
continuity.

Future Program Evaluations

Finally, we note a number of important implications for future evaluations of complex service programs for young children and their families:

1. Invest in thorough documentation of implementation fidelity and investigation of the contrast between the experiences of children and families in the intervention and control groups to support interpretation of the estimated impacts (or lack thereof).
2. Identify key subgroups of programs and families up front and plan for analyses of impacts within these subgroups.
3. Consider supplementing the main experimental analyses with additional exploratory analyses and careful nonexperimental analyses for investigating policy questions that fall outside the impact analyses.

Conclusions

The data described in this paper come from one of the many programs serving children who are most in need of support for realizing their potential. We hope that four conclusions, grounded in findings from the EHS program evaluation and its follow-up studies, will guide future policies for comprehensive programs serving low-income families and their children.

To maximize the benefits of early childhood programs in enhancing disadvantaged children's school readiness and later success in school, we need programs that (1) are of the highest possible quality and able to engage families fully in services, (2) begin at birth (or before), (3) either continue until the children enter kindergarten or provide for continuity of program services across programs throughout this 5-year period, and (4) work with the schools to ensure that educational and other services continue to support the learning and development of children from low-income families once the children are attending the schools.

ACKNOWLEDGMENTS

The findings reported here are based on research conducted as part of the national Early Head Start Research and Evaluation Project funded by the Administration for Children and Families (ACF), U.S. Department of Health and Human Services under Contract 105-95-1936 to Mathematica Policy Research, Princeton, New Jersey, and Columbia University's National Center for Children and Families, Teachers College, in conjunction with the Early Head Start Research Consortium (for the 0 to 3 phase) and under Task Order No. 32, Contract 282-98-0021, to Mathematica

Policy Research, Princeton, New Jersey, and grants for data collection with 15 university research partners (for the PreK follow-up). The Consortium consists of representatives from 17 programs participating in the evaluation, 15 local research teams, the evaluation contractors, and ACF. Research institutions in the Consortium (and principal researchers for conducting this research through 36 months of age) have included ACF (Rachel Chazan-Cohen, Judith Jerald, Esther Kresh, Helen Raikes, and Louisa Tarullo); Catholic University of America (Michaela Farber, Harriet Liebow, Nancy Taylor, Elizabeth Timberlake, and Shavaun Wall); Columbia University (Lisa Berlin, Christy Brady-Smith, Jeanne Brooks-Gunn, and Allison Sidle Fuligni); Harvard University (Catherine Ayoub, Barbara Alexander Pan, and Catherine Snow); Iowa State University (Dee Draper, Gayle Luze, Susan McBride, and Carla Peterson); Mathematica Policy Research (Kimberly Boller, Jill Constantine, Ellen Eliason Kisker, John M. Love, Diane Paulsell, Christine Ross, Peter Schochet, Susan Sprachman, Cheri Vogel, and Welmoet van Kammen); Medical University of South Carolina (Richard Faldowski, Gui-Young Hong, and Susan Pickrel); Michigan State University (Hiram Fitzgerald, Tom Reischl, and Rachel Schiffman); New York University (Mark Spellmann and Catherine Tamis-LeMonda); University of Arkansas (Robert Bradley, Richard Clubb, Andrea Hart, Mark Swanson, and Leanne Whiteside-Mansell); University of California, Los Angeles (Carollee Howes and Claire Hamilton); University of Colorado Health Sciences Center (Robert Emde, Jon Korfmacher, JoAnn Robinson, Paul Spicer, and Norman Watt); University of Kansas (Jane Atwater, Judith Carta, and Jean Ann Summers); University of Missouri–Columbia (Mark Fine, Jean Ispa, and Kathy Thornburg); University of Pittsburgh (Beth Green, Carol McAllister, and Robert McCall); University of Washington College of Education (Eduardo Armijo and Joseph Stowitschek); University of Washington School of Nursing (Kathryn Barnard and Susan Spieker), and Utah State University (Lisa Boyce, Catherine Callow-Heusser, Gina Cook, and Lori Roggman). We also are grateful to Rachel McKinnon of Columbia University for assistance in tracking down reference citations.

The content of this publication does not necessarily reflect the views or policies of the U.S. Department of Health and Human Services, nor does mention of trade names, commercial products, or organizations imply endorsement by the U.S. government.

NOTES

1. More details on the EHS findings can be found in the evaluation's technical reports (ACF, 2001, 2002a, 2006; Love et al., 2005; Love, Chazan-Cohen, Raikes, & Brooks-Gunn, in press).
2. We have participated in EHS evaluation activities across a number of contracts that the ACF has funded to evaluate the implementation and effectiveness of the program. In this chapter, we examine the key findings from the EHS evaluation through the months preceding children's entry into kindergarten (about age 5), with attention to how the earlier program impacts at age 3 relate to the later outcomes. The analyses were conducted by Mathematica Policy Research and Columbia University's National Center for Children and Families and our

collaborators from sister institutions in the EHS Research Consortium (ACF, 2002a, 2006; Love et al., 2005).

3. These analyses used the same regression-adjusted impact analyses with baseline controls, as described in note 4.

4. The ES was calculated by dividing the estimated impact per participant by the standard deviation of the outcome measure for the control group (Cohen's d; Cohen, 1988). We used two-tailed tests to gauge the statistical significance of the estimated impacts, without corrections for multiple comparisons. We report significant impacts when $p < .05$; we report impact estimates with $p < .10$ as approaching significance or as "trends" when they contribute to a conceptually consistent pattern of impacts across multiple outcomes or time points. We estimated separate models for each outcome measure and discuss results for each of the child, parent, and family domains we assessed.

5. Due to space limitations, we do not present tables of findings for all the subgroup analyses. These are available in the EHS national evaluation's technical reports (*www.acf.hhs.gov/programs/opre/ehs/ehs_resrch/index.html* and in a number of publications, primarily Love et al., 2005, 2009).

6. Families were not randomly assigned to the three program approaches; however, because programs serve families by identifying the mix of program services that would best meet families' needs, assigning families to those services at random would create an unrealistic situation that would not be generalizable to other EHS programs. However, a planned variation experiment could be very useful for documenting what services are most likely to impact children's outcomes for different types of families (and why).

7. Within the EHS low-income sample, we considered five risk factors: (1) single parent, (2) receiving public assistance, (3) neither employed nor in school or job training, (4) teenage parent, and (5) no high school diploma or graduate equivalency diploma (GED). Low-risk families were defined as having only one or two of these characteristics, moderate-risk families had any three, and high-risk families had any four or five risk characteristics.

REFERENCES

Administration for Children and Families. (2001, June). *Building their futures: How Early Head Start programs are enhancing the lives of infants and toddlers in low-income families.* Washington, DC: U.S. Department of Health and Human Services.

Administration for Children and Families. (2002a, June). *Making a difference in the lives of infants and toddlers and their families: The impacts of Early Head Start.* Washington, DC: U.S. Department of Health and Human Services.

Administration for Children and Families. (2002b, December). *Pathways to quality and full implementation in Early Head Start programs.* Washington, DC: U.S. Department of Health and Human Services.

Administration for Children and Families. (2006, April). *Research to practice: Preliminary findings from the Early Head Start prekindergarten followup.* Washington, DC: U.S. Department of Health and Human Services. Available at *www.acf.hhs.gov/programs/opre/EHS/EHS_resrch/reports/prekindergarten_followup/prekindergarten_followup.pdf*.

Administration for Children and Families. (2010, January). *Head Start impact study final report*. Washington, DC: U.S. Department of Health and Human Services.

Brooks-Gunn, J., Duncan, G. J., & Aber, J. L. (Eds.). (1997). *Neighborhood poverty: Context and consequences for children* (Volume 1). *Policy implications in studying neighborhoods* (Volume 2). New York: Sage.

Brooks-Gunn, J., Lebanon, P., Liaw, F., & Spiker, D. (1993). Enhancing the development of low-birthweight premature infants: Changes in cognition and behavior over the first three years. *Child Development, 64,* 736–753.

Brooks-Gunn, J., & Markman, L. (2005). The contribution of parenting to ethnic and racial gaps in school readiness. *The Future of Children, 15*(1), 138–167.

Campbell, F. A., & Ramey, C. T. (1995). Cognitive and school outcomes for high-risk African American students at middle adolescence: Positive effects of early intervention. *American Educational Research Journal, 32,* 743–772.

Campbell, F. A., Ramey, C. T., Pungello, E. P., Sparling, J., & Miller-Johnson, S. (2002). Early childhood education: Young adult outcomes from the Abecedarian Project. *Applied Developmental Science, 6,* 42–57.

Caspi, A., Moffitt, T. E., Newman, D. L., & Silva, P. A. (1996). Behavioral observations at age 3 predict adult psychiatric disorders: Longitudinal evidence from a birth cohort. *Archives of General Psychiatry, 53,* 1033–1039.

Chau, M., Thampi, K., & Wight, V. R. (2010). *Basic facts about low-income children, 2009, children under 3*. New York: National Center for Children in Poverty. Available at *www.nccp.org/publications/pub_971.html*.

Cohen, J. (1988). *Statistical power analysis for the behavioral sciences* (2nd ed.). Hillsdale, NJ: Erlbaum.

Currie, J. (2001). Early childhood education programs. *Journal of Economic Perspectives, 15,* 213–238.

Dishion, T. J., French, D. C., & Patterson, G. R. (1995). The development and ecology of antisocial behavior. In D. Cicchetti & D. J. Cohen (Eds.), *Developmental psychopathology: Vol. 2. Risk, disorder, and adaptation* (pp. 421–471). Oxford, UK: Wiley.

Drotar, D., Robinson, J., Jeavons, L., & Lester Kirchner, H. (2009). A randomized, controlled evaluation of early intervention: The Born to Learn curriculum. *Child: Care, Health & Development, 35*(5), 643–649.

Duncan, G. J., Brooks-Gunn, J., & Klebanov, P. K. (1994). Economic deprivation and early-childhood development. *Child Development, 65,* 296–318.

Duncan, G. J., Dowsett, C. J., Claessens, A., Magnuson, K., Huston, A. C., Klebanov, P., et al. (2007). School readiness and later achievement. *Developmental Psychology, 43,* 1428–1446.

Duncan, G., & Magnuson, K. (2005). Test score gaps: The contributions of family economic and social conditions. *The Future of Children, 15,* 35–52.

Duncan, G., Ziol-Guest, K., & Kalil, A. (2010). Early childhood poverty and adult attainment, behavior, and health. *Child Development, 81,* 306–325.

Heckman, J. (2006). Skill formation and the economics of investing in disadvantaged children. *Science, 312,* 1900–1902.

Heckman, J. J., & Masterov, D. V. (2004). *The productivity argument for investing in young children* (Working Paper No. 5). Washington, DC: Invest in Kids Working Group.

Hill, J., & Reiter, J. (2006). Interval estimation for treatment effects using propensity score matching. *Statistics in Medicine, 25*(13), 2230–2256.

Lally, R., Mangione, P., & Honig, A. (1988). The Syracuse University Family Development Research Program: Long-range impacts of an early intervention with low-income children and their families. In D. Powell (Ed.), *Parent education as early childhood intervention* (pp. 79–104). Norwood, NJ: Ablex.

Lambie, D., Bond, J. T., & Weikart, D. P. (1974). *Home teaching with mothers and infants: The Ypsilanti–Carnegie Infant Education Project, an experiment.* Ypsilanti, MI: High/Scope Educational Research Foundation.

Levenstein, P., & Levenstein, S. (2008). *Messages from home: The Parent–Child Home Program and overcoming educational disadvantage.* Philadelphia: Temple University Press.

Levenstein, P., Levenstein, S., Shiminski, J. A., & Stpolzberg, J. E. (1998). Long-term impact of a verbal interaction program for at-risk toddlers: An exploratory study of high school outcomes in a replication of the Mother–Child Home Program. *Journal of Applied Developmental Psychology, 19,* 267–285.

Leventhal, T., Dupéré, V., & Brooks-Gunn, J. (2009). Neighborhood influences on adolescent development. In L. Steinberg & R. Lerner (Eds.), *Handbook of adolescent psychology* (Vol. 2., pp. 411–443). New York: Wiley.

Love, J. M., Chazan-Cohen, R., Raikes, H., & Brooks-Gunn, J. (in press). What makes a difference?: Early Head Start evaluation findings in a developmental context. *Monographs of the Society for Research in Child Development.*

Love, J. M., Kisker, E. E., Ross, C., Raikes, H., Constantine, J., Boller, K., et al. (2005). The effectiveness of Early Head Start for 3-year-old children and their parents: Lessons for policy and programs. *Developmental Psychology, 41,* 885–901. Available at *www.apa.org/journals/releases/dev416885.pdf.*

Love, J. M., Vogel, C. A., Chazan-Cohen, R., Raikes, H. H., Kiser, E. E., & Brooks-Gunn, J. (2009, April). *The Early Head Start evaluation: Impacts at the end of the program, two years later, and the context for ongoing research.* Poster presented at the biennial meeting of the Society for Research in Child Development, Denver, CO.

Magnuson, K. A., & Waldfogel, J. (2005). Early childhood care and education: Effects on ethnic and racial gaps in school readiness. *The Future of Children, 15*(1), 169–196.

McCartney, K., & Phillips, D. (Eds.) (2006). *Blackwell handbook of early childhood development.* Oxford, UK: Blackwell.

McCormick, M. C., Brooks-Gunn, J., Buka, S. L., Goldman, J., Yu, J., Salganik, M., et al. (2006). Early intervention in low birth weight premature infants: Results at 18 years of age for the Infant Health and Development Program. *Pediatrics, 117,* 771–780.

Moore, K. A., Redd, Z., Burkhauser, M., Mbwana, K., & Collins, A. (2009). *Children in poverty: Trends, consequences, and policy options* (Research Brief No. 2009-11). Washington, DC: Child Trends.

Olds, D. L., Kitzman, H., Hanks, C., Cole, R., Anson, E., Sidora-Arcoleo, K., et al. (2007). Effects of nurse home visiting on maternal and child functioning: Age-9 follow-up of a randomized trial. *Pediatrics, 120,* e832–e845.

Phillips, M., Brooks-Gunn, J., Duncan, G. J., Klebanov, P. K., & Jencks, C. (1998). Family background, parenting practices, and the black–white test score gap. In C. Jencks & M. Phillips (Eds.), *The black–white test score gap* (pp. 103–145). Washington, DC: Brookings Institution.

Pianta, R. C., Cox, M. J., & Snow, K. (Eds.). (2007). *School readiness and the transition to kindergarten* (pp. 283–306). Baltimore: Brookes.

Reynolds, A. J., Wang, M. C., & Walberg, I. J. (Eds.). (2003). *Early childhood programs for a new century.* Washington, DC: Child Welfare League of America.

Rouse, C., Brooks-Gunn, J., & McLanahan, S. (2005). School readiness: Closing racial and ethnic gaps. *The Future of Children, 15*(1), 5–14.

Shonkoff, J. P., & Phillips, D. A. (Eds.). (2000). *From neurons to neighborhoods: The science of early childhood development.* Washington, DC: National Academy Press.

St. Pierre, R. G., Layzer, J. I., Goodson, B. D., & Bernstein, L. (1997). *National impact evaluation of the Comprehensive Child Development Program: Final report.* Cambridge, MA: ABT.

Wagner, M., Clayton, S., Gerlach-Downie, S., & McElroy, M. (1999). *An evaluation of the northern California Parents as Teachers demonstration.* Menlo Park, CA: SRI International.

CHAPTER 14

Research-Based Approaches for Individualizing Caregiving and Educational Interventions for Infants and Toddlers in Poverty

Judith J. Carta, Charles Greenwood, Kathleen Baggett, Jay Buzhardt, and Dale Walker

Developmental science has long known that poverty has a profound and lasting impact on children's development (Aber, Bennett, Conley, & Li, 1997; Bradley & Corwyn, 2002; Duncan, Brooks-Gunn, & Klebanov, 1994). In the last quarter-century, we have come to know that growing up in environments with limited resources can affect children as young as 9 months. As a result, an emphasis of intervention science has been the creation of systems of support to poor families and the crafting of specific strategies to prevent the adverse effects of poverty on infants and toddlers and their caregivers. Greater numbers and evermore sophisticated studies have been generated over the last two decades that demonstrate the efficacy of interventions aimed at infants and toddlers in poverty (Landry, Smith, & Swank, 2006; Love et al., 2005; Ramey & Campbell, 1991). Yet, finding ways to carry out interventions so that they are effective, efficient, and have long-lasting effects remains an elusive goal. Even the most effective interventions struggle to show effects on a significant segment of the population of children and families they attempt to reach. This chapter discusses some recently developed strategies for identifying infants and toddlers who are at highest risk for not benefiting from preventive interventions and then delivering more intensive strategies to promote their development and readiness for school.

In this chapter, we briefly describe some of the factors related to poverty that are known to influence the outcomes of young children and discuss the ways in which specific poverty-related mechanisms might affect the behavior of infants and toddlers. We then describe an approach that programs can use to identify infants and toddlers who may need more than the general intervention or curriculum aimed at preventing developmental delays and how programs can provide additional caregiving support specifically to those children and their families. We provide an example of how an approach like this is helping Early Head Start programs individualize their level of support to promote children's language development and include some preliminary data showing the effects of this individualization on children's language outcomes. We conclude with a discussion of approaches that help program staff individualize intervention and/or teaching strategies based on children's need, and the way such individualization can increase the overall effectiveness of prevention intervention programs.

What Do We Know about Poverty and Its Effect on Children's Outcomes?

Almost one-half of all infants and toddlers in the United States in 2009 were living in low-income families and more than one in four were growing up in families at or below the poverty line (Chau, Thampi, & Wight, 2010). Proportions of children living in poverty have been growing steadily in the last decade. While the effects of poverty can be apparent quite early in life, many studies have also documented the disparity in school readiness in children from low and middle-income families (e.g., Entwistle, Alexander, & Olson, 2005; Lee & Burkham, 2002). This begins an achievement gap as early as kindergarten that increases as children move through the school system (Zigler, Gilliam, & Jones, 2006).

Several researchers have described the various pathways through which poverty influences children's development and educational outcomes (Brooks-Gunn & Duncan, 1997; Conger, Ge, Elder, Lorenz, & Simons, 1994). Developmental systems theories (Bronfenbrenner, 1994; Sameroff, 2000) posit multiple mechanisms through which poverty may affect children's outcomes and these have recently been summarized as (1) the direct effects of poverty, (2) the moderated effects of poverty, (3) the mediated effects of poverty, and (4) the transactional effects of poverty (Engle & Black, 2008). First, poverty influences children's outcomes directly. For example, inadequate food security affects health outcomes (Cook et al., 2006), limited exposure to talking and to new words by caregivers affects vocabulary development (Hart & Risley, 1995) and school readiness (Walker, Greenwood, Hart, & Carta, 1994), and infrequent opportunities to share in book reading with family members or other caregivers affect literacy (Snow, Burns, & Griffin, 1998).

Second, the effects of poverty are also moderated or influenced in either positive or negative ways by families. For example, families that have limited resources but value education or are striving to obtain a higher degree of education may engage in more cognitively stimulating activities with their children and ultimately have positive effects on children. Conversely, families that are poor, have limited education, and have reduced decision-making skills may have difficulty protecting their children from the adverse effects of poverty, ultimately leading to more deleterious effects on these children. In summary, these parental characteristics moderate the effects of poverty.

Third, sometimes the impact of poverty is mediated or exacerbated by the effect that limited resources have on a family's functioning and these negative family outcomes have an influence on their children. For example, families in poverty that struggle to meet their children's caregiving needs often experience stress and co-occurring emotional and mental health problems. These family characteristics are known to increase the probability of harsh parenting, which results in developmental and behavioral problems for their children (Dodge, Pettit, & Bates, 1994). Finally, it is important to realize the transactional nature of the effects of poverty by understanding the two-way nature of the influence of poverty in the way limited resources may shape parents' behaviors toward their children and also in the manner in which children growing up in poverty may affect their parents (Sameroff & Chandler, 1975). For example, parents who are experiencing high levels of stress may have a difficult time coping with a child with behavioral problems and language delays caused by untreated ear infections. However, if these same parents have a child who gets timely intervention for health issues, that might lower the incidence of their child's behavior and developmental problems. Also, if the child gets regular progress monitoring in communication and behavior, then parents may have a greater understanding of their child and how to respond and promote his or her communication. Clearly, in this model, quality early child care and intervention can act as a moderator by helping children directly or by supporting parents to be more responsive and stimulating caregivers.

How Do We Structure Programs for Infants and Toddlers in Poverty to Maximize Outcomes for All Children?

Programs aimed at promoting the development of infants and toddlers typically focus on both sides of the transactional relationship concentrating primarily on children but also on the quality of the interactions that children receive from their caregivers. Programs for all infants and toddlers emphasize that caregivers must be responsive, interact individually, and help children learn about their environments and learn from peers. High-quality programs make sure interactions occur across caregiving and social routines that take place throughout the day. Staff in such programs make a point of teaching children new words and helping children learn to label their emotions and feelings. But infants and toddlers from families in poverty who are at highest risk are less likely to benefit from even high-quality programs such as Early Head Start (see Knitzer & Lefkowitz, 2006). Recent studies have examined the effects of multiple or cumulative risks on children's outcomes. For example, in the recent Early Head Start national evaluation, children who had four or more risk factors (e.g., having a teenage parent, a parent without a high school diploma, a parent who was unemployed) failed to show benefits from the program (Kisker, Raikes, Cohen, Carta, & Puma, 2009; Love et al., 2005). Similarly, we know that children growing up in environments with specific risks such as having a depressed parent or a parent who is involved with substance abuse may be less likely to benefit from high-quality programs (Malik et al., 2007). Therefore, even high-quality programs face the challenge of identifying the children who may need more intensive supports to promote their development. One approach to identification is based on family characteristics or number or type of risk. It is important to remember, however, that developmental literature on risk and children's trajectories provides information about the probability that a child may be affected by one or more risks but fails to account for how individual children will actually respond to risks. We know, for example, that multiple risks do not always lead to adverse outcomes for some children and that instead some of them succeed or develop normally in what many would consider a "toxic environment" (Garbarino, 1995). While some may describe these "at-risk" children as "resilient," that is, on track for beating the odds (Masten, 1994), and others may point to protective factors that moderate the effects of risk factors (Werner, 1993), the important consideration is that there is not a uniform response to growing up with risks. Therefore, programs seeking to identify children who need additional support should use child behavior or child performance as an important indicator of a need for greater intensity of intervention.

How Can Programs Individualize to Provide Children and Their Families with the Needed Level of Intervention Intensity?

In recent years researchers have developed new approaches for identifying infants and toddlers who are showing signs of atypical or delayed development in communication and social–emotional abilities. As noted, these are infants and toddlers who will benefit from individualized support. Such support could be indicated through a system of universal screening delivered in a tiered or hierarchical manner by employing an approach for monitoring children's progress and supplying data from which to make decisions, and incorporating evidence-based intervention practices that specifically support the acquisition of the skills targeted for individual children. Each of these features and the reasons they are especially critical in programs for infants and toddlers are described in the subsequent sections.

Hierarchical Models of Intervention and Caregiving

While hierarchical intervention models of service have been a staple of kindergarten through high school education, practitioners have only recently begun to implement this model with children in the PreK years (Coleman, Buysse, & Neitzel, 2006; Fox, Dunlap, Hemmeter, Joseph, & Strain, 2003; Greenwood et al., 2011), and their application for infants and toddlers has rarely occurred (Carta, Hemmeter, Broyles, & Baggett, 2009; Hunter & Hemmeter, 2009; Squires & Bricker, 2007). An example of a hierarchical approach to intervention for preschool children is the pyramid model (Fox, Carta, Strain, Dunlap, & Hemmeter, 2009; see Figure 14.1), which has been designed to address challenging behavior of young children. The pyramid model focuses on a tiered framework of evidence-based interventions that are differentiated based on levels of intensity for promoting the social, emotional, and behavioral development of young children. Like other multi-tiered systems of support, the tiers in the pyramid model incorporate three different levels of intervention practice: universal promotion, secondary prevention, and intensive or tertiary intervention.

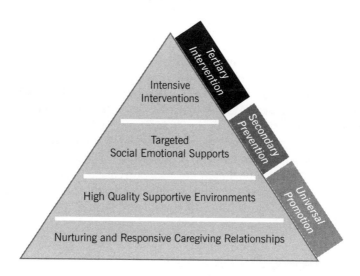

FIGURE 14.1. The pyramid model: An example of a tiered model of support to promote social–emotional outcomes. From Fox, Carta, Strain, Dunlap, and Hemmeter (2009).

Universal Promotion for All Children

This level incorporates caregiving or instructional practices known to be foundational for supporting the development of *all* children. In the pyramid model, these foundational components include (1) caregivers who sustain nurturing and responsive relationships with children (Dunst & Kassow, 2008), (2) high-quality environments that feature consistency and predictability (National Research Council, 2001), and (3) highly engaging activities that promote children's social interaction. The focus is on promotion of social competence and prevention of challenging behaviors rather than relying on procedures that are reactions to behavior problems.

Secondary Prevention

This level of the pyramid model incorporates the systematic and targeted teaching of social skills and emotional competencies to address the needs of children at risk for social–emotional challenges. While all children need some adult guidance and intentional teaching to learn social problem-solving strategies and self-regulation, a smaller proportion of children may need more systematic and focused instruction to acquire social–emotional skills. These children might need focused instruction on skills such as expressing emotions, self-regulation, initiating and maintaining interactions, cooperative responding, strategies for handling disappointment and anger, and friendship skills (Denham et al., 2003).

Intensive or Tertiary Intervention

At this level of the hierarchy in the pyramid model, comprehensive interventions are provided for children who have persistent challenging behavior. These are a set of strategies developed to resolve problem behavior and support the development of new skills. At this level, an individual plan is designed that can be applied within all natural contexts for a specific child by the child's everyday caregivers, and is focused on supporting the child in developing new skills (Dunlap & Fox, 2009; Lucyshyn, Dunlap, & Albin, 2002). The behavior support plan includes prevention strategies to address the triggers of challenging behavior, replacement skills that are alternatives to the challenging behavior, and strategies that ensure challenging behavior is not reinforced or maintained.

Systems for Ongoing Universal Screening

An essential element for individualizing programs for infants and toddlers is having an efficient and easy-to-use means of identifying children who need extra support. While screening instruments have been available for young children for many years, programs that seek to individualize for infants and toddlers face the special challenge of the rapidity with which children at the very youngest ages grow and change. Thus, programs need measures that can be used to screen children on an ongoing basis to be sure that no child within the program begins to fall behind and remains unidentified. So, measures used for progress monitoring infants and toddlers must be repeatable, brief, easy to use and score, inexpensive, and sensitive to short-term growth (Carta et al., 2002). But besides these practical features, these measures also must be reliable and valid and capable of *identifying* children who are not following a typical trajectory of development. Once a child is taking part in a more intensive tier of intervention, measures must be sensitive enough for *monitoring children's progress* within these interventions and for capturing children's change in response to the intervention.

All of the features listed above are incorporated into an assessment system called the Individual Growth and Development Indicators (IGDIs; Carta, Greenwood, Walker, & Buzhardt, 2010). IGDIs are brief, frequently administered assessments of an individual child's progress toward specific outcomes, such as learning to communicate or move in the environment. In design, an IGDI is an indicator of short-term progress and rate of growth. However, unlike most measurement in early childhood, IGDIs are not intended to be comprehensive measures of what a child knows and can do, but simply "indicators"—quick status checks of where a child is with respect to a broader outcome. While IGDIs have been designed to measure early literacy and language in preschool-age children (Missall & McConnell, 2010), of particular importance for those who wish to individualize programs for the youngest children are IGDIs for infants and toddlers (Carta et al., 2010; Walker, Carta, Greenwood, & Buzhardt, 2008). Specific IGDIs for children between 6 and 36 months have been developed to measure language (the Early Communication Indicator), movement (the Early Movement Indicator), social interaction (the Early Social Indicator), cognitive development (the Early Problem-Solving Indicator), and caregiver–child interaction (the Indicator of Parent–Child Interaction). Each of these is brief (from 6 to 10 minutes) and is carried out in a standardized but child-friendly situation. For example, the Early Communication Indicator provides a quick check on how well a child expresses wants and needs by counting a child's communicative attempts in a 6-minute interaction with a familiar adult in a play situation. The assessment employs a familiar adult as the child's partner who follows the child's lead during play activity. The child's expressive communication score is a count of his or her total number of gestures, vocalizations, single words, or multiple-word utterances. This score can be compared to normative levels of growth in communication. The idea is similar to plotting a child's height and weight as an index to his or her physical growth and development using the standard pediatric height and weight charts. Figure 14.2 depicts an actual web-generated report that an interventionist might access when monitoring the progress of a child. Each point on the graph is one child's total communication score

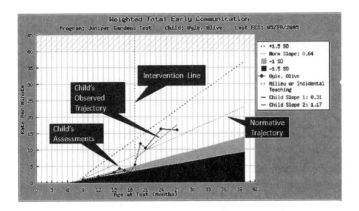

FIGURE 14.2. Example of a web-generated report of Early Communication Indicator progress monitoring data. From Juniper Gardens Children's Project, University of Kansas (*www.igdi.ku.edu*). Reprinted by permission.

that was obtained through a 6-minute assessment (beginning at 9 months of age and continuing through 27 months). The graph shows that even at the earliest assessment points, this child was in the "gray" area labeled "slightly below benchmark" meaning she was between 1 and 1.5 standard deviations below the normative trajectory. This lower-than-average performance alerted the interventionist at 15 months to monitor the child more frequently (monthly), and at 18 months a decision was made to begin more intensive Tier 2 intervention. This additional support for the child consisted of the home visitor engaging the parent in the use of language intervention strategies derived from milieu, prelinguistic milieu, and responsive teaching interventions (e.g., Alpert & Kaiser, 1992; Tannock, Girolametto, & Siegel, 1992; Warren, Yoder, Gazdag, Kim, & Jones, 1993) for promoting more communication at home with similar strategies being suggested for her caregivers in her infant/toddler center. The graph shows how the slope of the line depicting the child's total communication growth became much steeper with the implementation of intervention at 18 months and how the level of her communication was no longer in the "gray" area of concern. This type of information generated by the Early Communication Indicator was maximally helpful to the interventionist for the following reasons:

1. She could quickly see when the child's level of communication was in an area of concern.
2. She could see how changes in the child's growth corresponded to the changed level of intensity of strategies she was using.
3. She could get this information easily using a web-based system.

An approach employing technology for providing data in real time is described below.

Web-Based Progress Monitoring Systems

Practical experience in early intervention programs indicates that just having progress monitoring data alone without suggestions for how to use the data to modify interventions results in very infrequent changes in children's programs or in children's rates of progress (Walker, Greenwood, et al., 2008). For data to be accessible and ultimately used for individualizing intervention, the following features are important:

1. Data must be available to interventionists in a timely manner.
2. Data must be easy to interpret and decision-making guidelines must be available to help practitioners understand when a change in intervention is necessary (such as greater instructional or caregiving intensity).
3. Information and resources should be readily available for selecting specific evidence-based instructional strategies based on a child's level of performance.

One approach that incorporates these features is the Making Online Decisions (MOD) System (*www.igdi.ku.edu*), a web-based progress monitoring system for IGDIs in language and communication that recommends specific language-promoting intervention strategies (Buzhardt et al., 2010). The MOD gives interventionists data-based guidance and support for working through the steps of determining (1) which children need individualized support, (2) what individualized support should be provided, and (3) when the intervention is working (or not working). Based in part on Tilley's (2008) decision-making model (see Figure 14.3), and supported by data collected from regular Early Communication Indicator progress monitoring screening, the key decision-making steps are:

1. *Is there a problem?* Is the child's performance at least 1 *SD* below benchmark for the child's age?
2. *Why is it happening?* What might be causing this lower-than-typical performance?
3. *What should be done?* What Tier 2 intervention strategies can be implemented to individualize this child's program and address the delayed performance?
4. *Is it being done?* Is the intervention being implemented with fidelity?
5. *Is it working?* Is the child's performance closer to benchmark since beginning the intervention, and/or does the child's performance show a change in slope (growth)?
6. *And, if not:* What might be contributing to the child's lack of response to the intervention and how can the intervention be modified?

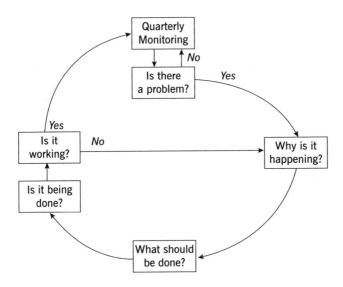

FIGURE 14.3. An instructional decision-making model. Based on Tilly (2008). From Juniper Gardens Children's Project, University of Kansas (*www.igdi.ku.edu*). Reprinted by permission.

While this approach to supporting interventionists is still experimental, we expect that an approach such as this, which guides practitioners' decision making, will lead to more timely decisions to provide children with needed additional levels of intervention intensity and result in trajectories in communication development that are more similar to those of typically developing children. Within the medical literature, there have been over 100 studies of technology-based clinical decision-making support systems (Ahmadian et al., 2011; Garg et al., 2005), the majority of which resulted in improved practitioner decision-making performance and patient outcomes relative to a comparison condition. Buzhardt et al. (2011) recently demonstrated that children whose home visitors had been randomly assigned to a group that had access to a web-based system for making intervention decisions (the MOD program) had higher levels of growth in communication than a comparison group without the web-based support. The home visitors assigned to the MOD were prompted by the MOD to monitor children's growth more frequently, received MOD-recommended intervention strategies individualized to the child's Early Communication Indicator performance, were prompted by the MOD to monitor and report implementation fidelity of the intervention, and received reports from the MOD regarding the child's Early Communication Indicator growth since beginning the intervention. These results show great promise for assisting practitioners in individualizing their services based on child response to specific educational or caregiving interventions.

Evidence-Based Approaches for Providing Tier 2 and Tier 3 Levels of Support

Certainly identifying children who need greater levels of intervention intensity is important but a critical aspect of individualization is providing intentional instruction to address children's areas of need. Numerous instructional strategies have been developed over the last two decades that have been demonstrated as effective for increasing children's growth in communication, social–emotional competence, movement, and cognitive outcomes. Many of these strategies are designed to be implemented by parents and caregivers in children's natural environments. For example, the responsive interaction intervention strategies (Tannock et al., 1992) and incidental teaching (Hart & Risley, 1975) milieu and prelinguistic milieu interventions (Kaiser, Ostrosky, & Alpert, 1993; Yoder & Warren, 1998) have been the backbone of language-promoting strategies used by Walker and colleagues (Walker, Bigelow, & Harjusola-Webb, 2008). This set of intervention procedures for increasing children's expressive communication skills includes strategies such as imitating and expanding on what a child says, providing choices to a child (who will be prompted to communicate a choice), and asking open-ended questions (i.e., those which have greater probabilities of longer and more complex responses than close-ended responses that require only a single-word utterance in reply). In a randomized trial, Walker and her colleagues (Walker, Bigelow, et al., 2008) have demonstrated that children in an intervention group whose caregivers use these language-promoting strategies with a high degree of fidelity in community-based child care were more likely to demonstrate higher rates of growth than children in a control group. Similar results have been demonstrated when using the intervention model in homes with parents of toddlers with disabilities (Walker et al., 2010). Other intervention strategies focusing on other areas such as children's social–emotional development have been developed and are also being used in tiered approaches to intervention (e.g., Hunter & Hemmeter, 2009).

How Can We Move Evidence-Based Practices for Individualizing Caregiving Support to Infants and Toddlers into Wide-Scale Practice?

While a number of these evidence-based strategies exist for individualizing caregiving support, the challenges of translating these approaches into wide-scale practice in child care are profound. While a 20-year lag time has been documented between the availability of evidence-based practices and their use in wide-scale practice in education settings (Walker, 2006), this time lag in translating research to practice is even greater in infant and toddler programs where the quality of caregiving is most often lower than adequate (National Association of Child Care Resource and Referral

Agencies, 2006). In addition, staff turnover rate in child care is extremely high, thereby increasing the need for ongoing training on practices documented to be evidence based.

One approach to overcoming the challenges in getting evidence-based strategies for individualization implemented in child care is through the use of the Internet for delivering professional development (Kinzie et al., 2006). One of the greatest obstacles in providing high-quality training to child care providers is that time for training is rarely built into their schedules. A second challenge is the need to personalize professional development so that practitioners can get information that will inform their practice and help them make data-based decisions. Baggett and colleagues (2010) are using a web-based professional development approach called Infant-Net for training difficult-to-reach parents. This multimedia instructional approach developed around the Play and Learning Strategies (PALS) curriculum (Landry, Smith, Swank, & Guttentag, 2008) is designed to increase parent sensitivity and responsiveness as well as improve child trajectories of social and communication development. The Infant-Net program incorporates a self-paced instructional presentation of the PALS concepts, behaviors, and skills via video examples and prompts the parent to create a 5-minute computer-collected video of parent–infant interactions for later remote coviewing by coach and parents. Over the telephone, the coach contacts the parent, and they both discuss the parent–infant video from the play session between the parent and child. Through this process, the coach provides individualized support for the acquisition and practice of parenting skills. This same web-based approach to professional development is also currently being developed and tested for use by child care providers as a means of increasing responsive caregiving interactions to promote infant social–emotional development. The web-based approach is promising because of two features: (1) it is efficient, relying on the use of remote skills training through brief tutorials with individual sessions requiring approximately 20 minutes to complete; (2) it is flexible, with coaching adaptable to different formats; and (3) it is accessible, with 24-hour access to the training on the Web and availability regardless of the trainee's location. Technological resources are starting to become available for helping early interventionists monitor children's progress, identify children needing additional support, obtain suggestions for strategies to increase instructional or caregiving intensity, and receive on-demand professional training. These are all exciting new developments for promoting individualized approaches for children who need them most.

Conclusions

In this chapter, we have outlined key strategies for individualizing programs for infants and toddlers who are at developmental risk due to poverty and other circumstances. Some of these strategies are "tried and true," whereas others are incorporating newly developed technology that may provide a virtual infrastructure for guiding intervention in real time. Clearly, more research is needed to advance many of these ideas and apply them broadly to programs serving infants and toddlers. Yet, whether applying old or new technology for differentiating caregiving and instruction to infants and toddlers, the benefits of employing these individualization strategies are many and include the strategies below.

First, screening all children to find those children who need more intensive instruction in the earliest years is an important step in narrowing the achievement gap and preventing failure in the later years. Identifying children early who can benefit from additional support will be a cost-effective way of reducing the number of children who might eventually require special education and other services (Diefendorf & Goode, 2005). Second, giving practitioners the tools they need to identify children expands the number of individuals who can recognize children experiencing difficulties, which in turn will result in more timely receipt of services. Finally, giving practitioners the skills and support for individualizing interventions empowers them as professionals to become instructional decision makers and to enrich and enhance caregiving and education they provide to our most vulnerable children.

REFERENCES

Aber, L., Bennett, N., Conley, D., & Li, J. (1997). The effects of poverty on child health and development. *Annual Review of Public Health, 18,* 463–483.

Ahmadiana, L., van Engen-Verheula, M., Bakhshi-Raieza, F., Peeka, N., Corneta, R., & de Keizera, N. (2011). The role of standardized data and terminological systems in computerized clinical decision support systems: Literature review and survey. *International Journal of Medical Informatics, 80,* 81–93.

Alpert, C., & Kaiser, A. (1992). Training parents as milieu language teachers. *Journal of Early Intervention, 16*(1), 31–52.

Baggett, K. M., Feil, E. G., Davis, B., Sheeber, L., Landry, S., Carta, J., et al. (2010). Technologies for expanding the reach of evidence-based interventions: Preliminary results for promoting social–emotional development in early childhood. *Topics in Early Childhood Special Education, 29,* 226–238.

Bradley, R. H., & Corwyn, R. F. (2002). Socioeconomic status and child development. *Annual Review of Psychology, 53,* 371–399.

Bronfenbrenner, U. (1994). Ecological models of human development. In T. Husen & T. N. Postlethwaite (Eds.), *The international encyclopedia of education* (2nd ed., pp. 1643–1647). New York: Elsevier Science.

Brooks-Gunn, J., & Duncan, G. J. (1997). The effects of poverty on children. *The Future of Children, 7,* 55–71.

Buzhardt, J., Greenwood, C. R., Walker, D., Anderson, R., Howard, W., & Carta, J. J. (2011). Effects of web-based support on Early Head Start home visitors' use of evidence-based intervention decision making and growth in children's expressive communication. *NHSA Dialog: A Research-to-Practice Journal for the Early Childhood Field, 14,* 121–146.

Buzhardt, J., Greenwood, C. R., Walker, D., Carta, J., Terry, B., & Garrett, M. (2010). A web-based tool to support data-based early intervention decision-making. *Topics in Early Childhood Special Education, 29,* 201–213.

Carta, J., Greenwood, C., Walker, D., & Buzhardt, J. (Eds.). (2010). *Individual growth and developmental indicators: Tools for monitoring progress and measuring growth in young children.* Baltimore: Brookes.

Carta, J. J., Greenwood, C. R., Walker, D., Kaminski, R., Good, R., McConnell, S., et al. (2002). Individual growth and development indicators (IGDIs): Assessment that guides intervention for young children. *Young Exceptional Children Monograph Series 4,* 15–28.

Carta, J., Hemmeter, M. L., Broyles, L., & Baggett, K. (2009). *The pyramid framework within early intervention programs: Promoting the social development of infants and toddlers.* Webinar presented on September 9, 2009, for the Technical Assistance Center for Social Emotional Intervention. Available at *www.challengingbehavior.org/explore/webinars/9.9.2009_tacsei_presentation_teleconference.htm.*

Chau, M., Thampi, K., & Wight, V. R. (2010). *Basic facts about low-income children, 2009: Children under age 3.* New York: National Center for Children in Poverty, Columbia University Mailman School of Public Health.

Coleman, M. R., Buysse, V., & Neitzel, J. (2006). *Recognition and response: An early intervening system for young children at risk for learning disabilities.* Chapel Hill: The University of North Carolina at Chapel Hill, FPG Child Development Institute.

Conger, R. D., Ge, X., Elder, G. H., Jr., Lorenz, F. O., & Simons, R. L. (1994). Economic stress, coercive family process and developmental problems of adolescents. *Child Development, 65,* 541–561.

Cook, J. T., Frank, D. A., Levenson, S. M., Neault, N. B., Heeren, T. C., & Black, M. M. (2006). Child food insecurity increases risks posed by household food insecurity to young children's health. *Journal of Nutrition, 136,* 1073–1076.

Denham, S. A., Blair, K. A., DeMulder, E., Levitas, J., Sawyer, K., Auerbach-Major, S., Frank, D. A., Levenson, S. M., Neault, N. B., Heeren, T. C., Black, M. M., et al. (2003). Preschool emotional competence: Pathway to social competence? *Child Development, 74,* 238–256.

Diefendorf, M., & Goode, S. (2005). The long-term economic benefits of high-quality early childhood intervention programs: A mini-bibliography. Retrieved from *www.nectac.org/~pdfs/pubs/econbene.pdf.*

Dodge, K. A., Pettit, G. S., & Bates, J. E. (1994). Socialization mediators of the relation between socioeconomic status and child conduct problems. *Child Development, 65,* 649–665.

Duncan, G. J., Brooks-Gunn, J., & Klebanov, P. K. (1994). Economic deprivation and early childhood development. *Child Development, 65,* 296–318.

Dunlap, G., & Fox, L. (2009). Positive behavior support and early intervention. In W. Sailor, G. Dunlap, G. Sugai, & R. Horner (Eds.), *Handbook of positive behavior support* (pp. 49–72). New York: Springer.

Dunst, C. J., & Kassow, D. Z. (2008). Caregiver sensitivity, contingent social responsiveness and secure infant attachment. *Journal of Early and Intensive Behavior Intervention, 5*(1), 40–56.

Engle, P. L., & Black, M. M. (2008). The effect of poverty on child development and educational outcomes. *Annals of the New York Academy of Sciences, 1136,* 243–256.

Entwistle, D., Alexander, K., & Olson, L. (2005). First grade and educational attainment by age 22: A new story. *American Journal of Sociology, 110,* 1458–1502.

Fox, L., Carta, J. J., Strain, P. S., Dunlap, G., & Hemmeter, M. L. (2009). *Response to intervention and the pyramid model.* Tampa, FL: University of South Florida, Technical Assistance Center on Social Emotional Intervention for Young Children.

Fox, L., Dunlap, G., Hemmeter, M. L., Joseph, G. E., & Strain, P. E. (2003). The teaching pyramid: A model for supporting social competence and preventing challenging behavior in young children. *Young Children, 58*(4), 48–52.

Garbarino, J. (1995). *Raising children in a socially toxic environment.* San Francisco: Jossey-Bass.

Garg, A. X., Adhikari, N. K. J., McDonald, H., Rosas-Arellano, M. P., Devereux, P. J., Beyene, J., et al. (2005). Effects of computerized clinical support systems on practitioner performance and patient outcomes. *Journal of the American Medical Association, 293,* 1223–1238.

Greenwood, C. R., Bradfield, T., Kaminski, R., Linas, M., Carta, J. J., & Nylander, D. (2011). The response to intervention (RTI) approach in early childhood. *Focus on Exceptional Children, 43*(9), 1–22.

Hart, B., & Risley, T. R. (1975). Incidental teaching of language in the preschool. *Journal of Applied Behavior Analysis, 8,* 411–420.

Hart, B., & Risley, T. R. (1995). *Meaningful differences in the everyday experience of young American children.* Baltimore: Brookes.

Hunter, A., & Hemmeter, M. L. (2009). The Center on the Social Emotional Foundations for Early Learning: Addressing challenging behavior in infants and toddlers. *Zero to Three Journal, 29,* Washington, DC: Zero to Three.

Kaiser, A. P., Ostrosky, M. M., & Alpert, C. L. (1993). Training teachers to use environmental arrangement and milieu teaching with non-vocal school children. *Journal of the Association for Persons with Severe Handicaps, 18,* 188–199.

Kinzie, M. B., Whitaker, S. D., Neesen, K., Kelley, M., Matera, M., & Pianta, R. C. (2006). Innovative web-based professional development for teachers of at-risk preschool children. *Educational Technology and Society, 9,* 194–204.

Kisker, E. E., Raikes, H., Cohen, R., Carta, J., & Puma, J. (2009, April). *Assessing program impacts on the highest risk families in Early Head Start.* Paper presented at the Society for Research in Child Development Conference, Denver, CO.

Knitzer, J., & Lefkowitz, J. (2006). Pathways to early school success: *Helping the most vulnerable infants, toddlers, and their families* (Issue Brief No. 1). Retrieved from *www.nccp.org/publications/pub_669.html.*

Landry, S. H., Smith, K. E., & Swank, P. R. (2006). Responsive parenting: Establishing early foundations for social, communication, and independent problem solving. *Developmental Psychology, 42,* 627–642.

Landry, S. H., Smith, K. E., Swank, P., & Guttentag, C. (2008). A responsive parenting intervention: The optimal timing across early childhood for impacting maternal behaviors and child outcomes. *Developmental Psychology, 44,* 1335–1353.

Lee, V. E., & Burkham, D. T. (2002). *Inequality at the starting gate.* Washington, DC: Economic Policy Institute.

Love, J., Kisker, E., Ross, C., Raikes, H., Constantine, J., Boller, K., et al. (2005). The effectiveness of Early Head Start for 3-year-old children and their families: Lessons for policy and programs. *Developmental Psychology, 41,* 885–901.

Lucyshyn, J. M., Dunlap, G., & Albin, R. W. (2002). *Families and positive behavior support: Addressing problem behavior in family contexts.* Baltimore: Brookes.

Malik, N. M., Boris, N. W., Heller, S. S., Harden, B. J., Squires, J., Chazan-Cohen, R., et al. (2007). Risk for maternal depression and child aggression in Early Head Start families: A test of ecological models. *Infant Mental Health Journal, 2,* 171–191.

Masten, A. (1994). Resilience and individual development: Successful adaptation despite risk and adversity. In M. C. Wang & M. W. Gordon (Eds.), *Educational resilience in inner-city America: Challenges and prospects* (pp. 3–26). New York: Routledge.

Missall, K., & McConnell, S. R. (2010). Early literacy and language IGDIs for preschool-aged children. In J. Carta, C. Greenwood, D. Walker, & J. Buzhardt (Eds.), *Individual growth and developmental indicators: Tools for monitoring progress and measuring growth in young children* (pp. 181–201). Baltimore: Brookes.

National Association of Child Care Resource and Referral Agencies. (2006). *We can do better: NACCRRA's ranking of state child care center standards and oversight.* Available at *www.naccrra.org/policy/recent_reports/scorecard. php.*

National Research Council. (2001). *Eager to learn: Educating our preschoolers. Committee on Early Childhood Pedagogy.* Washington, DC: National Academy Press.

Ramey, C. T., & Campbell, F. (1991). Poverty, early childhood education, and academic competence: The Abecedarian experiment. In A. Huston (Ed.), *Children in poverty: Child development and public policy* (pp. 190–221). New York: Cambridge University Press.

Sameroff, A. (2000). Ecological perspectives on developmental risk. In J. Osofsky & H. Fitzgerald (Eds.), *WAIMH handbook of infant mental health* (Vol. 4, pp. 4–33). New York: Wiley.

Sameroff, A. J., & Chandler, M. J. (1975). Reproductive risk and the continuum of caretaker casualty. In F. D. Horowitz (Ed.), *Review of child development research* (Vol. 4, pp. 187–204). Chicago: University of Chicago Press.

Snow, C., Burns, M., & Griffin, P. (1998). *Preventing reading difficulties in young children.* Washington, DC: National Academy Press.

Squires, J., & Bricker, D. (2007). *An activity-based approach to developing young children's social emotional development.* Baltimore: Brookes.

Tannock, R., Girolametto, L., & Siegel, L. S. (1992). Language intervention with children who have developmental delays: Effects of an interactive approach. *American Journal on Mental Retardation, 97,* 145–160.

Tilly, W. D. (2008). The evolution of school psychology to a science-based practice: Problem solving and the three-tiered model. In A. Thomas & J. Grimes (Eds.), *Best practices in school psychology V* (Vol. 1, pp. 17–36). Washington, DC: National Association of School Psychologists.

Walker, D., Bigelow, K., & Atwater, J., Gilson, M., Johnson, L., Patrick, K., et al. (2010, October). *Building the capacity of parents and early educators to use intentional communication interventions with infants and toddlers with disabilities.* Paper presented at the International Conference of the Division for Early Childhood, Kansas City, MO.

Walker, D., Bigelow, K., & Harjusola-Webb, S. (2008). Increasing communication and language-learning opportunities for infants and toddlers. *Young Exceptional Children Monograph Series, 10,* 105–121.

Walker, D., Carta, J. J., Greenwood, C. R., & Buzhardt, J. F. (2008). The use of individual growth and developmental indicators for progress monitoring and intervention decision making in early education. *Exceptionality: A Special Education Journal, 16,* 33–47.

Walker, D., Greenwood, C., Buzhardt, J., Carta, J., Baggett, K., & Higgins, S., et al. (2008, July). *Developing and testing a model for the use of progress monitoring measures for infants and toddlers.* Paper presented at the OSEP Project Directors' Meeting, Washington, DC.

Walker, D., Greenwood, C., Hart, B., & Carta, J. (1994). Prediction of school outcomes based on early language production and socioeconomic factors. *Child Development, 65,* 606–621.

Walker, H. (2006). *Addressing social behavior needs of students with disabilities and those at-risk through classroom, program, and school-wide systems of support.* OSEP Project Director's Meeting report, Institute on Violence and Destructive Behavior, University of Oregon.

Warren, S. F., Yoder, P. J., Gazdag, G. E., Kim, K., & Jones, H. A. (1993). Facilitating prelinguistic communication skills in young children with developmental delay. *Journal of Speech and Hearing Research, 36,* 83–97.

Werner, E. E. (1993). Risk, resilience, and recovery: Perspectives from the Kauai Longitudinal Study. *Development and Psychopathology, 5,* 503–515.

Yoder, P. J., & Warren, S. F. (1998). Maternal responsivity predicts the prelinguistic communication intervention that facilitates generalized intentional communication. *Journal of Speech, Language, and Hearing Research, 41,* 1207–1219.

Zigler, E., Gilliam, W., & Jones, S. (2006). *A vision for universal preschool education.* New York: Cambridge University Press.

CONCLUSION

CHAPTER 15

Translating Contemporary Developmental and Health Science

Designing an Early Childhood Program for Young Children and Their Families Living in Poverty

Samuel L. Odom, Elizabeth P. Pungello, and Nicole Gardner-Neblett

Almost every culture has a proverb, saying, or *dichos* (as noted by Cabrera, Chapter 11, this volume) about the value of early childhood experience for later development and life outcomes: *It is easier to straighten a tree during its nursery stage* [Ethiopian]; *Good work should begin as early as possible* [Indian]; *An ounce of prevention is worth a pound of cure* [American]; *Learning when young is like carving in stone* [Egyptian] (Odom & Kaul, 2003). This nearly universal belief is now substantiated by the science of brain development in early childhood that is documenting the toxic effects of risks associated with an economically impoverished environment and the benefits of environments that provide nurturance and care (Shonkoff & Phillips, 2000). Knowledge about the features of early child care and education (ECCE) programs that generate these benefits are informed by an active developmental and health science that has accrued over the past 40–50 years, since the classic and pioneering early education programs of the 1960s and 1970s. The purpose of this book has been to highlight the implications from the current scientific literature for designing a model of early care, intervention, and education that would positively affect life outcomes for the infants, toddlers, and their families experiencing the highest risks. In this chapter, we draw on the science reported by chapter authors, as well as other sources, to describe the implications of developmental and health science for infant/toddler/family care and intervention. We propose a model that is cross-disciplinary, center and home based, and could be individualized for infants/toddlers and families in poverty.

A Rationale for Focusing Early on Children and Families at Highest Risk Due to Poverty

As well stated by several authors of chapters in this book, during the prenatal, infancy, and toddler periods, formative features of health and development occur that have lifelong effects. Early brain development, beginning prenatally and advancing through the first 3 years of life (and beyond), is affected by maternal nutrition and health (Whitaker & Gooze, Chapter 9, this volume; Zuckerman, Chapter 10, this volume), the early social, linguistic, and physical environment (Bauer, Chapter 3, this volume), and the potentially toxic effect of stress (Shonkoff & Bales, 2011). Significant health events occur during that period, such as critical immunizations, nutrition and nutritional practices, and injury prevention (Zuckerman, Chapter 10, this volume; Whitaker & Gooze, Chapter 9, this volume). In addition, during the infant and toddler years, secure attachment to primary caregivers is formed (Berlin, Chapter 8, this volume), early cognitive skills and self-regulatory skills are established (Bauer, Chapter 3, this volume; Blair, Berry, & Friedman, Chapter 6, this volume; Columbo, Kannass, Walker, & Brez, Chapter 2, this volume), and language emerges (Hirsh-Pasik & Golinkoff, Chapter 4, this volume). Although subsequent life events will affect all of these features of development, the life events occurring between conception and the age of 3 have major effects on the course of development during later childhood, adolescence, and into adulthood (Aber, Chapter 1, this volume). All of the features of health, development, and learning, just noted, are affected by risks associated with poverty.

Infants, Toddlers, and Families at Highest Risk

Early care and intervention programs for very young children already exist, with the most scaled-up program being Early Head Start (EHS). Love et al. (Chapter 13, this volume) concluded that EHS has positive effects for many young children and families, especially when the programs are implemented well enough to meet quality standards set by the agency (Love et al., 2005). However, they also noted that infants and families at highest risk did not benefit significantly, as compared to the control group, which has two implications. First, a different and potentially more intensive model of early care, education, and intervention may be necessary for the most severely stressed children and families. Second, this raises a question concerning the identification of risk and the conceptualization of risk that is most likely to be useful for identifying potential nonresponders to typical early care and intervention programs.

Current theoretical perspectives elucidate the mechanisms by which risk factors play a role in human development and help to address these two issues (i.e., the possible need for different models for differentially stressed families and the identification and conceptualization of risk). Jones Harden, Monahan, and Yoches (Chapter 12, this volume) describe several types of risk models. Risk indicators include both biological and environmental variables associated with poor outcomes, such as lack of prenatal care, low birthweight, maternal education, teenage parenting, and poor quality of child care environment. An additive risk model suggests that risk variables have unique effects (Ackerman, Izard, Schoff, Youngstrom, & Kogos, 1999), while a cumulative risk model suggests that as the number of risks (regardless of their nature) increases the general risk to development increases (Rutter, 1979). Scientists have also proposed a transactional risk model (Belsky, Bakermans-Kranenburg, & van IJzendoorn, 2007; Sameroff & Chandler, 1975). In this view, children with certain biological risk conditions (e.g., low birthweight) may respond differently than the general population of infants to the accumulation of risks.

The psychobiological systems view of development (Gottlieb, Wahlsten, & Lickliter, 2006) describes the mechanisms by which children with differing risk factors may respond differentially to early learning environments. This theoretical perspective holds that development is characterized by probabilistic epigenesis, the emergence of new structures and functions in the developing child due to dynamic interactions between and within genetic, neurological, behavioral, and environmental activity, which in turn results in increased complexity and organization over time. Thus, poverty influences development via these dynamic interactions among environmental risk factors and the individual behavioral, neurological, and genetic levels of the unique developing child. Due to the increased complexity that is resulting over time, this perspective also elucidates why beginning earlier in the lifespan is more effective than at later stages.

An ecological risk perspective, based on Bronfenbrenner's (Bronfenbrenner & Morris, 1998) ecological systems model and extended by Conger and Donnellan (2007) to a "family stress" model, suggests development occurs in the context of dynamic interactions among multiple, interdependent environmental levels, with more distal environmental levels (e.g., factors associated with poverty) influencing the more immediate environments of the developing child (e.g., family and care/educational settings) via their influence on proximal processes. Development occurs via these proximal processes, increasingly complex reciprocal interactions between the developing child and people and objects in his or her immediate environment. To effectively promote development, this "interaction must occur on a fairly regular basis over extended periods of time" (p. 797). Further, risks residing within "microsystems" (e.g., family, child care setting) may potentially be moderated by "protective" influences at a "mesosystem" level (e.g., a high-quality child care program might moderate the influence of a high-stress family and/or home environment).

Some empirical research supports this theoretical proposition of potential moderating effects of protective environmental influences. In their study with the NICHD Early Child Care Research Network, Watamura, Phillips, Morrissey, McCartney, and Bub (2011) highlighted the deleterious effect for children in high-stress homes/poor-quality child care settings and the compensatory effects that could occur through high-quality child care. Some researchers find that children and/or families experiencing relatively greater risks may respond more strongly to treatment than children and families whose risks are less (Burchinal, Roberts, Zeisel, Hennon, & Hooper, 2006; see Pungello & Gardner-Neblett, in press). However, not all studies find this moderation effect (see Pungello & Gardner-Neblett, in press). For example, Love et al. (Chapter 13, this volume) found that the highest-risk families did not benefit from participation in EHS. The implication from these contrasting findings is that in designing an effective program for infants/toddlers/families in poverty, determining those who are not currently responding to standard, well-implemented early care and development programs is critical in order to provide an intervention that is intensive and well designed enough to work for them. To accomplish such a purpose, the current risk models need to be "translated" into operationalized procedures that can accurately predict high-risk infants/toddlers/families who are likely to be nonresponders to standard care already provided and procedures that will provide early intervention that will be most effective for them.

Center- and Home-Based Model

Although in their evaluation of EHS programs Love et al. (Chapter 13, this volume) could not make conclusive statements about the model of early child care that would be most effective, there is good reason to believe that a center-based model that has a significant home and family component may be very applicable for the highest-risk children and families. Several authors in this volume have noted that programs for this population should be "two-generational" in that they should provide health and developmental services for children and family members (primarily mothers and fathers). High-quality center-based care for infants and toddlers, as Watamura et al. (2011) noted, may benefit those children who are in highly stressed family situations. For some families, removing child care responsibility for part of the day may provide opportunities for the caregiver to look for work if needed or participate in social services if needed (e.g., job training, mental health services). In addition, a center-based program that is cross-disciplinary could be located where health care and social services may be accessed or provided.

A two-generational program would also include a significant home/family component. Such a comprehensive program would ideally begin prenatally with health care and social services for the mother and involve other family members. After the child is born, program staff would create a system for sharing information about programming at the center, plan a nutritional system that supports breast feeding and other appropriate nutrition, provide early parenting education (if needed), and involve the family members, as feasible in programs that occur at the center. The center–family linkage is a critical one. The acknowledged challenge will be to foster parental access and use of the program, because for the highest-risk parents an issue exists with child attendance (i.e., which could be addressed by providing programs in proximity to the home or transportation) and parent's utilization of services (Jones Harden et al., Chapter 12, this volume).

Drawing Implications from Developmental Health Sciences

The studies that documented the effects of the Perry Preschool Project (Schweinhart, Berrueta-Clement, Barnett, Epstein, & Weikart, 1985), the Abecedarian Project (Ramey & Campbell, 1984), and the Chicago Child Parent Centers (Reynolds, Temple, Ou, Arteaga, & White, 2011)—the pioneering early childhood education programs—are approaching middle age. These early experiments, designed for a different generation of children and parents, demonstrated that early learning environments can have significant long-term effects for children. Since that time, a great deal of basic research in health and developmental science has taken place. Work is now needed that applies these current findings to programs that serve families facing the adversity and stress of poverty. The chapters in this book highlighted the science that has unfolded in the decades after the pioneering programs were implemented. In this section, we discuss implications from the health and developmental science that would extend the important and foundational work conducted by the pioneering program developers.

Health and Nutrition

Following a cumulative risk model, Zuckerman (Chapter 10, this volume) proposes that individual risks related to poverty link together into a "chain" in which each risk "modifies and potentiates the other" (p. 241). As the persistence and number of risk factors mount, they establish an "allocastic load" that builds through repeated responses to stressors. This is the mechanism by which poverty "gets under the skin" of infants and toddlers, through the production of cortisol and debilitating sequalea of other physiological reponses to stress (Blair et al., Chapter 6, this volume). For the child, this load begins to accumulate as early as conception, with the mother's health having immediate impact during pregnancy. A two-generational feature of a comprehensive intervention model affecting the highest-risk children would address the mother's (and other caregivers') physical and mental health as the focus of the model as well as the child's health. Health-related features of such a model would include prenatal medical visits and care, well-baby checks, and immunizations at appropriate times. Zuckerman (Chapter 10, this volume) notes that health-related behaviors have lifelong effects beginning in childhood. Efforts to incorporate health care and early childhood developmental programming are the Healthy Steps program (Zuckerman, Parker, Kaplan-Sanoff, Augustyn, & Barth, 2004) that combines home visiting as follow-up to pediatric visits and the Medical–Legal Partnership (*www.medical-legalpartnership. org*) program that assists families in civil matters related to poverty (e.g., housing, accessing financial support). Certainly, models for incorporating medical and health care into a comprehensive prevention/early intervention program exist (Mendelsohn et al., in press), but they are not widespread.

A key feature of early health care is the role of nutrition and physical activity. For children and families living in poverty, there is the paradoxical concern about both undernutrition and obesity. Supplemental nutrition programs, like Women, Infants and Children (WIC), are universal in communities, but issues related to food insecurity continue to exist for many children and families in the United States (Fiese, Gundersen, Koester, & Washington, 2011). Providing adequate nutrition is a key feature of center-based programs, and assisting families in accessing adequate nutritional resources is a needed complement.

In parallel, early child care and intervention programs can play a major role in establishing healthy nutritional habits for children and their families and preventing obesity. Whitaker and Gooze (Chapter 9, this volume) note that obese children become obese adults, and they propose valuable principles for early child care and intervention programs. These include responsive feeding in which adults control proportion and children indicate how much food they want, small utensils, practices that promote breast feeding, and parent education about healthy food. They note that child care providers may need training to recognize signals of hunger and satiation in infants and very young children, and that child care workers should model moderation and healthy food choices.

In combination with nutritional routines, early child care programs should foster physical activity and motor development (McWilliams et al.,

2009). Intentionally organizing space that requires physical activity, placing infants in prone positions and allowing exploration, planning activities involving physical activity, and incorporating daily routines that foster physical activity should be an essential feature of early child care programs. Whitaker and Gooze (Chapter 9, this volume) note the relationship between short sleep duration and obesity, and offer valuable recommendations for sleep routines both in child care centers and at home.

Child Care Program Features

Developmental science has much to offer in designing an early child care treatment and intervention program for infants and toddlers living in poverty. Both basic and applied science has articulated features of early development that inform practice and assist in monitoring children's progress. One of the principles of child development is that the abilities we sometimes think of as relatively distinct in later childhood (e.g., cognition, language, social competence) are closely integrated in the infant/toddler years. Their differentiation is a characteristic of development across childhood. Yet, basic developmental science, by necessity, focuses on early developmental strands such as cognition (e.g., attention, memory), language (e.g., vocabulary development, syntax), social relationships and abilities (e.g., attachment, temperament), and self-regulation (being one ability that crosses strands).

Early Cognitive Skills

In the last 40 years, much has been learned about attention, memory, and self-regulation. Attention, in particular, is a key ability that early on affects the development of other cognitive processes. Infants and toddlers must be able to focus attention as well as shift attention in order for them to benefit from a rich learning environment. Columbo et al. (Chapter 2, this volume) note a developmental shift in attention abilities that occurs during early infancy, with infants younger than 6 months more often becoming fixated on objects with more volition in attentional shift emerging later in the first year. Young infants' attention is drawn to adults when adult speech is high pitch, slow rate, and accompanied with gestures (i.e., motherese). Later in the first year, a more productive strategy for fostering attention may be for the adult to "follow" the attentional lead of the child. Contingent adult attention (i.e., an adult action that routinely follows a child action) and response-contingent toys and games (i.e., noted as stimulus synchrony) may also be attention-facilitative strategies. Joint attention (in which the child shows interest by shifting his/her attention from an object to an adult) is a key component of vocabulary learning. A key skill that child care providers need is recognition of children's states of arousal in order to determine when is the best time to engage the child in a task that encourages attention and when the child is overstimulated.

Early memory development also is a cognitive capacity that develops across the early years and is related to attention (i.e., emerging memory abilities may allow the child to overcome object fixation during the first year). Bauer (Chapter 3, this volume) notes that early memory skills may be enhanced by use of multistep imitation, as may occur in caregiver–infant games. She also highlights the importance of consolidation on early memory development in that young children will have better retention of information presented if they have a period of time after the presentation to process the information and establish the memory. Consolidation and memory are enhanced through repetition, with the repetition including similar elements with elaborations (i.e., slight difference). This pattern has implications for building a curriculum for children in a "spiral" manner, in which concepts are related and elaborated across time.

Self-Regulation

In infancy and very early childhood, self-regulation stretches across cognitive and social domains. It has clear linkages to cognition in that early sustained attention in infants predicts later self-regulation. In addition, self-regulation has been proposed as a precursor to later executive function, and the absence or delays in self-regulation is associated with behavior problems in later life. Blair et al. (Chapter 6, this volume) propose that high-quality child care may positively affect self-regulation, which in turn may affect children's reaction to stress. Because of its centrality across domains, a strong argument exists for making self-regulation a central emphasis in early child care and intervention programs. This is bolstered by the fact that these abilities appear to be amenable to change. As Blair et al. note, several interventions have been developed for promoting mothers' support of infants' self-regulations (Landry, Smith, Swank, & Guttentag, 2008; van den Boom, 1994), and this training could well be extended for child care providers in center-based programs.

Language and Communication

The development of language and communication is one of the hallmark achievements of infancy and early childhood. Children's vocabulary at age 3 predicts language competence (Hart & Risley, 1995) and reading performance in later childhood (Dickinson, Golinkoff, & Hirsh-Pasek, 2010). A variety of factors associated with poverty conspire to produce poor language outcomes for infants and children from poor environments, yet with proper early child care and intervention the trajectory for language development is malleable (Landry, Smith, & Swank, 2006). The program of research conducted by Hirsh-Pasek and Golinkoff (Chapter 4, this volume) indicates that children learn words that they hear most and events that interest them, benefit from contingent responsiveness of caregivers, and are limited by prohibitors (i.e., negative directives from caregivers). The range of research cited by Hirsh-Pasek and Golinkoff indicates that infants benefit greatly from language-rich, responsive environments in which caregivers engage children in communicative interactions and elaborate the communicative efforts of the child. In fact, Hirsh-Pasek and Golinkoff cite David Dickinson et al.'s advice to "strive for five," meaning five communicative turns during an interaction sequence with children in which the adults elaborate the language concepts with each turn. Although five turns may be a lot for very young children, the strategy of repetition and elaboration is similar to Bauer's (Chapter 3, this volume) recommendation for memory development. Certainly establishing a style of interaction between caregiver and/or parents and their very young children that reflects these features of interaction will enhance language development and eventually the early literacy skills of infants and toddlers. Similarly, early literacy activities may enhance language development as well. The strategies of singing, oral narratives, nursery rhymes, repeated story reading, linkage of vocabulary to pictures in storybooks, and following the child's interests in storybook pictures through elaboration all may take place in center care or home settings.

Because of immigration to the United States, family members in many homes now speak a language other than English, and authors greatly debate the way in which language should be introduced and fostered for very young children in bilingual or non-English-speaking households. The research by Hoff and Place (Chapter 5, this volume) indicates that infants and toddlers living in non-English-speaking homes can indeed learn both the home language and English, although the acquisition of the two languages will be somewhat slower than for children only learning a single language. For these very young bilingual language learners, later developing expressive language may mask the cognitive or receptive language skills of the child, which should be a cue for care providers to guard against underestimating children's ability. Also, an important recommendation by Hoff and Place is that for infants and toddlers enrolled in a center-based setting and whose caregivers in the home have limited English, the home caregiver (e.g., mother, grandmother) should communicate with the infant/ toddler in the home language rather than modeling a less-than-fluent form of English.

Social Abilities: Temperament

Bates (Chapter 7, this volume) describes temperament as an early appearing, stable style of reacting to the environment. Temperament is thought to be biologically based, featuring an epigenetic overlay in its potential inter-actions with the environment. Decades of research (e.g., Chess & Thomas, 1984) has revealed reliable temperament styles, and whereas alone a child's temperament does not determine eventual outcomes, the ways in which caregivers respond to children's temperament are related to outcomes. For example, infants with difficult temperament, which Bates has identified as negative emotionality (e.g., irritable, frustrated, fearful), will respond dif-ferently to caregivers' responses (e.g., firm parenting, "not-so-nice" par-enting). If the style of caregiving is consistent across time, it will lead to different long-term outcomes.

The research by Bates (Chapter 7, this volume) and other temperament researchers has strong implications for an early child care and interven-tion program for very high-risk infants and toddlers. First, children with certain types of risks, such as very low birthweight or prenatal exposure to cocaine/crack, are more likely to exhibit temperaments that are difficult for caregivers. Second, and fortunately, caregivers (either parents or child care providers) can respond to information about temperament by chang-ing their parenting styles. Third, Bates's research has identified styles of caregiver responding that are likely to generate positive outcomes for chil-dren's temperamental styles. Certainly, early assessment of temperament may help caregivers plan such styles of interactions. His practical advice that caregivers' responses be predictable, that their general quality be warm and responsive (with some variations depending on the child's tempera-ment), and that for children who are temperamentally difficulty taking a "tag-team" approach (i.e., when there are multiple caregivers available who can share the responsibility) are all important.

Social Abilities: Attachment

Somewhat like the development of language, another important achieve-ment of infancy is establishing a secure attachment with at least one famil-ial caregiver, who is usually the mother. The importance of attachment for an early intervention program for very high-risk infants is underscored by the higher prevalence of insecure attachment for children living in poverty (Berlin, Chapter 8, this volume), and a great deal of research speaks to the poor long-term outcomes for children who have insecure attachments (Thompson, 2008). In addition, although there was once the belief that participation in infant/toddler child care interfered with the formation of an attachment relationship between familial caregivers (usually the mother) and their children, current research indicates that such interference does not necessarily happen (NICHD Early Child Care Research Network, 1997). Berlin notes that the literature is beginning to suggest a genetic predisposi-tion to insecure attachment that may be associated with child temperament and style of caregiving received (discussed above).

For a comprehensive ECCE program for infants/toddlers from low-income families, supporting the development of a secure attachment between the child and the mother/familial caregiver is important and substantiates the importance of having a family/home component. Berlin (Chapter 8, this volume) notes that Dozier et al. (2009) has developed an effective intervention program that consists of four features: parent nurturance, following the child's lead, nonthreatening caregiving, and "overriding" the parents own history of growing up in a non-nurturing environment (if it exists). Berlin notes that such training might be appropriate for child care center providers as well. In addition, child care providers may ease the strains of attachment by planning with the parent the infant's transition into the center (i.e., in terms of their initial attendance) and also the "drop-off" and "pick-up" transitions that occur daily.

Curriculum Model

In the traditional sense, an empirically based "curriculum" for infants and toddlers does not exist and would be a key feature of a comprehensive early child care program for children living in poverty. As suggested in the previous sections, such a curriculum would contain activities that foster sustained attention, build memory skills, promote early language development and self-regulation skills, and has opportunities for physical activities. Moving from more adult-directed activities for very young infants to more child-directed activities in which the adults' role is to elaborate, reinforce, and/or apply words to the activities of interest to the child would be important. Language-rich activities focusing on key concepts that are repeated and elaborated would promote language development. Associated early literacy (e.g., book reading) would be one fertile class context for such activities.

Parent and Family Services

One feature of the family dimension of a comprehensive ECCE program would focus on health care, nutrition, and potentially employment training services that might alleviate some of the economic stress that families experience. However, a second feature of the family component should focus on parental caregiving and the home environment when needed.

Using the NICHD Study of Early Child Care database, McCartney, Dearing, Taylor, and Bub (2007) found that in low-socioeconomic status (SES) households, positive caregiving occurred for 39% of the families, and the developmental outcomes for children living in low-SES homes in which there are non-nurturing environments are bleak. Jones Harden et al. (Chapter 12, this volume) note the potential protective effect of high-quality child care, but also stipulate that such care may not work for the highest-risk families because they may not utilize the service for their children. They propose that parenting programs need to accompany child care programs for the highest-risk families. The Dozier et al. (2009) early intervention parent education model, noted previously, is one example of a complementary program that could enhance responsive caregiving and secure attachment between child and family. Similarly, the Play and Learning Strategies (PALS) program developed by Landry et al. (2006) could complement the learning experiences very young children receive in a center-based context. These are but two of a growing number of programs designed to teach responsive interactions to caregivers in home settings. Importantly, Jones Harden and Nzinga-Johnson (2006) emphasized that such programs need to be grounded in the cultural context, with interventions applied in laboratory or clinical settings adapted for homes and home culture. The implications drawn by Jones Harden et al. and Cabrara (Chapter 11, this volume) provide a starting point in considering adaptations for African American and Latino families living in poverty, respectively. Cabrara also makes the very important point that caregiving in some homes and cultures extends beyond the mother, with fathers as well as other extended family members making potentially important and unique contributions to caregiving in the home and community.

Technology

A generational change that affects most aspects of children's (and adults') lives is the development and ubiquity of technology. Given the lag between research and publication, and the speed with which web and smart technology (e.g., iPads and other tablets, smartphones, iTouches) is advancing, the literature may just be beginning to reveal implications for ECCE programs. For example, images on visual displays have attention-evoking quality. Such images can be programmed to be "response contingent" and they can be organized into a pattern of presentations that allows a period of consolidation and subsequent elaborated content. In early child care programs, there are appropriate attempts to limit "screen time" for children (i.e., the showing of television programs or movies as a way of occupying young children's time). Those forms of visual display are different from carefully designed instructional technology that could introduce cognitive and language concepts, for example, on an iPad and with the adult potentially being a facilitator of the learning experience. However, the scientific evaluations of such innovations for infants and toddlers in child care centers are still in the future.

Web technology has been put to great use to assist EHS practitioners in monitoring children's progress and introducing educational plans when development lags. Carta, Greenwood, Baggett, Buzhardt, and Walker (Chapter 14, this volume) describe a web-based system, Making Online

Decisions (MOD) (*www.igdi.ku.edu*), that builds on the authors' previous identification of Individual Growth and Development Indicators (IGDIs) for language development. The language IGDIs system is an efficient assessment of children's early language development. With the MOD, teachers enter the IGDIs language data for children; the system calculates the growth trajectory for children, and the MOD recommends language learning activities when children lag behind in expected growth (Buzhardt et al., 2010). Buzhardt et al. (2011) report positive effects of the MOD for children enrolled in EHS.

The use of web-based technology to coach parents in the use of an intervention at home or teachers in the use of specific teaching approaches in a center-based setting is also evolving. Carta et al. (Chapter 14, this volume) describe the Infant-Net program designed by Baggett et al. (2010). Basing their work on the previously mentioned PALS program (Landry et al., 2006), Baggett and colleagues developed a self-paced set of activities and lessons for promoting infant–caregiver interactions that parents could employ (with some guidance) at home. An important part of that system was a video-sharing feature in which the computer could videotape the parents' interactions with their child at home, and parent and early child care professionals would jointly view and discuss the video at a later time. Using a somewhat similar strategy with young children with autism and their families, Vismara, Young, Stahmer, Griffith, and Rogers (2009) have delivered information about an intervention approach that would be used in the home (e.g., the Early Start Denver Model), observe parent–child interactions through a telemedicine format, and provide feedback to parents immediately after a play session. As the video capacities and utility of the smart technology continues to develop (e.g., better cameras in iPhones and iPads), the applications to early child care will emerge, perhaps at a faster pace than science can determine the impact.

Child Care Personnel and Professional Development

Recruiting effective teachers and other personnel for very early child care and education programs for at-risk infants and toddlers and their families is a continuing challenge. Berlin (Chapter 8, this volume) proposed that for practitioners to promote attachment for mothers and infants, they (child care providers) should feel comfortable with or confront their own attachment relationship. Reflecting on characteristics of the workforce, Bates (Chapter 7, this volume) suggests that potential teacher beliefs about the value of caregiver–infant interactions and the sensitive/responsiveness of potential teachers in those interactions be screened. Like infants, teachers bring with them temperamental styles that may be expressed through their caregiving.

Summary: Developing and Implementing a Model

Incorporating the implications from the chapters in this book into a vision for an effective early care and education program is a challenge. The adage that "The future looks a lot like the past" will be true in some ways, in that we have known, for example, about the value of attachment, parent–child interactions, temperament, and language development. Developmental and health science, however, is providing important new information about the importance of certain cognitive process (e.g., attention, memory), key features of the social environment for promoting language development, and epigenetic influences suggested by the interaction of temperament and caregiver style. Current science also indicates the importance of a language-rich environment and the effect of learning two (or more) languages at once in early childhood, "second-generation" influences of insecure attachment, the longitudinal consequences of early obesity, and the differences in family structure and caregiving among different linguistic and culture groups.

Following a "Back to the future" approach, the literature suggests that a high-quality center-based model of early child care and education can have significantly positive effects on children's development (Watamura et al., 2011) but also that there are critically important features of the home environment (i.e., parent–child interaction and caregiving) that can be addressed effectively through a well-implemented home-based program (Berlin, Zeanah, & Lieberman, 2008; Landry et al., 2008). A structural framework exists, emanating from EHS, for a center- and home-based combination (Love et al., Chapter 13, this volume), although a more significant health feature of such a model might be incorporated. A theoretical framework for such an early care and education program could be based on a Bronfenbrener-like ecological systems model, as can be seen in Figure 15.1. In this figure, the features residing within the child (i.e., cognitive and language abilities, self-regulation and social skills, temperament, gender, race) are the biosystem to which Bronfenbrenner and Morris (1998) refer; this system is represented by the baby icon. The child (biosystem) participates in microsystem environments such as the class–center, home, and the pediatric practice; the literature suggests features of a model important in each. The interactions and communications that exist among the center staff, family, and pediatric care staff represent Bronfenbrenner's mesosystem and should have reciprocal effects on actions within those ecological contexts and on the child. The center, home/family, and pediatric care service are also affected by regulations and other factors operating outside of these immediate ecological contexts but that still exert a primary influence on practice; these represent exosystem factors in Bronfenbrenner's model. All of these ecological systems are affected by more distal (from the child) factors such as the economy, cultural values, and technological innovations that Bronfenbrenner characterized as macrosystem influences.

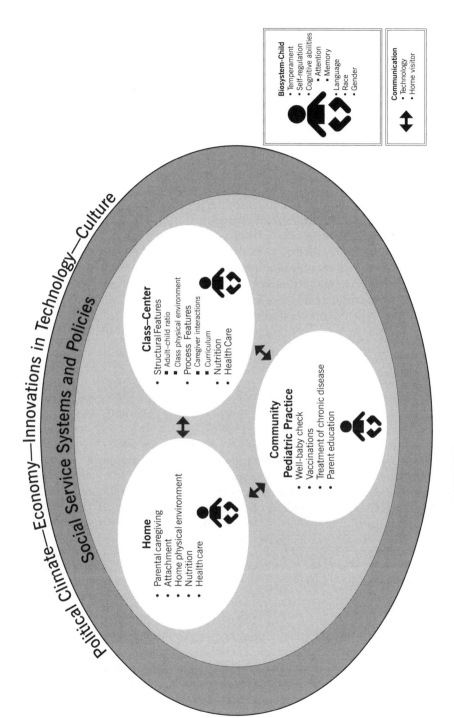

FIGURE 15.1. Early intervention conceptual model.

Political Climate—Economy—Innovations in Technology—Culture

Social Service Systems and Policies

Home
- Parental caregiving
- Attachment
- Home physical environment
- Nutrition
- Health care

Class—Center
Structural Features
- Adult–child ratio
- Class physical environment
Process Features
- Caregiver interactions
- Curriculum
- Nutrition
- Health Care

Community
Pediatric Practice
- Well-baby check
- Vaccinations
- Treatment of chronic disease
- Parent education

Biosystem–Child
- Temperament
- Self-regulation
- Cognitive abilities
  - Attention
  - Memory
- Language
- Race
- Gender

Communication
- Technology
- Home visitor

367

Such a model for early child care and education is ambitious and organizationally very challenging. Such a model, we propose, would offer child care, education, nutrition, health, and family education services in one location close to the families served. A primary issue with families facing the highest risks is their accessing services available (Jones Harden et al., Chapter 12, this volume), and proximity to services may well affect families' active use. Also, in addition to high-quality child care, it would offer intervention in the home focusing on sensitive and responsive caregiving, a safe home environment, nutrition, and mental health services for family members if necessary, and accessing vocational training and jobs if needed. Although such a model would focus on the prenatal to age 3 range, continuity into Head Start or preschool settings is critical (Love at al., Chapter 13, this volume), so proactive transition planning for children in the center, for parents, and for teachers in the next setting would be important.

In conclusion, although not widespread, examples exist of some programs that approximate this model. For example, a key feature of the Educare Centers (*www.educareschools.org*), child care centers serving families living in poverty in a small number of communities in the United States, is the provision of family support services. Family support specialists at each center provide programming within the center to promote and enhance the parent–child relationship. They also encourage parents to become engaged in their children's early education in the center and to make connections to needed services for families and children within the wider community (e.g., mental health services). On a wider community scale is the example of the Harlem Children's Zone (*www.hcz.org*), currently being replicated in other underresourced communities across the United States through the "Promise Neighborhoods" initiative by the federal government (*www2. ed.gov/programs/promiseneighborhoods*). This model operates at the neighborhood level, providing and coordinating a comprehensive system of programs to support children and families, beginning with "The Baby College" (a series of workshops for parents of children ages 0 to 3) and continuing with best-practice programs for children through college (including services in school, in after-school programs, social services, and health and community-building programs). Although larger in scope than the current model being proposed, the concept of coordinating services across early learning and community environments is similar, as is the tenant of beginning as early in the lifespan as possible. These examples provide some of the structural features that could be employed to develop a comprehensive model of early care and education. The science reviewed in this book and the implications from that science provide a basis for filling in the content. Another adage to which most readers who have worked in child care would resonate is that "The devil is in the details." Although this book has not removed the devil completely, the authors have offered implications for future practice that could enhance and elaborate, and dare we say, provide a more divine vision of early care and education for infants and young children from poor families.

REFERENCES

Ackerman, B. E., Izard, C. E., Schoff, K., Youngstrom, E. A., & Kogos, J. (1999). Contextual risk, caregiver emotionality, and the problem behaviors of six- and seven-year-old children from economically disadvantaged families. *Child Development, 70,* 1415–1427.

Baggett, K. M., Feil, E. G., Davis, B., Sheeber, L., Landry, S., Carta, J., et al. (2010). Technologies for expanding the reach of evidence-based interventions: Preliminary results for promoting social–emotional development in early childhood. *Topics in Early Childhood Special Education, 29,* 226–238.

Belsky, J., Bakermans-Kranenburg, M., & van IJzendoorn, M. (2007). For better and for worse: Differential susceptibility to environmental influences. *Current Directions in Psychological Science, 16*(6), 300–304.

Berlin, L. J., Zeanah, C. H., & Lieberman, A. F. (2008). Prevention and intervention programs for supporting early attachment security. In J. Cassidy & P. R. Shaver (Eds.), *Handbook of attachment: Theory, research, and clinical applications* (2nd ed., pp. 745–761). New York: Guilford Press.

Bronfenbrenner, U., & Morris, P. (1998). The ecology of developmental processes. In R. M. Lerner (Ed.), *Handbook of child psychology* (5th ed.) Vol. 1. *Theoretical models of human development* (pp. 993–1028). New York: Wiley.

Burchinal, M., Roberts, J. E., Zeisel, S. A., Hennon, E. A., & Hooper, S. (2006). Social risk and protective child, parenting, and child care factors in early elementary school years. *Parenting: Science and Practice, 6,* 79–113.

Buzhardt, J., Greenwood, C. R., Walker, D., Anderson, R., Howard, W., & Carta, J. J. (2011). Effects of web-based support on Early Head Start home visitors' use of evidence-based intervention decision making and growth in children's expressive communication. *NHSA Dialog: A Research-to-Practice Journal for the Early Childhood Field, 14,* 121–146.

Buzhardt, J., Greenwood, C. R., Walker, D., Carta, J., Terry, B., & Garrett, M. (2010). A web-based tool to support data-based early intervention decision-making. *Topics in Early Childhood Special Education, 29,* 201–213.

Chess, S., & Thomas, A. (1984). *Origins and evolution of behavior disorders.* New York: Brunner/Mazel.

Conger, R. D., & Donnellan, M. B. (2007). An interactionist perspective on the socioeconomic context of human development. *Annual Review of Psychology, 58,* 175–199.

Dickinson, D., Golinkoff, R., & Hirsh-Pasek, K. (2010). Speaking out for language: Why language is central to reading development. *Educational Researcher, 39,* 305–310.

Dozier, M., Lindhiem, O., Lewis, E., Bick, J., Bernard, K., & Peloso, E. (2009). Effects of a foster parent training program on young children's attachment behaviors: Preliminary evidence from a randomized clinical trial. *Child and Adolescent Social Work Journal, 26,* 321–332.

Duncan, G., Ludwig, J., & Magnuson, K. (2007). Reducing poverty through preschool interventions. *The Future of Children, 17*(2), 143–160.

Fiese, B. H., Gundersen, C., Koester, B., & Washington, L. (2011). Household food insecurity: Serious concerns for child development. *SRCD Social Policy Report, 25*(3), 1–19.

Gottlieb, G., Wahlsten, D., & Lickliter, R. (2006). Biology and human development. In W. Damon & R. M. Lerner (Eds.-in-Chief) and R. M. Lerner (Vol. Ed.), *Handbook of child psychology: Vol. 1. Theoretical models of human development* (6th ed., pp. 210–257). Hoboken, NJ: Wiley.

Hart, B., & Risley, T. (1995). *Meaningful differences in the everyday lives of American children.* Baltimore: Brookes.

Jones Harden, B., & Nzinga-Johnson, S. (2006). Young, wounded and black: The maltreatment of African-American children in the early years. In R. L. Hampton & T. P. Gullotta (Eds.), *Interpersonal violence in the African-American community* (pp. 17–46). New York: Springer.

Landry, S. H., Smith, K. E., & Swank, P. R. (2006). Responsive parenting: Establishing early foundations for social, communication, and independent problem-solving skills. *Developmental Psychology, 42,* 627–642.

Landry, S. H., Smith, K. E., Swank, P. R., & Guttentag, C. (2008). A responsive parenting intervention: The optimal timing across early childhood for impacting maternal behaviors and child outcomes. *Developmental Psychology, 44,* 1335–1353.

Love, J. M., Kisker, E. E., Ross, C., Raikes, H., Constantine, J., Boller, K., et al. (2005). The effectiveness of Early Head Start for 3-year-old children and their parents: Lessons for policy and programs. *Developmental Psychology, 41,* 885–901.

McCartney, K., Dearing, E., Taylor, B., & Bub, K. (2007). Quality child-care supports the achievement of low-income children: Direct and indirect pathways through caregiving and the home environment. *Journal of Applied Developmental Psychology, 28,* 411–426.

McWilliams, C., Ball, S. C., Benjeman, S. E., Hales, D., Vaughn, A., & Ward, D. S. (2009). Best practice guidelines for physical activities at child care. *Pediatrics, 124,* 1650–1659.

Mendelsohn, A. L., Huberman, H. S., Berkule-Silberman, S. B., Brockmeyer, C. A., Morrow, L. M., & Dreyer, B. P. (in press). Primary care strategies for promoting parent–child interactions and school readiness in at-risk families: Early findings from the Bellevue Project for Early Language, Literacy and Education Success (BELLE). *Archives of Pediatrics and Adolescent Medicine.*

NICHD Early Child Care Research Network. (1997). The effects of infant child care on infant–mother attachment security: Results of the NICHD Study of Early Child Care. *Child Development, 68,* 860–879.

Odom, S. L., & Kaul, S. (2003). Early intervention themes and variations from around the world. In S. Odom, M. Hanson, J. Blackman, & S. Kaul (Eds.), *Early intervention practices around the world* (pp. 333–346). Baltimore: Brookes.

Pungello, E. P., & Gardner-Neblett, N. (in press). Family factors, child care quality, and cognitive outcomes. In V. Maholmes & R. B. King (Eds.), *The Oxford handbook of poverty and child development*. New York: Oxford University Press.

Ramey, C. T., & Campbell, R. A. (1984). Preventative education for high risk children: Cognitive consequences of the Carolina Abecedarian Project. *American Journal on Mental Deficiency, 88,* 515–523.

Reynolds, A. J., Temple, J. A., Ou, S. R., Arteaga, I. A., & White, B. A. (2011). School-based early childhood education and age-28 well-being: Effects by timing, dosage, and subgroups. *Science, 333,* 360–364.

Rutter, M. (1979). Protective factors in children's responses to stress and disadvantage. In M. W. Kent & J. E. Rolf (Eds.), *Primary prevention of psychopathology: Vol. 3. Social competence in children* (pp. 49–74). Hanover, NH: University Press of New England.

Sameroff, A. J., & Chandler, M. J. (1975). Reproductive risk and the continuum of caretaking causality. In F. Horowitz, M. Hetherington, S. Scarr-Salapatek, & G. Sigel (Eds.), *Review of child development research* (Vol. 4, pp. 187–244). Chicago: University of Chicago Press.

Schweinhart, L. J., Berrueta-Clement, J. R., Barnett, W. S., Epstein, A. S., & Weikart, D. P. (1985). Effects of Perry Preschool Program on youths through age 19: A summary. *Topics in Early Childhood Special Education, 5*(2), 26–35.

Shonkoff, J. P., & Bales, S. N. (2011). Science does not speak for itself: Translating child development research for the public and policymakers. *Child Development, 82,* 17–32.

Shonkoff, J. P., & Phillips, D. A. (2000). *Neurons to neighborhoods: The science of childhood development*. Washington DC: National Academy Press.

Thompson, R. A. (2008). Early attachment and later development: Familiar questions, new answers. In J. Cassidy & P. R. Shaver (Eds.), *Handbook of attachment: Theory, research, and clinical applications* (2nd ed., pp. 348–365). New York: Guilford Press.

van den Boom, D. C. (1994). The influence of temperament and mothering on attachment and exploration: An experimental manipulation of sensitive responsiveness among lower-class mothers with irritable infants. *Child Development, 65,* 1457–1477.

Vismara, L. A., Young, G., Stahmer, A. C., Griffith, E. M., & Rogers, S. J. (2009). Dissemination of evidence-based practice: Can we train therapists from a distance? *Journal of Autism and Developmental Disorders, 39,* 1636–1651.

Watamura, S., Phillips, D., Morrissey, T., McCartney, K., & Bub, K. (2011). Double jeopardy: Poorer social–emotional outcomes for children in the NICHD SECYD experiencing home and child-care environments that confer risk. *Child Development, 82*(1), 48–65.

Zuckerman, B., Parker, S., Kaplan-Sanoff, M., Augustyn, B., & Barth, M. C. (2004). Healthy Steps: A case study of innovation in pediatric practice. *Pediatrics, 114*(3), 820–826.

Index